MENTAL HEALTH AND PALESTINIAN CITIZENS IN ISRAEL

INDIANA SERIES IN MIDDLE EAST STUDIES

Mark Tessler, *editor*

MENTAL HEALTH AND PALESTINIAN CITIZENS IN ISRAEL

Edited by Muhammad M. Haj-Yahia,
Ora Nakash, and Itzhak Levav

INDIANA UNIVERSITY PRESS

This book is a publication of

Indiana University Press
Office of Scholarly Publishing
Herman B Wells Library 350
1320 East 10th Street
Bloomington, Indiana 47405 USA

iupress.indiana.edu

Library of Congress Cataloging-in-Publication Data

Names: Yahia, Mohammed Haj, editor. | Nakash, Ora, editor. | Levav, Itshak,
editor.
Title: Mental health and Palestinian citizens in Israel / edited by Muhammad
M. Haj-Yahia, Ora Nakash, and Itzhak Levav.
Description: Bloomington, Indiana : Indiana University Press, [2019] |
Series: Indiana series in Middle East studies | Includes bibliographical
references and index.
Identifiers: LCCN 2018049697 (print) | LCCN 2018050669 (ebook) | ISBN
9780253043092 (e-book) | ISBN 9780253043061 (cl : alk. paper) | ISBN
9780253043078 (pb : alk. paper)
Subjects: | MESH: Mental Disorders—ethnology | Arabs—psychology | Minority
Health—ethnology | Social Determinants of Health | Social Alienation |
Israel
Classification: LCC RC455.4.E8 (ebook) | LCC RC455.4.E8 (print) | NLM WA 305
JI9 | DDC 362.2089—dc23
LC record available at https://lccn.loc.gov/2018049697

1 2 3 4 5   24 23 22 21 20 19

CONTENTS

FOREWORD

A NATIONAL MINORITY IS DEFINED AS A GROUP of people within a given nation-state that is numerically smaller than the rest of the population. However, the use of the word "minority" is controversial because many scholars refer to power differences among groups rather than differences in population size. A group may be defined as a minority because its culture, language, or religion is distinct from that of the majority of the population or simply because it does not hold a dominant position in society. Joe R. Feagin, a US sociologist and social theorist, states that a minority group has five characteristics: (1) it suffers discrimination and subordination; (2) it has physical and/or cultural traits that set it apart and that are disapproved of by the dominant group; (3) it shares a sense of collective identity and common burden; (4) its socially shared rules about who belongs and who does not determine minority status; and (5) there is a tendency to marry within the group (Feagin & Feagin, 2011).

Because of these common characteristics, minorities are especially vulnerable, and this vulnerability is often reflected in their health status (physical, mental, and social), which may be ranked lower than the rest of the population. This book focuses on Palestinian citizens in Israel, a minority group that may be subject to an additional vulnerability: suffering from mental ill health.

Addressing the issue of mental health among minorities is important and timely for two main reasons:

1. The mental health risks intrinsic to minorities are not sufficiently studied. As a consequence, needs and specificities of vulnerable populations are ignored when planning interventions aimed at preventing mental ill health and treating mental disorders.
2. The growing interest in a new discipline such as global mental health (Patel & Prince, 2010) should include the study and research findings about mental health of minorities, simply because minority groups are increasingly widespread on the global scene. A better knowledge of their needs and specificities should make a fundamental contribution to the global mental health discourse.

Being a Palestinian citizen in Israel means being exposed to specific sociopolitical determinants of mental health and experiencing specific gender- and family related conditions. Domestic violence occurs everywhere and in all human groups, but every group has its own sociocultural contexts; suicides and suicide attempts as well as smoking and other addictions are also affected by cultural and social specificities. Finally, attitudes toward and beliefs about psychiatric disorders require deep analysis and understanding that obviously need reliable epidemiological data about the prevalence of mental disorders and assessment of service response and therapeutic interventions.

As Giora Kaplan, Itzhak Levav, and Ora Nakash write in chapter 11, devoted to reviewing community studies on the psychiatric epidemiology of Palestinian citizens in Israel: "Despite major health gains, the social stresses of being a minority that is undergoing major social changes may explain the greater emotional distress among Palestinians. A combination of cultural and political factors, including the perceptions of mental disorder, psychiatric care, and stigma, as well as a lesser availability of culturally tailored services, may account for the marked treatment gap among Palestinians."

This important book, the product of a collective effort, addresses all these issues and in so doing represents an informed and concrete answer to the UN Human Rights Council's call for better understanding of minorities to promote dialogue and cooperation on issues pertaining to national or ethnic, religious, and linguistic minorities.

In 2007 the Human Rights Council established a forum on minority issues in recognition that, within the UN system, it is essential to have a platform for discussing minority issues and the rights of minorities. The forum aims to identify and analyze best practices, challenges, opportunities, and initiatives for the further implementation of the Declaration on the Rights of Persons Belonging to National or Ethnic, Religious and Linguistic Minorities (UN General Assembly, 1992).

This book honors not only science and public health but also the UN's call for a global commitment on the rights of minorities.

Benedetto Saraceno, MD, HonFRCPsych
Gulbenkian Professor of Global Health
Faculty of Medical Sciences
NOVA University of Lisbon
Formerly, Director, Mental Health
and Substance Abuse,
World Health Organization, Geneva

MENTAL HEALTH AND PALESTINIAN CITIZENS IN ISRAEL

INTRODUCTION

Muhammad M. Haj-Yahia, Ora Nakash, and Itzhak Levav

ISRAEL, WITH AN ESTIMATED POPULATION OF 8,793,000 (ISRAEL Central Bureau of Statistics, 2018), is a mosaic of ethnic, national, religious, and cultural identities that embraces diverse groups:

- Palestinian citizens of Israel, 20.8% of the total population, are mostly Muslim (about 17.8%), including Bedouins. Palestinians also include the relatively smaller Christian (1.5%) and Druze (1.5%) communities (Israel Central Bureau of Statistics, 2018).
- Jewish Israelis comprise 74.8% of the total population (Israel Central Bureau of Statistics, 2018).
- A heterogeneous group, usually identified as "Others" in the demography reports of the Israel Central Bureau of Statistics, makes up 4.4% of the total population (2018).

This book addresses mental health–related themes concerning the Palestinian population, a piece of the Israeli mosaic that, while interacting with one or more of the other ethnic, national, religious, or cultural entities, has its own past and recent history, language, national status, origin, traditions, social organization, and aspirations. Simply stated, the Palestinian minority's identity encompasses all those components that have contributed to building its distinctiveness over the years, as portrayed in different chapters in the book focusing on sociocultural, economic, educational, demographic, and political environments and their impacts on mental health.

As expected, the century-long conflict between Jewish Israelis and Palestinians, more acutely involving Palestinians residing outside the state of Israel, has left its mark on all communities involved. The scholars in this book integrate scholarly research with ideologies and observations as they passionately discuss the narrative of the Palestinian citizens of Israel and the impact of their circumstances on mental health. As required by academic standards, each author assumes total responsibility for his or her own contribution, and the editors have carefully observed the principles of academic freedom. Further, all translations are by authors. The three editors of this book agree that recognizing the impact of the Palestinian narrative in Israel, on both collective and individual levels, should facilitate the understanding of the complex general scenario. The different chapters highlight the predicaments facing service users, their families, and the general community in their contacts with the curative and rehabilitation services and their exposure to mental health promotion and primary prevention programs. In this particular context, the sociopolitical and historical narratives of both minority and majority groups are acknowledged but are nevertheless secondary to the common pursuit of mental health objectives for the benefit of both populations. Indeed, mental health action does not stop at the borders, internal or external, as witnessed by the shared efforts reflected in the preparation of this book.

The editors (from the fields of social work, psychology, and psychiatry) aim to highlight and make gradually accumulating critical information accessible to all mental health agents and other relevant stakeholders. In this way, we seek to upgrade the mental health care provided to Palestinian citizens in Israel with information that is evidence based. The contributors emphasize selected issues in their respective chapters, such as the importance of the sociopolitical history and context, the particular social organization and values of the Palestinian communities, and the central role of the family with its age-old traditions, among other thematic domains. Interestingly, this collective frame of reference arose in the conception of the chapters without prompting by the editors.

Admittedly, to reach all stakeholders in Israel requires providing information in Arabic and Hebrew. We have opted to first publish this text in English to ensure that at least a common language is established. In addition, the selection of English enables reaching the widest readership interested in the nascent global mental health movement in the Middle East and beyond. Yet the current effort will need to be supplemented in the future with Arabic and Hebrew versions.

Some repetitions, albeit minor, have been left in the text to facilitate the independent reading of each chapter. The five sections of the book comprehensively cover different themes related to mental health among Palestinian citizens in Israel.

Part I covers cultural and sociopolitical determinants of mental health. As'ad Ghanem and Ibrahim Khatib have contributed "Palestinian Citizens in Israel: Sociopolitical Status as a Mental Health Determinant"; Sfaa Ghnadre-Naser has written "Between Past and Present: Psychological Effects of the Nakba among Palestinian Citizens in Israel"; Adel Manna has contributed "The Nakba and Its Repercussions on Palestinian Citizens in Israel"; Mahmoud Mi'ari and Nazeh Natur have coauthored "Collective Identity and Mental Health among Palestinian Citizens in Israel"; and Nohad 'Ali has written "Palestinian Citizens in Israel: A Sociological Portrait."

This group of studies highlights a number of issues that are intimately related to the history of the Jewish-Palestinian conflict over the years, with all its painful ramifications for Palestinians before and after 1948, when the state of Israel was established and open warfare followed. At this time, additional adverse factors came into play for Palestinians, such as living for a number of years under military control. The effects of the conflict on the mental health of the population require research based on empirical data, with an emphasis on vulnerability and resilience factors.

As an illustration, Mi'ari and Natur have noted: "No studies have been carried out on Palestinian citizens in Israel to examine the impact of identity level on mental health." In light of the scarcity of empirical studies on the impact of the political trauma on mental health, the study reported by Ghnadre-Naser in chapter 2 should be highlighted. Ghnadre-Naser retrospectively explores the subjective meanings and psychological effects of the Nakba ("catastrophe," the term Palestinians use for the 1948 war) for its first survivors among the Palestinian population living in Israel. She concludes that "working through the trauma and confronting its psychological consequences may persist as a journey that younger generations must embark on. Issues of familial dynamics, identity formation, and vulnerability versus resiliency should be addressed professionally."

Chapter 5 closes part I with a history of the pains associated with the development of Palestinian society since 1948, including the current trend toward modernization. 'Ali reviews issues of conflict and coexistence in a number of domains. These provide the stage for adverse socioenvironmental factors such as discrimination and exclusion. All these factors require appreciation by mental health agents.

Part II includes three chapters covering mental health issues related to the family and gender and discusses milestones in the life cycle. Chapter 6, "The Palestinian Family in Israel: Its Collectivist Nature, Structure, and Implications for Mental Health Interventions" by Muhammad M. Haj-Yahia, is of particular interest. In contrast to Western values that predicate individual responsibility for one's well-being and decisions regarding care, the Palestinian community expects the family to be actively and primarily involved. Bridging the communication gap between the culture and sociopolitical background of the treating agent and the service user is a major challenge that this chapter intends to meet. In the author's own words: "Considering the collectivistic nature of the Palestinian family, exclusive emphasis on individualistically oriented goals may endanger the intervention and its outcomes." It is thus not surprising that Haj-Yahia, when he refers to siblings, for example, adds: "Because siblings constitute a source of different types of tangible and intangible resources, the importance of this source of support in the intervention cannot be underestimated or ignored."

Chapter 7, "Mental Health Issues among Palestinian Women in Israel" by Sarah Abu-Kaf, dovetails closely with the previous chapter. In Abu-Kaf's words, "Appropriate answers to the mental health needs of Palestinian women must consider the Arab culture as an integral part of every individual's development, mental health problems, and healing/care practices. For example, being familiar with the cultural dynamics that influence the professional/client relationship and behaving in a manner that enhances the mental health professional/patient relationship and employs a preferred pattern of communication may lead to more effective interventions and lower dropout rates." The recognition and understanding of diversity in cultures is critical. The mental health agent may care for women that live in a polygamous family, for example, such as among Bedouins of the Negev. The agent may intervene as the "transition from monogamous to polygamous family structure can be a traumatic change for the senior wife, eliciting reactions similar to those that follow divorce, with mourning and low self-esteem being common." As the author states: "Polygamy may contribute to mental health adversities through the family environment."

Part II closes with Rabia Khalaila's chapter, "Mental Health in Older Adult Palestinian Citizens in Israel." Of the many different subjects covered in this chapter, it is noted here that abuse of older adults (later chapters address this as well) is a problem in the Palestinian community despite traditional values of respect for this age group. The author notes: "These [relatively high rates found in a community study] were attributed to the modernization process and the consequent family disruptions experienced by the Palestinian minority over the four decades prior to the study." Interestingly, the increasing recognition of mental disorders among older adults meets obstacles raised by limited mental health literacy, including stigma, that are particularly problematic for this age group.

Part III includes chapters covering psychiatric and behavioral health disorders among Palestinian citizens in Israel. In chapter 9, "Attitudes, Beliefs, and Stigma toward Mental Health Issues among Palestinian Citizens in Israel," Alean Al-Krenawi notes that, for many Palestinian citizens in Israel, "cultural beliefs may contend that mental illness is caused by evil spirits and is related to delusions of possession and control. Muslim Arabs believe that there are two spirits; one is good, and the other, called *Iblis* (the devil), is bad. . . . The bad spirit seduces humankind to commit sins against God, and therefore the sinners are punished physically and psychologically. . . . This belief can be demonstrated in everyday language—a common Arabic term used to describe mental illness is *majnun*, which is derived from the term *jinn*, meaning, 'a supernatural spirit.'" This set of beliefs often leads service users to look for traditional healers that adhere to those beliefs rather than to Western-oriented pratitioners. Al-Krenawi discusses the magnitude of stigma in the population and its impact on help seeking.

In chapter 10, "Mental Health Status, Service Use, and Help-Seeking Practices of Children and Adolescents among Palestinian Citizens in Israel," Ivonne Mansbach-Kleinfeld and Raida Daeem address findings acquired in community epidemiological studies. Those findings are of high interest and relate to the prevalence rates of internalizing and externalizing mental disorders, among other issues: "The rate of internalizing disorders among Palestinian adolescents was 9.1%, a nonstatistically significant difference from the 7.9% rate among Jewish adolescents. Externalizing disorders were significantly lower for Palestinian adolescents than for Jewish adolescents (1.9% vs. 5.7%, respectively). Risk factors for an externalizing disorder were being male, living with a divorced or single parent, and having only one or no siblings. These risk factors may explain some of the variance between Jewish and Palestinian adolescents as most of the latter live in two-parent families and have many siblings." The authors quote researchers who have argued that the strong family values and a community orientation [among Palestinians], favor control and surveillance over children's behavior, so that they conform to group norms (Sagy, Orr, Bar-On, & Awwad, 2001).

The next group of epidemiological studies was conducted among adults. Each chapter offers information that could be used profitably in mental health service planning. Chapter 11, "The Psychiatric Epidemiological Portrait of Palestinian Citizens in Israel: A Review of Community Studies," reports on data from the World Mental Health Survey conducted by the World Health Organization (WHO) and Harvard University in the United States. Of the twenty-eight participating countries (the respective research teams continue analyzing data and publishing findings), three are from the Middle East: Israel, Iraq, and Lebanon. This is the first time that a critical comparison of mental health metrics has been possible at an international level. As Giora Kaplan, Itzhak Levav, and Ora Nakash report, in Israel the rates of common mental disorders were higher among Palestinian citizens of Israel (11.1%, 95% confidence interval [CI], 8.7–14.2) than among Jewish Israelis (9.3%, 95% CI, 8.3–10.3), and higher among women than among men.

In chapter 12, Ido Lurie and Anat Fleischman's "Psychiatric Hospitalization among Palestinian Citizens in Israel: A Historical Cohort Study," the authors compare the distinctive patterns of psychiatric hospitalization among Palestinian citizens in Israel versus among Israeli Jews. The most striking finding is the lower rate for Palestinian women, an indication that this service is regarded as unsuitable for this group.

In chapter 13, "Smoking among Palestinian Citizens in Israel," Lital Keinan-Boker and Yael Bar-Zeev report that "in Israel, smoking rates in Palestinian males are the highest, while in Palestinian females smoking rates are the lowest, creating a unique population group where about half the men actively smoke while women, mostly nonsmokers, and children are heavily exposed to [passive smoking]." They have further noted that, "in contrast to the Jewish population, smoking rates in Palestinian men have not decreased, regardless of their educational level. . . . Social and cultural factors may explain this—for example, smoking is considered a positive social norm in Palestinian society, and these positive norms prevent smoking cessation." The authors add: "Going against the norm in a more collective and traditional society may be more difficult than in a more individualistic society."

Like other societies, the Palestinian community in Israel is not free from violence directed at others but, in contrast, is characterized by remarkably low rates of self-inflicted violence, including suicide. Part IV covers themes related to violent behavior and mental health among Palestinian citizens in Israel. Chapters 14 and 15 address violence toward the young. In "Child Abuse and Neglect among Palestinian citizens in Israel," Haneen Elias and Raghda Alnabilsy highlight "the need for governmental ministries to adopt policies and allocate adequate resources to reduce the [relatively high] incidence [rates] of child abuse and neglect in Palestinian society." The authors note that the "risk factors are diverse and complex and . . . are related to various levels of individual and family life, as well to the lives of the

Palestinian population and its status as an indigenous minority in Israel. Poverty, unemployment, and discrimination in services are examples of sociopolitical risk factors that may account for the problem."

The school is another locus of potential exposure to violence against children. This theme is covered in Mona Khoury-Kassabri's chapter, "Palestinian Children in Israel: Involvement in School Violence as Victims and Perpetrators." Of the many subjects the author addresses, perpetration of violence is of the highest concern. Indeed, "about one in two Palestinian students in Israel (52.5%) reported carrying out at least one aggressive act against a peer, and 20.0% reported acting aggressively toward a teacher at least once in the month prior to the study." Research on this subject has advanced, and Khoury-Kassabri discusses possible interventions.

Additional chapters in this section address violence among adults and the elderly. In chapter 16, "Intimate Partner Violence against Palestinian Women in Israel and the Relevance of the Sociocultural and Sociopolitical Context," Raghda Alnabilsy and Haneen Elias present many findings and relevant insights. They note: "These findings support the argument . . . that societies with relatively high rates of [intimate partner violence] against women, such as the Palestinian society, are characterized by a patriarchal culture in terms of gender roles; emphasis on the values of family unity; priority of the national group over the emotional and physical well-being of the individual and over human and civil rights; social exclusion; and high rates of problems such as unemployment, poverty, and community violence."

The subject of abuse of older adults is the focus of Samir Zoabi's chapter, "Abuse of Older Adults among Palestinian Citizens in Israel: Social, Economic, and Family Related Factors." In the study reported on in the chapter, Zoabi found that abuse of older adults affected 4% of the older Palestinians living in the north of Israel and was higher (4.9%) among urban residents. He notes that, similar to the findings in the previous chapter, the "difference was explained mainly by the impact of modern living conditions and changes in the social and family support networks, a trend found to be strong[er] in the large cities" than in other settings.

Self-directed violence is addressed in chapter 18, "Suicide and Suicide Attempts among Palestinian Citizens in Israel" by Anat Brunstein-Klomek et al. Reporting on data from the national databases of suicide (1999–2011) and suicide attempts (2004–2012), this study shows that suicide rates are relatively low among Palestinian citizens in Israel, although there is some intergroup variability. Suicide rates were lowest among Muslims (2.5 per 100,000 population) and highest among the Druze (8.7 per 100,000 population). Suicide rates were higher for Palestinian males than females and highest for the 15- to 24-year-old age group. The frequency of suicide attempts was highest among Muslims (84.8 per 100,000 population). Suicide attempts were more frequent among women than among men in all groups except for the Druze population.

Part V concludes the book with three chapters that address interventions on issues related to the restoration of the mental health of affected individuals, their families, and communities. In chapter 19, "Psychotherapy for Palestinian Citizens in Israel," Nazeh Natur raises several culture-related issues in the delivery of psychotherapy. He states that in order to "provide culturally relevant services, practitioners need to dismantle the secular terminology and repackage it with precepts in terminology that reflect Islamic teaching." Unsurprisingly, Natur further points out that "psychodynamic approaches may not be as effective as cognitive approaches when dealing with Muslim service users. The difficulty in adopting this type of therapy with Palestinians stems . . . from the fact that most of them are traditional, are members of patriarchal and hierarchical families, and may reject liberal individualistic values." This poses a challenge to non-Palestinian therapists, who are likely to require both training and supervision to feel comfortable dealing with users from this culture. A need for the development of evidence-based culturally responsive treatments is eminent. To that effect, the author proposes solutions to improve psychotherapy effectiveness with Palestinian citizens in Israel.

"From Psychoanalysis to Culture-Analysis: Culturally Sensitive Psychotherapy for Palestinian Citizens in Israel" by Marwan Dwairy further elaborates on and illustrates the difficulties in the psychotherapeutic encounters between minority service users and culturally dissonant therapists. Dwairy notes three major assumptions of Western psychotherapy that do not hold true for most or all Palestinian service users in Israel: "(1) individuals are independent entities and possess autonomous selves or personalities; (2) intrapsychic processes and conflicts explain and predict behavior and symptoms; and (3) psychotherapy helps generate new intrapsychic order by bringing repressed unconscious content to consciousness. This new order enables self-control and self-actualization." Dwairy proposes the application of "culture-analysis [which] is an approach and technique that directs therapists to employ the client's culture to bypass . . . resistance and facilitate change while avoiding confrontation with the family."

The book closes with a discussion and illustration in chapter 21, "Psychiatric Rehabilitation in the Context of Palestinian Citizens in Israel." David Roe, Paula Garber-Epstein, and Anwar Khatib follow the results of the rehabilitation law approved in Israel in 2000. This legislation was designed to fulfill objectives for psychiatric care by addressing psychosocial needs that enable full participation in society. The law complies with the UN Convention on the Rights of Persons with Disabilities, which Israel has signed and ratified.

The editors thank the contributors, each of whom shares responsibility for this book and has contributed generously with both knowledge and time. Without their efforts, this publication would not have been possible. Further special thanks go to the Israeli Institute for Health Services Research and the Paul Barrwald School of Social Work and Social Welfare at the Hebrew University of Jerusalem, which generously supported the work of editing and indexing the book with unrestricted grants. Finally, we thank Barbara Doron and Shir Zur for their professional and diligent editorial work. Our recognition goes as well to the two anonymous reviewers for their insightful comments and to Indiana University Press, which provided us with its expertise and reputation.

References

Feagin, J. R., & Feagin, C. B. (2011). *Racial and ethnic relations.* (9th ed.). Upper Saddle River, NJ: Pearson.

Israel Central Bureau of Statistics. (2018). Demographics. Retrieved from https://www.cbs.gov.il /he/publications/DocLib/2018/shnaton69/shnaton69.pdf.

Patel, V., & Prince, M. (2010). Global mental health: A new global health field comes of age. *JAMA, 303*(19), 1976–1977.

Sagy, S., Orr, E., Bar-On, D., & Awwad, E. (2001). Individualism and collectivism in two conflicted societies: Comparing Israeli-Jewish and Palestinian-Arab high school students. *Youth & Society, 33*(1), 3–30.

UN General Assembly. (1992). *Resolution 47/135: Declaration on the rights of persons belonging to national or ethnic, religious and linguistic minorities.* Geneva: United Nations. Retrieved from http://www.un-documents.net/a47r135.htm.

PART I
CULTURAL AND SOCIOPOLITICAL DETERMINANTS OF MENTAL HEALTH

1

PALESTINIAN CITIZENS IN ISRAEL

Sociopolitical Status as a Mental Health Determinant

As'ad Ghanem and Ibrahim Khatib

T HE SITUATION OF THE PALESTINIAN MINORITY IN ISRAEL is complex, with several intertwined sets of political and psychological dimensions. Understanding the status and politics of these people requires understanding how they are affected by three domains:

1. National clashes: Waged in the political field, the struggle between Palestinians and Israelis, especially Zionists, involves both national identities in their attempts to possess and control historical Palestine and its inhabitants.

Zionism, in its political practical stage, began with the migration of Jews to Palestine during the nineteenth century and with the establishment of settlement outposts such as Tel Aviv, Nahalal, Petah Tikva, and others. By the time of the Palestinian expulsion in 1948 (during the Nakba), there were 312 Jewish settlements in Israel, including 26 cities, towns, and villages; 44 *moshavim* (working villages); 148 *kibbutzim* (collectivistic communities); and 94 small settlement outposts. Approximately 650,000 Jewish residents controlled about 7% of the land (Yiftachel, 2006).

The Arab-Israeli War (1947–1949) broke out in the wake of the proposed UN partition plan, which aimed to set up two states: a Jewish state covering 55% of the land of Mandatory Palestine and a Palestinian state covering about 45% of the territory. During this war, more than 700,000 Palestinians became refugees, and Israel took control of more than 78% of Mandatory Palestinian land (Khalidi, 1997). The borders of this area, known as the Green Line, demarcate Israel from its neighbors. One hundred sixty thousand Palestinians remained in Israel and were granted citizenship. A decade later, Israel had taken in about 800,000 Jewish refugees and immigrants. In contrast, Palestinian refugees were denied the right to return. Most of these have remained scattered all over the world, including in neighboring Arab states. Following the 1967 war, Israel occupied the rest of Mandatory Palestine. The state and its colonial branches started the settlement process hesitantly at first, then unrestrainedly. Settlers eventually seized more than 40% of the West Bank territories.

Israel's successes and victories have not ended the Palestinians' struggle for land, rights, and recognition of their right for self-determination and return from forced exile by Israel. Palestinians continue to engage in bitter opposition against Israel and maintain strong positions within historical Palestine. This has prevented Israel from achieving its national goal of total control. Importantly, Palestinian citizens in Israel have taken a decisive role in this clash, thus becoming an essential part of the Israel-Palestine conflict, although not all have supported this effort.

Accordingly, Palestinian citizens in Israel constitute a target of Israeli policies and security concerns. Security resources, including surveillance and dispersal and demoralization tactics, are employed to observe and control them so that they do not form an effective component of the general struggle between Israel and the Palestinians (see, for example, Ghanem & Mustafa, 2011; Lustick, 1980). The deployment of such policies has intensified with the growing awareness of Palestinian national identity concomitant with the rise of the Israeli extreme right to power and its widening base.

2. Type of minority: The civil status of minorities in general is influenced by the type of minority—that is, indigenous versus immigrant (Ghanem, 2012; Kymlicka, 1995). For Palestinians in Israel, their citizenship is based on the dissonant relationship between an indigenous minority and the colonial entity that has taken over the land.

"Indigenous minority" is a modern political term that refers to the remaining members of a population group who continue to live in their homeland despite its occupation by immigrant groups that have come to establish a new state over its ruins. This process turns them into a numerical and political minority (Jamal, 2011). Palestinian citizens in Israel are classified as an indigenous minority in both definition and form. As such, this group meets most of the criteria that define indigenous people set by the UN Sub-Commission on Prevention of Discrimination and Protection of Minorities (United Nations, 2013, pp. 6–10): historical continuity; voluntary preservation of cultural identity; self-identification as indigenous; and facing subjugation, marginalization, expulsion, exclusion, and discrimination by the dominant community. In addition, indigenous status is based on the conditional relations between the existence of a group of people as a community and their link to a specific place (Jamal, 2011; Pappé, 2011).

What concerns us in this context is how this indigenous minority maintains its political, social, and cultural specificity. Its collective rights to distinction from the dominant majority are confirmed in the International Labor Organization (ILO) Convention 169 on Indigenous and Tribal Peoples in Independent Countries (1989) in various articles: Article 2(2) mandates "promoting the full realization of the social, economic and cultural rights of these peoples with respect for their social and cultural identity, their customs and traditions and their institutions." Article 3(2) states, "No form of force or coercion shall be used in violation of the human rights and fundamental freedoms of the peoples concerned." Article 5(a) states, "The social, cultural, religious and spiritual values and practices of these peoples shall be recognized and protected, and due account shall be taken of the nature of the problems which face them both as groups and as individuals" (see International Labour Organization, 1989). Note as well that Article 1 of the 1992 UN Declaration on the Rights of Persons Belonging to National or Ethnic, Religious and Linguistic Minorities determines, "States shall protect the existence and the national or ethnic, cultural, religious and linguistic identity of minorities within their respective territories and shall encourage conditions for the promotion of that identity" (United Nations, 1992).

According to the Palestinian narrative, Israel is the product of a colonial oc-cupation by population groups of heterogeneous origins of a land that does not belong to them. This narrative has provoked broad debate among Israeli academics since Israeli researcher Gershon Shafir (1989) published a book about the colonial nature of the Zionist project in Palestine. Shafir and Peled consider colonialism the most appropriate theoretical framework to understand and deeply analyze the development of Israeli society from 1882 to the present (Peled & Shafir, 2005; Shafir & Peled, 2002). Other researchers consider the colonial nature of Israel to be the key to understanding Israeli society, which is based on the expulsion of the Palestinians (Pappé, 2007).

3. Character of the regime: Israel has generally been presented by the Israeli and Western academic establishment as being a normal state established on the ba-sis of the Jewish national (Zionist) demand for the right to self-determination. This vision has received international political support from UN resolutions, the most important being the partition plan in 1947, as well as strong support from a large number of states. This position is also backed by public opinion and the political elite in Israel, as well as some of the local Palestinian elite.

In addition, the Israeli regime is usually presented as being a stable democracy with the basic advantages of the Western democratic system. It has been analyzed using theoretical frameworks developed in the Western world to understand the structures of states and their changes (see, for example, Peled & Shafir, 2005; Ram, 1995). Some researchers even characterize the Israeli regime as one of the world's liberal democracies. They employ these theoretical frameworks to respond to claims that cast doubt on this view (Yakobson & Rubinstein, 2003). Israeli social scientists have dedicated enormous efforts to showing Israel—state and community—as a liberal democratic system that has a policy of assimilating minorities, both indig-enous residents and immigrants, using similar methods to those adopted by the open systems in Europe, the United States, and Canada. According to this concept, Israel belongs to the club of so-called enlightened states that include the aforemen-tioned states (for more details, see Ram, 1995; Shafir & Peled, 2002).

In contrast, other researchers have developed a different understanding, arguing that Israel is a state established by a colonizing process and maintained by a regime based on ethnicity that relies on preferential treatment for the group that founded it. For example, Zureik (1979), Nakhleh (1975, 1979), and Falah (1989) have published a series of studies that describe Israel as a clear demonstration of classic colonialism, one whose internal structure is a product of the paradoxes that accompany colonialism. Additionally, some researchers have analyzed the superstructure of the Israeli state and its relationship to groups. Ghanem (1998, p. 429) presents the regime in Israel as bearing the features of a "tyranny of the majority." Yiftachel and Ghanem (2004) have developed an alternative theoretical framework to understand Israel and other groups of international regimes that consider Israel an ethnocratic state.

An ethnocratic regime is based on a nationalist project that imposes the dominant national ethnicity's control over place through expansion and settlement. In the case of Zionism, the extension of place and control over space creates this ethnocratic regime (Yiftachel, 2004). Space is considered an essential aspect that aims to create a new ethnic political geography following these steps: colonial separation aimed at spreading the majority group in space, conversion of the minority into a threat to ethnic control over space, application of planning policies that include ethnic spatial control, and, finally, continuous structural discrimination in the fields of development and the distribution of resources (Yiftachel & Ghanem, 2004, p. 653).

Israel's treatment of the Palestinian minority in the period after 1948 was not based on democracy and citizenship but on colonial behavior toward the indigenous group. The structure applied to the Palestinian citizens in Israel has led to their marginalization. The Palestinian educational system is aimed at retaining control of Palestinian citizens in Israel (Al-Haj, 1995), and the Israeli political system seeks to exclude Palestinian citizens from political decision making—although they have representation in the Knesset (parliament)—and from control of the distribution of tangible and intangible resources (Ghanem, 2001). Palestinian participation in the Israeli economy is marginal and will remain so until there is a self-ruled autonomous Palestinian economy (Haidar, 1990). However, in light of the changes that began at the end of the 1990s and reached their climax in the second intifada (insurrection or uprising) in October 2000 and beyond, Palestinians have had to look for political tools and messages that take them from the "situation of following," the case for five decades, to a "process of starting," by redefining citizenship through a special Palestinian national agenda and new political tools (see Ghanem & Mustafa, 2018)

Recent Developments Assailing Palestinian Citizenship

During the past few years, political and legal efforts have been directed toward eroding the status and rights of Palestinian citizens in Israel. These attempts have been translated into practices and actions on the ground and fueled by official statements and legislation in the Knesset that reflect increased discrimination against Palestinian citizens. Indeed, reports have shown increasing inequality between the Jewish majority and the Palestinian minority in all areas of life in Israel (Adalah: The Legal Center for Arab Minority Rights in Israel [Adalah], 2012; Fuchs, Blander, & Kremnitzer, 2015).

These developments have been accompanied by a popular climate that largely supports strengthening the Jewish character of the state, even at the expense of democracy and the rights of Palestinian citizens. According to the *Democracy Index 2015* (Hermann, Heller, Cohen, & Bublil, 2015), an Israel Democracy Institute poll shows that many Jewish people oppose the inclusion of Palestinian citizens in Israel in decision making, while some Jewish Israelis actually support discrimination against Palestinians, including the desire to prevent Palestinians from living near them.

According to this study, most of the Jewish community (61%) also support depriving Palestinians of the right to vote unless they swear an oath of allegiance to the state as a Jewish state and to its symbols (Hermann et al., 2015). This response expresses a prevailing view within the Jewish community that Palestinians constitute a threat to the state as an entity and the state as it is defined.

A poll by the Pew Research Center (2016) indicates that Jewish Israelis hold a negative image of Palestinians and of their relationship to them. The poll showed that 48% of Israeli Jews support the expulsion of Palestinians from Israel. The respondents also felt that Jewish Israeli residents of different political and social backgrounds must remain united in the view that Israel is a nation for the Jewish people (Sudan, 2016).

This popular Israeli sentiment is fueled by the move to the extreme right of the political spectrum and the erosion of Palestinian citizenship. Official governmental and political bodies seek to strengthen this move through laws and statements aimed at advancing the status of the Jewish majority at the expense of the Palestinian minority. Such legislation has become increasingly common in recent years, particularly since Benjamin Netanyahu became prime minister. During Netanyahu's second term as prime minister, from 2009 to 2013, many undemocratic laws were approved, essentially aimed at undermining the equality of Palestinian citizens and fundamental democratic values (Fuchs et al., 2015).

Adalah (2015) maintains a database of discriminatory laws against Palestinians. Some of these laws dating from 2008 to 2015 relate to land issues and are meant to secure the Jewish character of the state and allow for the seizure of land owned by Palestinian refugees who left their land after the Nakba and the establishment of the state of Israel. These lands are now owned by the state; the Israel Land Authority, the governmental body that manages land allocation; and the Jewish Agency, a nonprofit organization promoting Jewish immigration. The new laws allow the privatization of state land and its use in ways that serve the state agenda; such as selling and exchanging land with the nonprofit organization the Jewish National

Fund. Eventually, these lands are made available exclusively for the use of the Jewish people. A recent law also guarantees representation of the Jewish National Fund on the Israel Lands Council, which sets land policies for the Israel Land Authority.

In addition, the Economic Efficiency Law, applied in 2009 and 2010, provides the state with unchecked discretion to classify some towns as national priority areas, granting them advantages in the allocation of facilities, including reduction in taxes and targeting them for economic stimulus programs. The law's wording does not spell out specific measures to determine which towns merit these privileges. In practice, it is predominantly Jewish Israeli towns that receive these benefits, while Palestinian towns that suffer from economic hardship are clearly discriminated against.

The Negev region, in the south of Israel, is currently a major focus of the struggle between Palestinian citizens and Israeli authorities. This conflict is manifested in the demolition of Bedouins' homes, which the government claims are built illegally; the confiscation of land; and the refusal to recognize dozens of settlements that existed before the establishment of the state. Amendment No. 4/2010 of the Negev Development Authority Law (Knesset, 2010) enables the Negev Development Authority to recommend land to be used to create additional settlements for Jews in the Negev. Currently, 60 Jewish settlements in the Negev have been individually built and legally approved. Yet, there is no recognition or even provision of basic facilities for villages inhabited by about 80,000 Palestinian Bedouins, all of whom have Israeli citizenship (Adalah, 2015).

Other Developments Undermining Palestinian Minority Rights

In addition, there is an attempt to erase the collective memory of Palestinian citizens in Israel. For example, an amendment to the Budgets Foundations Law known as the Nakba Law, approved by the Knesset in May 2011, gives the finance minister authority to cut government funding or support to institutions that conduct activities that reject the definition of the state of Israel as a democratic Jewish state or that commemorate Israel's Independence Day, the day the state was established, as Nakba Day, a day of sadness and mourning for Palestinians. The law is apparently aimed at criminalizing opposition to the Jewish definition of Israel by undermining freedom of expression and the need to debate and exchange views on political issues that concern all citizens, particularly Palestinian citizens. The law also attempts to cut the emotional ties Palestinian citizens in Israel have to their past and their people and to forcibly integrate them into the Israeli state system.

Conclusion

In our view, since the start of the peace process with the Palestinians that led to the signing of the Oslo Accords in 1993 that relegated the majority of Palestinians to living outside the Green Line, and after the 2000 intifada, Israel has officially moved to a new stage in its dealings with its Palestinian citizens. A series of laws and procedures, approved by the Jewish majority in the Knesset and carried out by official bodies, implicitly support the need to protect the ethnic superiority of Jews and set out a clearly discriminatory legal definition of the Jewish state.

These policies have been accompanied by inflammatory statements made by popular Israeli leaders that promote official animosity toward Palestinians, despite their legal status as citizens. One example is a statement made by Netanyahu on election day in 2015 that "Arab voters are heading to the polling stations in droves" (Zonszein, 2015). Netanyahu himself also warned Arabs against supporting their elected leaders and demanded that they break away from them, saying, "The leadership is causing a provocation" (Jabbour, 2015), and other statements and laws that show the Arabs as a threat to Israeli "national security paradigm" (Ghanem & Khatib, 2017). These statements have contributed to the ongoing degradation of Palestinians' rights as citizens. Palestinian leaders in Israel have pointed to the increasing trend toward using citizenship as a way of consolidating Jewish supremacy. The Israeli government still seeks to legislate limits on Palestinian citizenship that will fit its Zionist-Israeli aims and vision.

AS'AD GHANEM is Professor in the School of Political Science at the University of Haifa, Israel.

IBRAHIM KHATIB is an academic visitor conducting his postdoctoral research at the Oxford School of Global and Area Studies at the University of Oxford, United Kingdom.

References

Adalah: The Legal Center for Arab Minority Rights in Israel [Adalah]. (2012). *Report on inequality: Palestinian-Arab minority in Israel* [in Arabic]. Retrieved from https://www .adalah.org/uploads/oldfiles/Public/file/Inequality%20Report%20Arabic.pdf.

Adalah: The Legal Center for Arab Minority Rights in Israel [Adalah]. (2015). *Database of discriminatory laws* [in Arabic]. Retrieved from https://www.adalah.org/en/content/view /7771.

Al-Haj, M. (1995). *Education, empowerment and control: The case of the Arabs in Israel.* Albany: State University of New York Press.

Falah, G. (1989). *The forgotten Palestinian: The Arab Bedouins in the Naqab* [in Arabic]. Tayiba: Palestinian Heritage Center.

Fuchs, A., Blander, D., & Kremnitzer, M. (2015). *Anti-democratic legislation in the 18th Knesset (2009–2013)* [in Hebrew]. Jerusalem: Israel Democracy Institute. Retrieved from https:// www.idi.org.il/media/4058/anti_democratic_legislation.pdf.

Ghanem, A. (1998). State and minority in Israel: The case of ethnic state and the predicament of its minority. *Ethnic and Racial Studies, 21*(3), 428–448.

Ghanem, A. (2001). *The Palestinian-Arab minority in Israel, 1948–2000: A political study.* New York: State University of New York Press.

Ghanem, A. (2012). Understanding ethnic minority demands: A new typology. *Nationalism and Ethnic Politics, 18*(3), 358–379.

Ghanem, A. A., & Khatib, I. (2017). The nationalisation of the Israeli ethnocratic regime and the Palestinian minority's shrinking citizenship. *Citizenship Studies, 21*(8), 889–902.

Ghanem, A. & Mohanad M. (2018). *Palestinians in Israel: The politics of faith after Oslo.* Cambridge University Press.

Ghanem, A., & Mustafa, M. (2011). The Palestinians in Israel: The challenge of the indigenous group politics in the "Jewish state." *Journal of Muslim Minority Affairs, 31*(2), 177–196.

Haidar, A. (1990). *The Arab population in the Israeli economy.* Tel Aviv: International Center for Peace in the Middle East.

Hermann, T., Heller, E., Cohen, C., & Bublil, D. (2015). *The Israeli democracy index 2015* [in Hebrew]. Jerusalem: Israel Democracy Institute. Retrieved from http://www.idi.org.il/media/4254068/democracy_index_2015.pdf.

International Labour Organization. (1989). Indigenous and Tribal Peoples Convention. Geneva: International Labour Organization. Retrieved from https://www.ilo.org/dyn/normlex/en/f?p=NORMLEXPUB:12100:0::NO::P12100_ILO_CODE:C169.

Jabbour, A. (2015). Odeh: Netanyahu should be prosecuted for incitement. *NRG* [in Hebrew]. Retrieved from http://www.nrg.co.il/online/1/ART2/731/049.html.

Jamal, A. (2011). *Arab minority nationalism in Israel: The politics of indigeneity.* New York: Routledge.

Khalidi, R. (1997). *Palestinian identity: The construction of modern national consciousness.* New York: Columbia University Press.

Knesset. (2010). Amendment No. 4/2010 of the Negev Development Authority Law. Jerusalem: Knesset. Retrieved from http://negev.co.il/%D7%97%D7%95%D7%A7-.

Kymlicka, W. (1995). *Multicultural citizenship: A liberal theory of minority rights.* New York: Clarendon.

Lustick, I. (1980). *Arabs in the Jewish state: Israel's control of a national minority.* Austin: University of Texas Press.

Nakhleh, K. (1975). Cultural determinants of Palestinian collective identity: The case of the Arabs in Israel. *New Outlook, 18*(7), 31–40.

Nakhleh, K. (1979). *Palestinian dilemma: Nationalist consciousness and university education in Israel.* Shrewsbury, MA: Association of Arab-American University Graduates.

Pappé, I. (2007). *The ethnic cleansing of Palestine.* London: Oneworld.

Pappé, I. (2011). *The forgotten Palestinians: A history of the Palestinians in Israel.* London: Yale University Press.

Peled, Y., & Shafir, G. (2005). *Being Israeli* [in Hebrew]. Tel Aviv: Tel Aviv University Press.

Pew Research Center. (2016, March 8). *Israel's religiously divided society.* Retrieved from http://www.pewforum.org/2016/03/08/israels-religiously-divided-society/.

Ram, U. (1995). Zionist historiography and the invention of modern Jewish nationhood: The case of Ben Zion Dinur. *History and Memory, 7*(1), 91–124.

Shafir, G. (1989). *Land, labor and the origins of the Israeli-Palestinian conflict, 1882–1914.* London: University of California Press.

Shafir, G., & Peled, Y. (2002). *Being Israeli: The dynamics of multiple citizenship.* Cambridge: Cambridge University Press.

Sudan, O. (2016, March 8). Serious poll: Nearly half of Jews support expelling Arabs from Israel [in Hebrew]. *Maariv.* Retrieved from http://www.nrg.co.il/online/1/ART2/759/498.html.

United Nations. (1992). Declaration on the rights of persons belonging to national or ethnic, religious and linguistic minorities. Geneva: Office of the United Nations High Commissioner for Human Rights. Retrieved from https://www.ohchr.org/en/professionalinterest/pages/minorities.aspx.

United Nations. (2013). Declaration on the rights of indigenous peoples: A manual for national human rights institutions. Geneva: Office of the United Nations High Commissioner for Human Rights. Retrieved from https://www.ohchr.org/documents/issues/ipeoples/undripmanualfornhris.pdf.

Yakobson, A., & Rubinstein, A. (2003). *Israel and the family of nations* [in Hebrew]. Tel Aviv: Schocken.

Yiftachel, O. (2004). Contradictions and dialectics: Reshaping political space in Israel/Palestine. An indirect response to Lina Jamoul. *Antipode, 36*(4), 607–613.

Yiftachel, O. (2006). *Ethnocracy: Land and identity politics in Israel/Palestine*. Philadelphia: University of Pennsylvania Press.

Yiftachel, O., & Ghanem, A. (2004). Understanding "ethnocratic" regimes: The politics of seizing contested territories. *Political Geography, 23*(6), 647–676.

Zonszein, M. (2015). Binyamin Netanyahu: "Arab voters are heading to the polling stations in droves." *The Guardian*. Retrieved from https://www.theguardian.com/world/2015/mar/17/binyamin-netanyahu-israel-arab-election.

Zureik, E. (1979). *The Palestinians in Israel: A study in internal colonialism*. London: Routledge.

2

BETWEEN PAST AND PRESENT

Psychological Effects of the Nakba among Palestinian Citizens in Israel

Sfaa Ghnadre-Naser

If your past is an experience,
make tomorrow a meaning and a vision.

—Mahmoud Darwish, *Counterpoint for Edward Said*

THE 1948 WAR—THE NAKBA—IS CONSIDERED THE MOST SIGNIFICANT crisis point in the history of Palestinian people. For years, however, the wartime experiences and their lingering emotional and physical effects on the Palestinians were silenced and kept absent from public and academic discourse. This chapter attempts to shed some light on this much-neglected subject by presenting the main findings of a research project that retrospectively explored the subjective meanings and psychological effects of the Nakba on those who survived the ordeal among the Palestinian population living in Israel.[1]

Since World War II, studies reporting the severe consequences of wars and armed conflicts on the psychological world of the individual and on the individual's ability to function in different fields of life have multiplied (Eyber, 2002). Most documented effects refer to the development of posttraumatic symptoms and disorders such as anxiety, depression, and posttraumatic stress disorders (PTSDs) (Briere, 2004; Farhood & Dimassi, 2012; Jamil et al., 2002; Richards et al., 2011). Studies have also discussed the role of vulnerability and resiliency in the individual's ability to face those ordeals (Bonanno, Galea, Bucciarelli, & Vlahov, 2007; Porter & Haslam, 2005; Sossou, Craig, Ogren, & Schnak, 2008). These studies raise awareness of the psychological effects of war and the psychological dynamics that the population experiences while coping with them, highlighting the population's needs for care for policy makers.

One sad outcome of armed conflicts is that people are forcibly displaced. Over 65 million people have been displaced worldwide according to the recent report of the UN High Commissioner for Refugees (UNCHR) (2017). The psychological needs of these populations are considered a health priority; therefore, action is needed to identify, understand, and resolve these mental health issues. Refugees lose their homes, sources of income, and the social and cultural communities that have granted them a sense of belonging and stability (Fangen, 2006; Porter & Haslam, 2005). After arriving at their new destinations, refugees face continuing daily struggles, including psychological aftereffects and acculturation challenges. They are simultaneously expected to deal with the discontinuity of their previous lives and adjust to their new social and cultural realities (Bernardes et al., 2011; Bottura & Mancini, 2016).

High levels of psychological distress, anxiety, depression, and PTSDs have been documented among various refugee populations at different periods after they have been forced to leave their countries (Ai & Peterson, 2005; Jamil et al., 2002; Mollica, Caridad, & Massagli, 2007; Richards et al., 2011), as well as among internally displaced populations who have not crossed international borders seeking sanctuary (Araya, Chotai, Komproe, & de Jong, 2007; Schmidt, Kravic, & Ehlert, 2008). Exposure to war has been found to elevate anxiety and PTSD prevalence rates in multiple Arab countries, including Algeria, Iraq, Kuwait, Lebanon, Sudan, and Palestine (de Jong et al., 2001; Farhood & Dimassi, 2012; Tanios et al., 2009).

In recent decades, studies have been carried out among different groups of Palestinians. A significant body of literature addresses the effects of the prolonged occupation, military attacks, and wartime events on those living in the West Bank and the Gaza Strip (Hobfoll, Hall, & Canetti, 2012; Netland, 2013; Shehadeh, 2015), while others have investigated Palestinian refugees in Arab countries (Chatty, 2009; Feldman, 2008; Salih, 2013). Regarding Palestinians living in Israel, scholars have started to pay more attention to their distinctiveness in different fields of social and psychological research (Hamama-Raz, Solomon, Cohen, & Laufer, 2008; Somer, Maguen, Or-Chen, & Litz, 2009). Nonetheless, the sparse discourse about the Nakba remains mostly confined to sociohistorical fields of research (Al-Haj, 1986; Kabha, 2006; Kassem, 2011; Ram, 2009) and has neglected exploration of its psychological effects (Dwairy, 2010).

The Nakba and Palestinian Citizens in Israel

In November 1947, the proposed UN partition plan for Palestine recommended the creation of two states—Arab and Jewish. Harsh fighting and military operations took place for more than a year and a half, leading to the establishment of Israel and to the events of the Nakba—the catastrophe of the Palestinian people (for a detailed history of the events, see Abu-Sitta, 2004). Yet, in the words of Edward Said (1998), Palestine and Palestinians remain, despite Israel's concerted efforts from the beginning either to get rid of them or to circumscribe them so much as to make them ineffective. . . . There is no getting away from the fact that as an idea, a memory, and as an often buried or invisible reality, Palestine and its people have simply not disappeared.

The Syrian Lebanese intellectual Constantin Zureiq coined the term "Nakba" to convey the dreadful consequences of the 1948 war on the Palestinians (Ibn Khaldun Association, 2005). According to different estimates, by the end of the war, Israel controlled 78% of Palestine (instead of the 56% outlined in the partition plan) and had succeeded in emptying and destroying approximately 450 villages while expelling approximately 750,000 Palestinian inhabitants to bordering Arab countries (Abu-Sitta, 2004; Khalidi, 1997).

About 160,000 Palestinians remained in the territory that became Israel. Fifty percent of them were internally displaced persons (IDPs) who were prevented from returning to their villages or regaining possession of their property (Kabha & Barzilai, 1996; Wakim, 2001). At the time, the provisional government of Israel enacted the Defense (Emergency) Regulations of the British Mandate of 1945 that served as the legal basis for imposing martial law on Palestinian citizens, controlling every aspect of their lives for almost two decades (Ozacky-Lazar, 2002). Within a few months, Palestinians living in Israel became refugees in their own homeland, citizens in a country that initially disregarded their existence and continues to define itself as Jewish. This has been a further complicated and agonizing reality for the IDPs. Abu-Baker and Rabinowitz (2004) called the first generation of Palestinians who suffered the political, social, and cultural upheavals of the Nakba and became Israeli citizens "the survivors." For years, these survivors strived to rebuild their lives while dealing with their status as an oppressed minority, facing racism, poverty, discrimination, and insecurity (Al-Haj, 1986; Kabha & Barzilai, 1996).

The Nakba therefore resulted in the disintegration of Palestinian society, leaving it in a state of crisis and chaos (Abu-Lughod & Sa'di, 2007). As noted earlier, for years, researchers and scholars have ignored the consequences of the Nakba on its surviving population. Different rationales have been suggested for this void, starting with reasons related to the Palestinians themselves: to events they have experienced throughout their history and to faults in their documentation and research traditions. Suggested external reasons focus on the effect of sociopolitical agendas and power processes, such as the complicated relations within the Arab world, the pervasive Israeli narrative, and the prolonged military occupation (Abu-Lughod & Sa'di, 2007; Kabha, 2006; Ram, 2009).

As with many wars and traumatic events in human history, the Palestinian Nakba is an ongoing reality; the present remains tangled with the past. Palestinians living in Israel continue to encounter injustice, discrimination, and racism daily (Arab Association for Human Rights, 2016; Association for Civil Rights in Israel, 2016). Under these circumstances, the appropriate and safe conditions needed for Palestinians to think about and reflect on their past are impeded (Abu-Lughod & Sa'di, 2007; Kassem, 2011).

To this day, Israel and the majority of its Jewish population fail to acknowledge Palestinian suffering as a result of the 1948 war (Even-Tzur, 2016). The Palestinians' Nakba experience is deemed illegitimate and even dangerous for undermining the "rightful" existence of Israel (Abu-Lughod & Sa'di, 2007; Kassem, 2011) and thus is being suppressed by the popular narrative (Liem, 2007; Sawada, Chaitin, & Bar-On, 2004) of the victorious birth of the Israeli state: "The uprooting of the Palestinians in 1948 thus gets here a doubly layered meaning—first, their actual uprooting from the place, and second, the later ideational . . . uprooting from Israeli collective conscience for decades to come" (Ram, 2009, p. 370).

Psychological perspectives have recently been offered to explain this silencing of the Nakba in Israel by addressing the effects of group dynamics, emotional reactions, and defense mechanisms, such as repression and denial (Even-Tzur, 2016; Halperin, Bar-Tal, Sharvit, Rosler, & Raviv, 2010; Kleinot, 2011). Kemp (2011), for example, has analyzed the effect of guilt felt by Israelis that unconsciously sustains their denial of accountability and contributes to dehumanization of the Palestinians.

Intrapsychic dynamics may have also contributed to the absence of a coherent Nakba narrative. Defending themselves against facing hurtful memories (Nakhleh, 2009), survivors might activate avoidance and repression mechanisms. In this regard, scholars have identified a conspiracy of silence as a communication pattern among Holocaust and other trauma survivors, which refers to the unspoken agreement within the family to avoid talking about past traumatic experiences (Gheith, 2007; Kellermann, 2001; Tankink, 2004; Wiseman, Metzl, & Barber, 2006). Recently, Abu-El-Hija (2016) has reported similar results among Palestinian IDPs in Israel. His findings showed that forcibly displaced parents tended to keep silent about their traumatic experiences, sharing them less frequently with younger generations than parents who were not displaced during the Nakba.

A Psychological Perspective on the Nakba: The Birth of a Research Project

As a Palestinian living in Israel, I have been exposed to the relentless effort to suppress and erase my national identity and the collective history of my people. It started with the education system. In elementary school, I was taught an Israeli independence song, "بعيد استقلال بلادي غرد الطير الشادي" (At the independence holiday of my country the singing bird sang!). In high school, I studied and had my matriculation exams in Jewish history, which taught me such false aphorisms as "A land without a people for a people without a land," "Zionists who made the desert bloom," and "the Arabs who themselves ran away." Literature lessons included Jewish writers and poets (e.g., Rachel Blubshtein and Hayim Nahman Bialik) while Palestinian authors and poets (e.g., Mahmoud Darwish and Ghassan Kanafani) were absent.

I was raised in a politically involved family and community, and at home I was taught to acknowledge my national history and cultural heritage. My parents, who were young children during the Nakba, were expelled with the rest of my village population and started to walk toward the Lebanese border. A few weeks later, a combination of circumstances allowed them to return to the village, where they discovered that their homes had been robbed. Srouji (2004) painfully describes how he witnessed the expulsion of the people of my village, Rama: "Meanwhile this gunfire was continuing, clearly intending to get people moving. . . . Sobbing loudly, they passed in front of the Nakhle [family] houses. . . . They were setting off on a 'trail of tears' towards the Lebanese border. The most heartrending sight was the cats and dogs trying to follow their masters; I heard a man shout to his dog: 'Go back! At least you can stay!'" (p. 77).

While studying for my academic degree in clinical psychology, I became increasingly interested in the subjective experiences of the individual and in human feelings, thoughts, and psychic reality. Accordingly, I began raising questions about the psychological aspects of my people's existence, tracing back to the seminal event of their lives. The imbalance between the sociopolitical emphasis and the psychological disregard concerning the Nakba always bothered me. My curiosity regarding the private experiences of those who went through the Nakba paved the way to my doctoral thesis (Ghnadre-Naser, 2012), in which I was trying to reach a more balanced and integrated existence for myself while attempting to give voice to those who were usually silenced before it was too late.

In the following sections, I present selected aspects of this research, which appears to be the first to address not only the reported events of the Nakba and the subsequent uprooting but also its immediate and later psychological consequences among Palestinians living in Israel, applying a mixed methods examination.

Mixed Methods

This method involves collecting, analyzing, and integrating quantitative and qualitative data for a more comprehensive understanding of the research problem (Creswell, 2009; Morgan, 1998; Tashakkori & Teddlie, 2003). Using mixed methods enables the researcher to address a wider range of questions and provide stronger evidence for the conclusions (Johnson & Onwuegbuzie, 2004).

Sequential exploratory design (Creswell, 2009) was applied, consisting of two sequential phases. The first phase refers to a qualitative phenomenological exploration of the subjective experience of the IDPs and the uprooting of their villages during the Nakba. That is followed by a quantitative phase, which examined the relations between exposure to wartime events and loss of personal resources and the emotional consequences of war among the Palestinian population in Israel in general.

Researchers recommend using phenomenology to explore an uninvestigated phenomenon or population (Creswell, 1998, 2009; Moustakas, 1994). Thus, I applied a phenomenological method of inquiry in an attempt to bring the experience and its aftermath to life and capture its shared meaning among aging participants.

I designed the quantitative phase based on the identified themes of the first phase, hence allowing exploration of the generalizability of the results. The research hypotheses were grouped into three main clusters and identified a number of expectations.

1. Hypotheses regarding the period of the 1948 war: a relationship was expected to be found between the level of exposure to potentially traumatic events, the level of resource loss during the war, and posttraumatic symptoms experienced during the war and its aftermath and reported in the present.
2. Hypotheses regarding relations between participants' experiences of the 1948 war and their emotional state in the present: it was expected that reports of more difficult wartime experiences (according to the measures in the preceding cluster) would be connected to a poorer emotional state in the present, according to the measures of psychological distress and psychological well-being.
3. Hypotheses about differences between groups: it was expected that the experiences of the war and its consequences would be more severe among IDPs than among comparative populations who had not been uprooted (henceforth referred to as locals).

Participants

People who were contacted usually responded positively to the request to participate in a study about the 1948 war. Those who refused gave various reasons, primarily concerning health and age-related difficulties. A few were reluctant to talk about the 1948 war. Five other participants were excluded from the second phase for nonvalid questionnaires. Overall, the 131 participants of both phases of the study represent 71% of those initially contacted.

The qualitative phase included 10 participants, five women and five men originally from 10 different uprooted villages and now IDPs living in northern Israel. As recommended in phenomenological research, sampling was purposeful and aimed at a deliberate search for IDPs who had experienced the Nakba and were able to elaborate on their wartime experiences (Creswell, 1998; Morse, 2000).

The quantitative phase included 121 participants (60 women and 61 men) living in different villages and cities in northern Israel. Of these, 60 had been internally displaced and 61 were locals. The current age range of the participants was 69–93 ($M = 76.9$; $SD = 4.8$), while during the Nakba, the age range had been 7–31 ($M = 15.4$; $SD = 4.7$).

Matched sampling was used to minimize the effect of different background variables. For each internally displaced participant, a corresponding participant was recruited from the local group who was of the same gender, religion, and age range (± five years) and who was presently living in the same village or city. To ensure diversity of wartime experiences, the recruiting process for the study was designed to include participants from as many uprooted villages as possible. The 61 participants of the IDP group represented 28 uprooted villages in the north of Israel (e.g., Amqa, Bir'im, Hadatha, and Myjaydil).[2]

Measures

Semistructured in-depth interviews were conducted for phenomenological exploration during the first phase. Open-ended questions were designed to fully explore the participants' experiences of the Nakba and their uprooting from their villages: events and challenges they faced during and after the war; their personal reactions, thoughts, feelings and coping strategies; and their current understanding and personal meanings of their experiences.

Various questionnaires were administered during the quantitative phase:

- The Background and Nakba Questionnaire was composed for the study and included questions regarding demographic data (e.g., age, gender, education, economic state, number of children) alongside questions concerning the participants' personal history during the Nakba.
- The Harvard Trauma Questionnaire (HTQ) (Mollica et al., 1992) inquires about a variety of traumatic events, as well as the emotional symptoms considered to be uniquely associated with them. It has been used with various refugee populations around the world, demonstrating satisfactory reliability and validity for evaluating traumatic events and symptoms among different cultures (Shoeb, Weinstein, & Mollica, 2007), including studies in the Arab world (Farhood & Dimassi, 2012; Farwell, 2003; Slewa-Younan et al., 2012). Two parts of the HTQ were included for this study:
  - Traumatic events: 30 items describing potentially traumatic events of war, including exposure to dangerous situations (e.g., combat) alongside difficult life circumstances (e.g., lack of food or water).
  - Posttraumatic symptoms: 30 items evaluating posttraumatic symptoms following the war. The questionnaire includes 16 items derived from the American Psychiatric Association *Diagnostic and Statistical Manual* (*DSM*) criteria for PTSD and 14 other items describing symptoms related to refugee trauma.
- The Conservation of Resources Evaluation (COR-E) (Hobfoll & Lilly, 1993) evaluates the participants' loss of personal resources as a result of the 1948 war. The administered scale included 20 items (e.g., suitable house, family stability) chosen from the original 74-item COR-E according to the identified themes of the first phase.
- The Mental Health Inventory (MHI) (Veit & Ware, 1983) provides a measure of mental health according to two general dimensions: psychological well-being, describing positive aspects of mental health (e.g., cheerfulness, interest in and enjoyment of life), and psychological distress, describing negative aspects of mental health (e.g., anxiety and depression).

Analysis

Thematic analysis was applied to data derived from the interviews of the first phase (Creswell, 2009; Moustakas, 1994). Through inductive content analysis, meaningful segments were distilled from the participants' accounts, classified according to various units of meaning, then integrated into main themes describing their experience of the Nakba and the expulsion from their village.

The quantitative data of the second phase were processed statistically using SPSS for Windows. Preliminary analysis and descriptive statistics were completed. To investigate the research hypothesis, *t* test, multivariate analyses of variance (MANOVA), and Pearson correlation analyses were used.

Findings

The following summary of the results conveys the meanings and effects of the Nakba among Palestinians living in Israel. (For further detailed results, see Ghnadre-Naser, 2012; Ghnadre-Naser & Somer, 2016). Results are presented in an integrated statistics-by-themes manner. Each identified theme of the qualitative phase is described in combination with the relevant statistical findings from the quantitative phase, thus providing a more comprehensive and profound understanding of the Nakba experience. Two main aspects are presented, the stressors, such as exposure to potentially traumatic events and resource losses, followed by their immediate and long-term psychological repercussions.

THE NAKBA STRESSORS

Frightening suddenness characterized the participants' first encounter with the war. The rural inhabitants of the region were seemingly carrying on with their daily routines, unaware of the impending danger. They abruptly found themselves facing threats of direct gunfire, shelling, and armed attacks while their villages came under siege and military troops invaded their neighborhoods.

IDPs who participated in the qualitative phase recounted exposure to a wide range of potentially traumatic events including dangerous combat situations, forced evacuation, and even death of acquaintances or family members:

> When my father went into the garden . . . the airplane bombed for the second time . . . he was buried in the ground . . . we could see only his hair. I started screaming; I thought my son G. was with him. People started digging him out. I asked him where G. was. He said he wasn't with him. I told him: "No! You don't remember; you are confused now; he was with you . . . and people continued digging, looking for him, until my neighbor came with G. She had found him near the door. . . . What can I say . . . a horrible hour I went through. (Afifa)[3]

> They used to come and besiege the village, every day or two. . . . We would wake up in the morning and find the neighborhood surrounded. . . . They gathered us and put us in one place from the morning till evening; we were trapped. (Hoda)

I was 15 years old, hiding in a cave, watching people fleeing, running, people coming and going, terror, fear, chaos. (Kamal)

In contrast to these experiences, two participants described a quieter first encounter with the Israeli troops:

The Israeli soldiers went into the village and everyone welcomed them. . . . They did nothing in our village . . . like they were going on a trip." (Gassan)

However, this initial, fragile security would soon be challenged when the same welcomed troops drove the population out of their villages, leaving them feeling betrayed:

People were surprised. . . . We welcomed you [addressing the Jews] in our homes. For 15 days they ate and drank our water. . . . We believed you and you lied to us. (Gassan)

They deceived us, they expelled us even though we didn't fight them. There was no firing . . . we welcomed them and gave them food and they deceived us. (Nada)

Expelling the IDPs from their home villages further exposed these people to intimidation and adversities such as lack of the basic necessities and conditions required for survival. The uprooting from their home villages severed the IDPs from their stable and secure past, propelling them toward a frightening, insecure, and blurry future:

We had to run; we left without our clothes, without necessities, without anything; we left everything in our homes. . . . People wanted to save themselves. Of course, we were afraid; we had no weapons to protect us; it was horrifying. (Sami)

What can I say, very very very . . . I feel these painful hours, I feel the fatigue, the bitterness. . . . Do you know what it is like to have no water, no food? Nothing! The whole night people couldn't drink or eat, and were afraid to return; we went through difficult times and distress. (Gassan)

I swear to you our home was full, wheat, lentil, legumes. I told you we took some mattresses and left. . . . No money; nothing to eat. . . . "It is humiliating to complain to anyone but God" [quoting an Arabic proverb, الشكوى لغير الله مذلة]. (Hasan)

They demolished our homes; all of our belongings were there. . . . We went and found the whole village ruined. There was a Jewish guard from whom we used to run away. . . . We used to pick our olives and figs secretly. (Zahra)

Personal assets were lost, agricultural lands were confiscated, and family members and friends were scattered. These painful losses marked the beginning of a new era characterized by socioeconomic deterioration and daily struggles to restore their lives. The need to survive and provide for their families, combined with hard work, determination, and willpower, gradually helped the IDPs regain a sense of control and stability:

> We started to rebuild our lives from below zero. They brought us and threw us here with nothing. . . . This way we started below zero. . . . We lived in a shed. I bought some wooden boards and attached them and made a concrete floor and lived in it. (Gassan)

> Everyone tried to work . . . to provide for his family, to feed the children. I worked picking fruit, like other women, and my children were still young. What could I do? They needed to eat, needed to live. (Nada)

> We used to work at temporary jobs, eat day by day. I worked a lot. I wanted to live. What could I do? I needed to provide for my family; they needed to eat. (Sami)

Corresponding findings from the quantitative assessments further support the identified themes of the war stressors. Findings derived from the HTQ traumatic event report and COR-E measures indicated high levels of exposure to extreme violence and threatening events during the Nakba, together with high proportions of resources lost as a result of the war among the Palestinian population in general. For example, between 30% and 60% reported exposure to different life-threatening situations during the war, 64% reported lack of food or water, and more than 60% reported losing personal belongings, accompanied by losing their psychological resources of stability, predictability, and hope. As shown in table 2.1 and table 2.2, these events were commonly experienced in both groups of the study, the IDPs as well the locals, to varying degrees. Differences between the two groups are further highlighted in this discussion.

PSYCHOLOGICAL REPERCUSSIONS FOLLOWING THE NAKBA

The psychological effects of these traumatic experiences on participants can be readily identified in the previous themes. In the short term, these effects were manifested by symptoms of psychological distress, including intense fear, pain, and feelings of helplessness and despair:

> Look, when a person goes through difficult times his soul gets tired. This is a normal thing, and his morale breakdowns. (Kamal)

> What did I feel? I felt darkness, distress; what I felt! So much pain. . . . It was too much; we didn't expect them to be so cruel. (Gassan)

Table 2.1. Traumatic Events Reported Most Frequently (Percent)

	Traumatic events	Total (N = 121)	IDPs (N = 60)	Locals (N = 61)
1.	Lack of shelter	107 (88%)	55 (92%)	52 (85%)
2.	Lack of food or water	77 (64%)	44 (73%)	33 (54%)
3.	Confiscation or destruction of personal property	74 (61%)	56 (93%)	18 (30%)
4.	Forced to hide	70 (58%)	40 (67%)	30 (49%)
5.	Confined to home because of danger outside	62 (51%)	31 (52%)	31 (51%)
6.	Forced evacuation under dangerous conditions	55 (45%)	36 (60%)	19 (31%)
7.	Combat situation (e.g., shelling/grenade attacks)	54 (45%)	32 (53%)	22 (36%)
8.	Other forced separation from family members	35 (29%)	23 (38%)	12 (20%)
9.	Murder or death due to violence of other family member or friend	35 (29%)	22 (37%)	13 (21%)
10.	Present while someone searched for people or things in your home	24 (20%)	14 (23%)	10 (17%)
11.	Extortion or robbery	24 (20%)	18 (30%)	6 (10%)

Note. IDPs, internally displaced persons.
Source: S. Ghnadre-Naser. (2012). *Effects of the 1948 war on the mental health of Palestinians living in Israel: A retrospective qualitative and quantitative examination* (Unpublished doctoral dissertation). University of Haifa, Israel.

Table 2.2. Lost Resources Reported Most Frequently (Percent)

	Resources	Total (N = 121)	IDPs (N = 60)	Locals (N = 61)
1.	Financial assets (stocks, property, etc.)	76 (63%)	57 (95%)	19 (31%)
2.	Housing that suits my need	73 (60%)	54 (90%)	19 (31%)
3.	Financial stability	73 (60%)	50 (83%)	23 (38%)
4.	Adequate clothing	72 (60%)	46 (77%)	26 (43%)
5.	Adequate food	72 (60%)	43 (72%)	29 (48%)
6.	Adequate home furnishings	69 (57%)	51 (85%)	18 (30%)
7.	Time for adequate sleep	69 (57%)	40 (67%)	29 (48%)
8.	Family stability	64 (53%)	43 (72%)	21 (34%)
9.	Feeling that I am accomplishing my goals	55 (45%)	36 (60%)	19 (31%)
10.	Hope	54 (45%)	38 (63%)	16 (26%)
11.	Knowing where I am going with my life	53 (44%)	38 (63%)	15 (25%)

Note. IDPs, internally displaced persons.
Source: S. Ghnadre-Naser. (2012). *Effects of the 1948 war on the mental health of Palestinians living in Israel: A retrospective qualitative and quantitative examination* (Unpublished doctoral dissertation). University of Haifa, Israel.

We tried to comfort ourselves; what could we do! We felt helpless. . . . When those who harmed you are now controlling you, what could we say! (Nada)

Similarly, high levels of distress were found among the participants of the quantitative phase according to the HTQ symptoms scale. Distributions of the most reported symptoms reveal cautiousness and overwhelming feelings of insecurity. Table 2.3 presents the most-reported trauma symptoms among the participants.

Participants who retrospectively reported greater exposure to potentially traumatic events also reported higher incidence of posttraumatic symptoms ($r = .60$, $p < .001$). In addition, a strong positive correlation was found between resource loss and posttraumatic symptoms. Participants who retrospectively reported losing more resources as a result of the war reported higher levels of posttraumatic symptoms ($r = .84$, $p < .001$).

Comparing the Nakba experiences of the IDPs with the locals revealed crucial differences. For the IDP group, MANOVA detected a significant main effect of wartime experiences [$F(4, 115) = 18.26$, $p < .001$] and psychological consequences felt at the time [$F(4, 116) = 385.60$, $p < .001$]. As expected, IDPs were exposed to more traumatic events during the Nakba, lost more personal resources, and reported suffering from more posttraumatic symptoms. Table 2.4 shows means and standard deviations for both groups.

Table 2.3. Trauma Symptoms Reported Most Frequently (Percent)

	Trauma symptoms	Total (N = 121)	IDPs (N = 60)	Locals (N = 61)
1.	Feeling on guard	97 (80%)	53 (88%)	44 (72%)
2.	Recurrent thoughts or memories of the most hurtful or terrifying events	92 (76%)	49 (82%)	43 (71%)
3.	Spending time thinking why these events happened to you	74 (61%)	48 (80%)	26 (43%)
4.	Feeling as though the event is happening again	65 (54%)	40 (67%)	25 (41%)
5.	Feeling exhausted	62 (51%)	39 (65%)	23 (38%)
6.	Feeling irritable or having outbursts of anger	61 (50%)	38 (63%)	23 (38%)
7.	Feeling that you have no one to rely on	60 (50%)	36 (60%)	24 (39%)
8.	Avoiding thoughts or feelings associated with the traumatic or hurtful events	60 (50%)	36 (60%)	24 (39%)
9.	Feeling no trust in others	58 (48%)	33 (55%)	25 (41%)
10.	Feeling jumpy, easily startled	57 (47%)	33 (55%)	24 (39%)
11.	Feeling as if you don't have a future	56 (46%)	37 (62%)	19 (31%)

Note. IDPs, internally displaced persons.
Source: S. Ghnadre-Naser. (2012). *Effects of the 1948 war on the mental health of Palestinians living in Israel: A retrospective qualitative and quantitative examination* (Unpublished doctoral dissertation). University of Haifa, Israel.

Table 2.4. Comparison of Nakba Experiences between IDPs and Locals
(Means and Standard Deviations)

	IDPs		Locals		
	M	*(SD)*	*M*	*(SD)*	*F*
HTQ, events	8.67	(3.72)	5.88	(3.98)	16.68*
COR-E	36.75	(17.20)	14.57	(17.93)	47.81*
HTQ, symptoms	2.03	(0.58)	1.50	(0.51)	27.98*

Note. SD, standard deviation; HTQ, Harvard Trauma Questionnaire;
COR-E, Conservation of Resources Evaluation.
* $p < .001$.
Source: S. Ghnadre-Naser. (2012). *Effects of the 1948 war on the mental
health of Palestinians living in Israel: A retrospective qualitative and
quantitative examination* (Unpublished doctoral dissertation). University of Haifa, Israel.

Additionally, IDPs reported suffering from psychological distress for longer periods than locals did [t (72) = −4.02, $p < .001$]. In addition, 42 out of 58 (72.4%) IDPs claimed to have reexperienced these symptoms at subsequent periods during their lives compared to 12 out of 56 (21.4%) locals [$\chi^2(1) = 29.71, p < .001$].

BETWEEN PAST AND PRESENT: THE LONG-TERM EFFECTS OF THE NAKBA

While the IDPs have markedly improved their living conditions and external real-ity, internally their existence seems to have been frozen at the time of their expul-sion, as though decades have not passed. Personal distress and complicated feelings of pain, helplessness, guilt, and longing for lost home villages still accompany the IDPs' inner reality:

> We used to mix some mud and a few rocks and build little houses, whenever we went to the lands with our parents. We used to sit and play on the dirt pile, while our parents worked the land and gathered the harvest. I still feel myself as a baby, I still feel myself as that same child who used to play there at that time, I still feel that. (Gassan)

> Very very very much, as much as you can say it affected me. At night I go to sleep and I dream I'm still there. . . . Even now, when I go to the kitchen to cook or to do something else, I remember what I was doing then at this time, I think of and remember each day. (Afifa)

> This is the hardest thing ever and still aches my heart that I left my home and can't get in anymore, and I pass by it. I pass by my village and I'm not allowed to go inside. This is truly difficult, and it has affected my spirit. (Kamal)

The longing is always there, especially because I'm not so far from my village. This is harder than refugees outside of Palestine, because "no eye sees and no heart gets sad" [quoting an Arabic proverb, لا عين تشوف ولا قلب يحزن]. But you are a few kilometers away and are forbidden to go there, to live there. (Nabel)

The Nakba's unresolved experiences were revealed by yet another split existing between the pre-Nakba idealized past and the awful postwar reality. As the preceding themes indicate, experiences of loss, insecurity, struggles, and harsh work have colored the IDPs' perspectives on their lives since the uprooting. In contrast, their lives before the Nakba were portrayed as humble, peaceful, and satisfying, with close, harmonious relations:

Even though we worked hard on the lands, we felt peaceful; there was love and people loved each other and helped each other. (Kamal)

In the past people lived simpler lives . . . worked their land and were satisfied; people were happier . . . there was more love and close relations between people. (Salwa)

Our village was plentiful with goodness . . . with its fruits vegetables and land, with close relations between people. . . . It was like heaven. (Hasan)

Examining the relations between the different Nakba experiences and current psychological health in the second phase indicated mixed results. No correlations were found between exposure to potentially traumatic events during the Nakba and mental health measures at present. In contrast, significant correlations were found between the reported resource loss and current psychological health, as indicated by psychological well-being and psychological distress scales of the MHI. More resource losses were related to more psychological distress and to less well-being at present. In addition, trauma symptoms reported after the Nakba were found to be significantly related to current psychological health measures. No significant differences were found between the IDPs and the locals in psychological well-being and psychological distress measures of the present (table 2.5).

Discussion

The objective of the preceding study was to examine the psychological effects of the Nakba among Palestinians who had experienced it and are now living in Israel. We have an obligation to Palestinians in general, and to the Nakba's first generation in particular, now that most of them have passed away, to explore the Nakba's effects among the younger generation who were exposed to it.

The research findings generally support the determination that, for Palestinians living in Israel, the 1948 war was a sudden, traumatic experience that caused them severe emotional distress that persisted throughout their lives. This will come

Table 2.5. Correlations between Nakba Experiences and Present Mental Health

	Psychological distress	**Well-being**	**MHI**
HTQ—Events	.11	−.10	−.15
COR-E	.27*	−.25*	−.29*
HTQ—Symptoms	.39**	−.31**	−.39**

Note. MHI, Mental Health Inventory; HTQ, Harvard Trauma Questionnaire; COR-E, Conservation of Resources Evaluation.
* $p < .01$. ** $p < .001$.
Source: S. Ghnadre-Naser. (2012). *Effects of the 1948 war on the mental health of Palestinians living in Israel: A retrospective qualitative and quantitative examination* (Unpublished doctoral dissertation). University of Haifa, Israel.

as no surprise to the Palestinians, for it reflects a common knowledge passed from one generation to another. Yet the current findings make it possible to describe these long-held notions using academic concepts and theories, such as traumatic event exposure, resource loss, posttraumatic effects, and mental health.

High levels of exposure to potentially traumatic events during the Nakba were found among the Palestinian population, including life-threatening and violent events alongside predicaments related to difficult life circumstances. All at once, Palestinian inhabitants faced combat and life-or-death situations, direct fire and cross fire, property destruction, water or food shortages, and exile and hiding under dangerous conditions. These results replicate findings among other civilian populations facing wars and conflicts and were found to intensify the traumatic psychological effects of such violence (Ai & Peterson, 2005; Briere, 2004; Mollica et al., 2007; Richards et al., 2011). Further, these wartime events affected the entire Palestinian population, in particular the people that directly experienced expulsion from their villages. As such, they are similar to the experiences of other refugee populations (Araya et al., 2007; Porter & Haslam, 2005; Schmidt et al., 2008).

The distributions and frequencies of the reported traumatic events and resources lost show that most of the difficulties the population faced at that time were linked to the Nakba's effect on their daily lives and living conditions. Changes in the population's familial, social, and economic realities were main sources of stress, associated with the term "the survivors," as previously discussed (Abu-Baker & Rabinowitz, 2004). Studies among other populations have confirmed the centrality of these predicaments and have shown that improving these daily conditions usually alleviates the population's distress and increases its resiliency (Hamid & Musa, 2010; Horn, 2009; Porter & Haslam, 2005).

For the Palestinians living in Israel, the consequences of the Nakba did not receive the appropriate institutional care, and these effects were further intensified by the implementation of martial law restricting every aspect of their lives (Ozacky-Lazar, 2002). In addition, they were subjected to constant governmental neglect and discrimination, hindering any chance for restoration of their lives, physically as psychologically. Rehabilitation thus became a prolonged, private, and local community challenge.

The current study provides strong support for the conservation of resources theory (Hobfoll, 1989, 2001), which suggests that overwhelming loss of personal resources might develop into losing spirals that affect the immediate and long-term outcome of the original event (Hobfoll et al., 2012; Hobfoll, Mancini, Hall, Canetti, & Bonanno, 2011; Palmieri, Canetti-Nisim, Galea, Johnson, & Hobfoll, 2008). Severe loss of material resources as a result of the Nakba further developed into loss of psychological resources, such as feelings of stability and hope or the sense that one could accomplish one's goals. Over time, the remarkable and relentless efforts invested by the IDPs gradually allowed them to regain some of these resources and reestablish their resiliency.

This resiliency through the years could explain the lack of significant difference between the IDPs and the locals in current mental health measures. Studies show that psychic pain and psychological vulnerability following a traumatic experience may coexist alongside forces of endurance and fortitude, enabling processes of recovery and growth (Kellermann, 2001; Shmotkin, Blumstein, & Modan, 2003; Sossou et al., 2008). In addition, over the long term the accumulation of life events and experiences as a result of discrimination against the Palestinian minority might eventually have blurred the differences between the internally displaced and the locals.

The inability of the IDPs to regain their most valued resources (e.g., homes, land, and villages) continues to affect their intrapsychic domain. Themes of the first phase revealed the continuous gap that exists between their internal and external realities and the acute pain and longing the IDPs still feel over their lost past lives (Ghnadre-Naser & Somer, 2016). Homes, land, and the local communities constitute the private cosmos in which people manage their lives and find stability and sense of belonging. Losing these detached the IDPs from the basic elements that define their personal identity and have resulted in feelings of confusion and disintegration (Akhtar, 1995; Boğaç, 2009; Gosling & Williams, 2010). A new disintegrated identity of internally displaced people, or "present absentees,"[4] has emerged, where one pole represents strength, diligence, and resiliency, and the opposite pole continues to be tangled with feelings of traumatic loss, inequity, and vulnerability (Dwairy, 2010; Pérez-Sales, 2010; Qossoqsi, 2010).

These psychological findings are interconnected with the collective level of the Nakba narrative. Preserving the Nakba as representing the victimhood of the Palestinian people and the historical injustice imposed on them, highlights the weakness and helplessness pole, hence casting a shadow over the individual's opportunity to mourn private losses, achieve reconciliation, and, subsequently, position the individual as an active agent of his or her reality. Working through the trauma and confronting its psychological consequences may persist as a journey that younger generations must embark on. Issues of familial dynamics, identity formation, and vulnerability versus resiliency should be addressed professionally. In this regard, Volkan (2001) wrote: "The transgenerational transmission of a shared traumatic event is linked to the past generation's inability to mourn losses of people, land or prestige, and indicates the group's failure to reverse narcissistic injury and humiliation inflicted by another large group" (p. 87).

SFAA GHNADRE-NASER is a clinical psychologist and Lecturer at Oranim-Academic College of Education, Kiryat Tiv'on, Israel.

Notes

1. I conducted the research presented in this chapter during my doctoral studies in psychology at the University of Haifa, Israel. Dr. Michael Katz and Professor Eli Somer acted as advisors.
2. A full list of villages can be obtained from the author.
3. All names of participants have been changed to ensure anonymity and confidentiality.
4. "Present-absentees" is a controversial expression known in Israel, following the "present absentees' law" in the 1950s, allowing the confiscation of IDPs' property for they were "absent" from their villages after the Nakba, and yet, they were "present" in the region that became the Israeli state.

References

Abu-Baker, K., & Rabinowitz, D. (2004). *The stand-tall generation* [in Arabic]. Ramallah: Madar.

Abu-El-Hija, A. (2016). *The transgenerational impact of the Nakba* (Unpublished doctoral dissertation). University of Konstanz, Germany.

Abu-Lughod, L., & Sa'di, A. (2007). Introduction: The claims of memory. In A. Sa'di & L. Abu-Lughod (Eds.), *Nakba: Palestine, 1948, and the claims of memory* (pp. 1–24). New York: Columbia University Press.

Abu-Sitta, S. (2004). *Atlas of Palestine 1948*. London: Palestine Land Society.

Ai, A., & Peterson, C. (2005). Symptoms, religious coping, and positive attitudes of refugees from Kosovar war. In T. A. Corales (Ed.), *Focus on posttraumatic stress disorder research* (pp. 123–156). New York: Nova Science.

Akhtar, S. (1995). A third individuation: Immigration, identity, and the psychoanalytic process. *Journal of the American Psychoanalytic Association, 43*(4), 1051–1084.

Al-Haj, M. (1986). Adjustment patterns of the Arab internal refugees in Israel. *International Migration, 24*(3), 651–674.

Arab Association for Human Rights. (2016). *The Palestinian Arab minority in Israel: From marginalization to delegitimization*. Nazareth: Arab Association for Human Rights.

Araya, M., Chotai, J., Komproe, I. H., & de Jong, J. T. (2007). Effect of trauma on quality of life as mediated by mental distress and moderated by coping and social support among postconflict displaced Ethiopians. *Quality of Life Research, 16*(6), 915–927.

Association for Civil Rights in Israel. (2016). *Situation report: The state of human rights in Israel and the OPT*. Retrieved from http://www.acri.org.il/campaigns/report2016en/.

Bernardes, D., Wright, J., Edwards, C., Tomkins, H., Dlfoz, D., & Livingstone, A. (2011). Asylum seekers' perspectives on their mental health and views on health and social services: Contributions for service provision using a mixed-methods approach. *International Journal of Migration, Health and Social Care, 6*(4), 3–19.

Boğaç, C. (2009). Place attachment in a foreign settlement. *Journal of Environmental Psychology, 29*(2), 267–278.

Bonanno, G. A., Galea, S., Bucciarelli, A., & Vlahov, D. (2007). What predicts psychological resilience after disaster? The role of demographics, resources, and life stress. *Journal of Consulting and Clinical Psychology, 75*(5), 671–682.

Bottura, B., & Mancini, T. (2016). Psychosocial dynamics affecting health and social care of forced migrants: A narrative review. *International Journal of Migration, Health and Social Care, 12*(2), 109–119.

Briere, J. (2004). *Psychological assessment of posttraumatic states: Phenomenology, diagnosis, and measurement* (2nd ed.). Washington, DC: American Psychological Association.

Chatty, D. (2009). Palestinian refugee youth: Agency and aspiration. *Refugee Survey Quarterly, 28*(2–3), 318–338.

Creswell, J. W. (1998). *Qualitative inquiry and research design: Choosing among five approaches.* London: Sage.

Creswell, J. W. (2009). *Research design: Quantitative, qualitative, and mixed methods approaches* (3rd ed.). Thousand Oaks, CA: Sage.

de Jong, J. T., Komproe, I. H., Van Ommeren, M., El Masri, M., Araya, M., Khaled, N., . . . Somasundaram, D. (2001). Lifetime events and posttraumatic stress disorder in 4 postconflict settings. *JAMA, 286*(5), 555–562.

Dwairy, M. (2010, August). The human being, Palestinian society, and the Nakba. *Jadal, 7*, 1–6.

Even-Tzur, E. (2016). "The road to the village": Israeli social unconscious and the Palestinian Nakba. *International Journal of Applied Psychoanalytic Studies, 13*(4), 305–322.

Eyber, C. (2002). *Forced migration online thematic guide: Psychosocial issues.* Retrieved from https://www.alnap.org/system/files/content/resource/files/main/fm0004-forced -migration-online-series.pdf

Fangen, K. (2006). Humiliation experienced by Somali refugees in Norway. *Journal of Refugee Studies, 19*(1), 69–93.

Farhood, L. F., & Dimassi, H. (2012). Prevalence and predictors for post-traumatic stress disorder, depression and general health in a population from six villages in south Lebanon. *Social Psychiatry and Psychiatric Epidemiology, 47*(4), 639–649.

Farwell, N. (2003). In war's wake: Contextualizing trauma experiences and psychosocial well-being among Eritrean youth. *International Journal of Mental Health, 32*(4), 20–50.

Feldman, I. (2008). Refusing invisibility: Documentation and memorialization in Palestinian refugee claims. *Journal of Refugee Studies, 21*(4), 498–516.

Gheith, J. M. (2007). "I never talked": Enforced silence, non-narrative memory, and the Gulag. *Mortality, 12*(2), 159–175.

Ghnadre-Naser, S. (2012). *Effects of the 1948 war on the mental health of Palestinians living in Israel: A retrospective qualitative and quantitative examination* (Unpublished doctoral dissertation). University of Haifa, Israel.

Ghnadre-Naser, S., & Somer, E. (2016). "The wound is still open": The Nakba experience among internally displaced Palestinians in Israel. *International Journal of Migration, Health and Social Care, 12*(4), 238–251.

Gosling, E., & Williams, K. J. (2010). Connectedness to nature, place attachment and conservation behaviour: Testing connectedness theory among farmers. *Journal of Environmental Psychology, 30*(3), 298–304.

Halperin, E., Bar-Tal, D., Sharvit, K., Rosler, N., & Raviv, A. (2010). Socio-psychological implications for an occupying society: The case of Israel. *Journal of Peace Research, 47*(1), 59–70.

Hamama-Raz, Y., Solomon, Z., Cohen, A., & Laufer, A. (2008). PTSD symptoms, forgiveness, and revenge among Israeli Palestinian and Jewish adolescents. *Journal of Traumatic Stress, 21*(6), 521–529.

Hamid, A. A., & Musa, S. A. (2010). Mental health problems among internally displaced persons in Darfur. *International Journal of Psychology, 45*(4), 278–285.

Hobfoll, S. E. (1989). Conservation of resources: A new attempt at conceptualizing stress. *American Psychologist, 44*(3), 513–524.

Hobfoll, S. E. (2001). The influence of culture, community, and the nested-self in the stress process: Advancing conservation of resources theory. *Applied Psychology, 50*(3), 337–421.

Hobfoll, S. E., Hall, B. J., & Canetti, D. (2012). Political violence, psychological distress, and perceived health: A longitudinal investigation in the Palestinian authority. *Psychological Trauma: Theory, Research, Practice, and Policy, 4*(1), 9.

Hobfoll, S. E., & Lilly, R. S. (1993). Resource conservation as a strategy for community psychology. *Journal of Community Psychology, 21*(2), 128–148.

Hobfoll, S. E., Mancini, A. D., Hall, B. J., Canetti, D., & Bonanno, G. A. (2011). The limits of resilience: Distress following chronic political violence among Palestinians. *Social Science & Medicine, 72*(8), 1400–1408.

Horn, R. (2009). Coping with displacement: Problems and responses in camps for the internally displaced in Kitgum, northern Uganda. *Intervention, 7*(2), 110–129.

Ibn Khaldun Association. (2005). *Identity and belonging: The basic concepts project for Arab students* [in Arabic]. Tamra, Israel.

Jamil, H., Hakim-Larson, J., Farrag, M., Kafaji, T., Duqum, I., & Jamil, L. H. (2002). A retrospective study of Arab American mental health clients: Trauma and the Iraqi refugees. *American Journal of Orthopsychiatry, 72*(3), 355–361.

Johnson, R. B., & Onwuegbuzie, A. J. (2004). Mixed methods research: A research paradigm whose time has come. *Educational Researcher, 33*(7), 14–26.

Kabha, M. (2006). The challenges of writing Palestinian modern history: The emergency of writing a complete narrative. In M. Kabha (Ed.), *Towards a Historical Narrative of the Nakba, Complexities and Challenges* (pp. 5–25). Haifa: Mada al-Carmel: Arab Center for Applied Social Research.

Kabha, M., & Barzilai, R. (1996). *Refugees in their land—The internal refugees in Israel 1948–1996* [in Hebrew]. Givat Haviva: Institute for Peace Studies.

Kassem, F. (2011). *Palestinian women: Narrative histories and gendered memory.* London: Zed.

Kellermann, N. P. (2001). The long-term psychological effects and treatment of Holocaust trauma. *Journal of Loss & Trauma, 6*(3), 197–218.

Kemp, M. (2011). Dehumanization, guilt and large group dynamics with reference to the West, Israel and the Palestinians. *British Journal of Psychotherapy, 27*(4), 383–405.

Khalidi, W. (1997). *All that remains: The Palestinian villages occupied and depopulated in 1948.* Washington, DC: Institute for Palestinian Studies.

Kleinot, P. (2011). Transgenerational trauma and forgiveness: Looking at the Israeli–Palestinian families forum through a group analytic lens. *Group Analysis, 44*(1), 97–111.

Liem, R. (2007). Silencing historical trauma: The politics and psychology of memory and voice. *Peace and Conflict: Journal of Peace Psychology, 13*(2), 153–174.

Mollica, R. F., Caridad, K. R., & Massagli, M. P. (2007). Longitudinal study of posttraumatic stress disorder, depression, and changes in traumatic memories over time in Bosnian refugees. *The Journal of Nervous and Mental Disease, 195*(7), 572–579.

Mollica, R. F., Caspi-Yavin, Y., Bollini, P., Truong, T., Tor, S., & Lavelle, J. (1992). The Harvard trauma questionnaire: Validating a cross-cultural instrument for measuring torture, trauma, and posttraumatic stress disorder in Indochinese refugees. *The Journal of Nervous and Mental Disease, 180*(2), 111–116.

Morgan, D. L. (1998). Practical strategies for combining qualitative and quantitative methods: Applications to health research. *Qualitative Health Research, 8*(3), 362–376.

Morse, J. M. (2000). Determining sample size. *Qualitative Health Research, 10*(1), 3–5.

Moustakas, C. (1994). *Phenomenological research methods.* Thousand Oaks, CA: Sage.

Nakhleh, K. (2009, December 13). Another childhood Nakba memory. *Palestine Chronicle.* Retrieved from http://palestinechronicle.com/old/view_article_details.php?id=15611.

Netland, M. (2013). Exploring "lost childhood": A study of the narratives of Palestinians who grew up during the first intifada. *Childhood, 20*(1), 82–97.

Ozacky-Lazar, S. (2002). Martial law as a mechanisim of control over the Arab citizens: 1948–1958 [in Hebrew]. *The New East, 43*, 103–132.

Palmieri, P. A., Canetti-Nisim, D., Galea, S., Johnson, R. J., & Hobfoll, S. E. (2008). The psychological impact of the Israel–Hezbollah War on Jews and Arabs in Israel: The impact of risk and resilience factors. *Social Science & Medicine, 67*(8), 1208–1216.

Pérez-Sales, P. (2010). Identity and trauma in adolescents within the context of political violence: A psychosocial and communitarian view. *Clinical Social Work Journal, 38*(4), 408–417.

Porter, M., & Haslam, N. (2005). Predisplacement and postdisplacement factors associated with mental health of refugees and internally displaced persons: A meta-analysis. *JAMA, 294*(5), 602–612.

Qossoqsi, M. (2010, August). The Narrative of the Nakba and the politics of trauma. *Jadal, 7*, 1–4.

Ram, U. (2009). Ways of forgetting: Israel and the obliterated memory of the Palestinian Nakba. *Journal of Historical Sociology, 22*(3), 366–395.

Richards, A., Ospina-Duque, J., Barrera-Valencia, M., Escobar-Rincón, J., Ardila-Gutiérrez, M., Metzler, T., & Marmar, C. (2011). Posttraumatic stress disorder, anxiety and depression symptoms, and psychosocial treatment needs in Colombians internally displaced by armed conflict: A mixed-method evaluation. *Psychological Trauma: Theory, Research, Practice, and Policy, 3*(4), 384–393.

Said, E. (1998). Scenes from Palestine. *Al-Ahram.* Retrieved from http://weekly.ahram.org.eg/Archive/1998/1948/370_said.htm.

Salih, R. (2013). From bare lives to political agents: Palestinian refugees as avant-garde. *Refugee Survey Quarterly, 32*(2), 66–91.

Sawada, A., Chaitin, J., & Bar-On, D. (2004). Surviving Hiroshima and Nagasaki—Experiences and psychosocial meanings. *Psychiatry: Interpersonal and Biological Processes, 67*(1), 43–60.

Schmidt, M., Kravic, N., & Ehlert, U. (2008). Adjustment to trauma exposure in refugee, displaced, and non-displaced Bosnian women. *Archives of Women's Mental Health, 11*(4), 269–276.

Shehadeh, S. (2015). The 2014 war on Gaza: Engineering trauma and mass torture to break Palestinian resilience. *International Journal of Applied Psychoanalytic Studies, 12*(3), 278–294.

Shmotkin, D., Blumstein, T., & Modan, B. (2003). Tracing long-term effects of early trauma: A broad-scope view of Holocaust survivors in late life. *Journal of Consulting and Clinical Psychology, 71*(2), 223–234.

Shoeb, M., Weinstein, H., & Mollica, R. (2007). The Harvard trauma questionnaire: Adapting a cross-cultural instrument for measuring torture, trauma and posttraumatic stress disorder in Iraqi refugees. *International Journal of Social Psychiatry, 53*(5), 447–463.

Slewa-Younan, S., Chippendale, K., Heriseanu, A., Lujic, S., Atto, J., & Raphael, B. (2012). Measures of psychophysiological arousal among resettled traumatized Iraqi refugees seeking psychological treatment. *Journal of Traumatic Stress, 25*(3), 348–352.

Somer, E., Maguen, S., Or-Chen, K., & Litz, B. T. (2009). Managing terror: Differences between Jews and Arabs in Israel. *International Journal of Psychology, 44*(2), 138–146.

Sossou, M.-A., Craig, C. D., Ogren, H., & Schnak, M. (2008). A qualitative study of resilience factors of Bosnian refugee women resettled in the southern United States. *Journal of Ethnic & Cultural Diversity in Social Work, 17*(4), 365–385.

Srouji, E. (2004). The fall of a Galilean village during the 1948 Palestine war: An eyewitness account. *Journal of Palestine Studies, 33*(2), 71–80.

Tanios, C. Y., Abou-Saleh, M. T., Karam, A. N., Salamoun, M. M., Mneimneh, Z. N., & Karam, E. G. (2009). The epidemiology of anxiety disorders in the Arab world: A review. *Journal of Anxiety Disorders, 23*(4), 409–419.

Tankink, M. (2004). Not talking about traumatic experiences: Harmful or healing? Coping with war memories in southwest Uganda. *Intervention: International Journal of Mental Health, Psychosocial Work and Counselling in Areas of Armed Conflict, 2*(1), 3–17.

Tashakkori, A., & Teddlie, C. (2003). *Handbook on mixed methods in the behavioral and social sciences.* Thousand Oaks, CA: Sage.

UN High Commissioner for Refugees. (2017). *Global appeal: 2017 update.* Retrieved from http://reporting.unhcr.org/sites/default/files/ga2017/pdf/GA_2017%20Update%20Eng_Book_low-res.pdf.

Veit, C. T., & Ware, J. E. (1983). The structure of psychological distress and well-being in general populations. *Journal of Consulting and Clinical Psychology, 51*(5), 730–742.

Volkan, V. D. (2001). Transgenerational transmissions and chosen traumas: An aspect of large-group identity. *Group Analysis, 34*(1), 79–97.

Wakim, W. (2001). The "internally displaced": Seeking return within one's own land. *Journal of Palestine Studies, 31*(1), 32–38.

Wiseman, H., Metzl, E., & Barber, J. P. (2006). Anger, guilt, and intergenerational communication of trauma in the interpersonal narratives of second generation Holocaust survivors. *American Journal of Orthopsychiatry, 76*(2), 176–184.

3

THE NAKBA AND ITS REPERCUSSIONS
ON PALESTINIAN CITIZENS IN ISRAEL

Adel Manna

B Y THE END OF THE WAR IN PALESTINE in 1949, the newly established Jewish state had expanded its control over 78% of historical Palestine. Of the 900,000 Palestinians who had lived in their homeland for centuries, approximately 156,000 remained in Israel, while the rest became refugees. Palestine disappeared from the map, and new geographical terms were born—for example, the West Bank and the Gaza Strip. As a result, Palestinians lost their identity, their security, and their equality under the new rulers, and entire villages disintegrated and were scattered into separate communities that lacked self-determination. Furthermore, the displaced people lost homes, lands, and properties, and many endured miserable conditions in refugee camps in neighboring Arab countries and beyond. This, in short, is the meaning of the Nakba.

The Palestinians who experienced the Nakba and eventually became formal Israeli citizens suffer from a double marginality. They are neither full partners in the state and society where they live, nor are they fully accepted members of the Arab nations outside Israel. The feeling of being strangers in their homeland has become an important component of the sociopolitical identity of Palestinian citizens in Israel. They constitute a special case of a "trapped minority" (Monterescu & Rabinowitz, 2007; Rabinowitz, 2001, pp. 64–65). As such, Palestinian survivors have been compelled to prove their loyalty to the state of Israel that, by its own definition as "Jewish," cannot be loyal to them. In parallel, the Arab world, which boycotts Israel, looks on them with suspicion and mistrust merely for being Israeli citizens.

This chapter explores the story of the Palestinian citizens in Israel as a trapped minority, a status that constitutes a sociopolitical determinant of mental health among members of the community. The formative years of the 1950s anchored the status of Palestinian citizens in Israel as second-class citizens affected by their double marginality. In all likelihood, this situation has continued to heighten their feelings of insecurity and fear. In my opinion, the trauma of the 1948–1949 wartime events has not healed but rather has intensified as a result of the Palestinians' lack of full inclusion in the state of Israel. Indeed, they have witnessed the gradual transformation of their historical homeland into a Jewish landscape without being able to effectively resist the state policies of expropriation and colonization.

The policies established toward the Palestinian minority during the first decade of Israel (1948–1958) continue to shape their realities and current status. Demolishing Arab houses and confiscating Arab lands for the purpose of building new Jewish settlements were part and parcel of these policies. Palestinian citizens are asked to accept the inherent inequalities instituted by the Israeli settler system. Any opposition to the policies of the Israeli state may be criminalized and even treated as a security threat (Jiryis, 1966, 1976). Lingering early perceptions continue to shape the attitude of the Jewish majority toward Palestinian citizens. Admittedly, by accepting those discriminatory policies, Palestinians receive some socioeconomic benefits, but they are perceived as collaborators and are never offered the option of equal partnership and meaningful citizenship.

Because the current predicament of Palestinian citizens in Israel is rooted in the formative years of the first decade of the state, it is imperative to study and acknowledge the repercussions of the Nakba on this trapped minority to understand its social and psychological world of today. In my view, the traumas of the Nakba are not remote events. Furthermore, the recollections of those traumas (e.g., massacres, expulsions) are transmitted from Nakba survivors to the second and third generations. While this topic of transmission has not been adequately investigated, it can be inferred from the active role of the second and third generations of the "present absentees" in the ceremonies commemorating the loss of their villages in 1948 (Masalha, 2005, pp. 43–45).

In sum, the traumas of 1948–1949 and the 1950s remain open wounds for this community. The feelings of estrangement, deprivation, and insecurity born in 1948—subsequently silenced or openly acknowledged—have been intensified by overt and covert discriminatory policies imposed on the Arab localities by the military government in the early years of the state. People who lost their cherished lands and homes were not allowed to visit those sites of memory, including their parents' graves in the deserted localities. Israeli military authorities forced survivors to quell their grief and limit its expression to the private sphere.

A Story of Nakba and Survival

The Palestinian refugee problem was created in 1948–1949 when the state of Israel was established. Little is known about the predicament in the early years of the Palestinians who survived in the Jewish state and eventually became its citizens. Neither Arabs nor Jews were interested in the lot or study of the Palestinian survivors' realities in Israel after the Nakba. They were doubly marginal (Manna, 2017). The Nakba shattered their basic collective feelings of security and identity. As a result, members of this minority lost the option of equality, national identity, and dignity in their homeland. Israel has treated Palestinian citizens as remnants of its previous enemies, notwithstanding the fact that they were granted formal citizenship and promised full equality in the Israeli Declaration of Independence.

At the end of the 1948–1949 war and after signing the cease-fire agreements, about 750,000 Palestinians became refugees. As mentioned previously, only about 160,000 remained in Israel. This chapter highlights the story of the 100,000 who continued to live in the northern part of Israel (Haifa and the Galilee), where the traumatic events of the war were more salient than in other parts of Palestine. Recall here that most of the Galilee was meant to have been an integral part of the Arab state according to Resolution 181 of the UN partition plan, a scheme ultimately rejected by the Arab nations. Despite the UN resolution, Israel extended its occupation.

The formal citizenship status granted to the Palestinians who remained in Israel did not prevent their being suspected of disloyalty to the Jewish state. But being faithful to the state, its common good, and its policies meant betraying their own people and self-interests. Importantly, the change in the national landscape—the demography and the culture of the homeland—was a very painful experience for the Palestinian remnant. Survivors witnessed the elimination of Arab villages during the late 1940s and early 1950s and the establishment of new Jewish localities on their ruins. Many became "internal refugees" who had to keep silent while their own homes and lands were colonized by others (Cohen, 2000, pp. 44, 72). The constant feeling of helplessness after the catastrophe of the Nakba added to the agony of individual and national loss. Significantly, military administration of the Arab localities in Israel was formally established in October 1948 and continued until December 1966.

Palestinians who remained in Israel were cut off from the Arab world and their Palestinian brethren. Culturally and psychologically, these survivors felt that they had been left alone to face the conquerors of their homeland. The plight of the Palestinians in general and those who continued to live in Israel in particular did not heal in the aftermath of the armed conflict; rather it intensified under Israeli repression and the constant threats of expulsions, at least until 1956. Indeed, during the war that year against Egypt, the inhabitants of two Arab villages (Krad el-Baqqara and Krad el-Ghannameh) in the Hula Valley were expelled to Jordan and Syria. Thus, the Nakba is not an event but rather a process.

The postwar years (1949–1956) witnessed the institutionalization of Zionist ideologies and policies by the new Jewish state. The Law of Return, the Citizenship Law, and other legislation in the early 1950s turned survivors into "strangers in their homeland." These laws provided immediate and unconditional meaningful citizenship only for Jews. Palestinians, who were a vast majority of the country's population, turned into an undesired minority in the Jewish state (Kretzmer, 1990, pp. 35–38).

The situation became complex. Living under military control and policies that prevented the return of refugees meant living under constant fear of expulsion. Indeed, Israel did expel thousands of Palestinians in the early 1950s and during the war of 1956. It is estimated that over 20,000 Palestinians were forced out of their homes and localities (Manna, 2017, pp. 194–195). In addition, thousands of refugees crossed the borders and tried to join their families in the Galilee and elsewhere. Returnees were labeled as dangerous infiltrators, and Israel prevented their return and reunification with their families. While Israeli literature records those military operations as "Israel's border war" (Morris, 1996), from the Arab point of view, this was a war against relatives who had risked their lives trying to return to their ancestral homes.

Denial and Silencing of the Nakba

The impact of the Nakba on the Palestinian minority that remained in Israel after the 1948 war is rarely studied by mental health professionals. Most of the literature dealing with the tragedy has focused on the crisis of the refugees and the dismemberment of Palestinian society outside Israel. In contrast, the fate of the nonrefugees attracted little attention from UN institutions, the Arab states, and Israeli scholars, particularly in the 1950s. Hence, the history of Palestinian citizens in the Jewish state and their struggle for survival has been neglected and even silenced. In my view, without understanding what happened during the formative years of the state of Israel, it is impossible to grasp the complexities of later periods. This chapter looks at two situations: the present absentees and the unrecognized villages. Today, the issue of the unrecognized villages is related mainly to the more than 40 Arab settlements in the Negev. However, in the 1950s many other Arab villages in the Galilee were unrecognized and did not get basic services.

Importantly, the attitude toward Palestinian citizens contradicts democratic values and myths of Israeli achievements. Israel succeeded in marketing the new Jewish state as a Western democracy compensating the survivors of the Holocaust. The narrative of Palestinian citizens in Israel, victims of oppression and colonizing policies, does not fit this Zionist narrative. Hence, it has been silenced, and the socioeconomic realities of the Palestinian citizens under the military government is legitimized by security concerns.

Healing past wounds and building common ground for equal citizenship requires recognition, not denial. Acknowledgment of past wrongdoings and sincere attempts to heal the post-Nakba traumas is needed. Such a new policy should not be limited to apologies and symbolic gestures (e.g., Israeli president Reuven Rivlin's relatively recent visit to Kafr Qasim and his acknowledgement of the Israeli massacre that had occurred there on October 29, 1956). It should address solving real and urgent problems, such as those of the present absentees and the status of the unrecognized villages.

Memories of Deprivation and Historical Injustice

Palestinians who survived the Nakba are perceived today as relatively lucky. Most stayed in their localities and did not suffer expulsion and the misery of living in refugee camps. They continued living on part of their homeland and eventually became citizens of Israel. Nevertheless, the painful events of the Palestinian catastrophe became part of the survivors' identity. The agonizing experiences of the Palestinians in general and those who survived in Haifa and the Galilee in particular started in the spring of 1948. The fall of Tiberias and Haifa to the Israelis shocked many Palestinians in the northern part of the country. Tens of thousands of people were uprooted from their homes and lands and became refugees. In May 1948, the towns of Safad, Beisan, and Akka surrendered, and a new wave of Palestinians were expelled while Nazareth (and most of its neighboring villages) was spared the experience of the other northern Palestinian cities (Abbasi, 2014). The peaceful surrender of Nazareth in July 1948 marked a turning point in the history of nonexpulsion and survival. Twenty out of 24 villages of the district survived while four—Mjeidel, Ma'lul, Safuryye, and 'Ilut—were uprooted and destroyed. With regard to 'Ilut, 20 young men were killed and the entire population was expelled. However, the hundreds who took refuge in Nazareth were later allowed to return to their homes in early 1950.

The people of Nazareth were not the first to be allowed to stay by the Israeli government. Two months earlier, leaders of the Druze community in the Mount Carmel area and the western Galilee had signed an agreement that made the survival of all Druze localities possible (Firro, 1999). Druze fighters who had volunteered to protect the Galilee agreed to withdraw from the battle, and, in return, Jewish Israeli leaders from Haifa promised that no harm would be inflicted on members of the community. Indeed, after the fall of Acre, a few villages east of the city surrendered, and their residents were allowed to stay.

Palestinian leaders in the Galilee (Druze, Muslims, and Christians) chose to collaborate with the victors to secure survival of their respective communities (Al-Zu'bi, 1987). The population of this area constituted the core of the first survivors of the Nakba. The relatively positive experiences of Palestinians in and around Nazareth nourished hopes of nonexpulsion in the middle region and Upper Galilee. However, unlike their neighbors, the approximately 60,000 people living in that area suffered from brutal attempts to uproot most of them. The Israeli army conducted about 14 massacres against unarmed civilians in a clear attempt to push these Palestinians into Syria and Lebanon (Manna, 2017, pp. 106–107).

Notwithstanding, tens of thousands succeeded in keeping their homes and localities in the Upper Galilee. It is estimated that about half of the 60,000 original residents and refugees in this region remained following the Israeli assault while the other half became refugees in Syria and Lebanon (Manna, 2017, p. 112).

Others were removed from their homes by the army, which promised that they would be permitted to return home in a few weeks. However, these people were ultimately not allowed to return and became present absentees despite the Israeli High Court ruling in 1951 that their eviction had been illegal. While expulsions were conducted in the Galilee, the July 1948 survivors received Israeli citizenship and took part in the first parliamentary elections in 1949. The contradictory Israeli policies were confusing, but most survivors tried to adapt to the new realities and behave accordingly.

Israeli Policies Beyond 1948

As mentioned earlier, Israeli attempts to have as few Palestinians as possible in the Jewish state did not stop at the end of the Arab-Israeli War in early 1949 (Masalha, 1997). Palestinian survivors of the Nakba in Israel were governed by military control and the harsh conditions of life as set by the earlier 1945 British Mandatory Emergency Laws. Furthermore, a number of attempts were made to evict the Palestinians who had become citizens of the Jewish state. Undesired inhabitants in small villages, as well as in localities on the Lebanese border and in the southern part of Israel, were brutally expelled from their homes. One well-known case of expulsion in 1950 is the uprooting of a few thousand Palestinians from the township of Majdal (Ashkelon today), not far from the Gaza Strip. Much less known is the expulsion of a few thousand Palestinians from two villages (Krad el-Baqqara and Krad el-Ghannameh) in the Hula Valley in late 1956 (Rabin, 1979, p.97). Much of this story of expulsions, particularly of Bedouins from the Negev, has been silenced for decades.

The refugees who crossed the borders into Israel and found asylum among their families were a target of repeated expulsions. The families were trapped in an impossible situation: either they informed Israeli authorities of the border crossings or they would be blamed as partners in hiding so-called infiltrators. The criminalization of Palestinian citizens for attempting to support family members devastated the social fabric of the traumatized survivors.

Israel not only prevented the return of Palestinian refugees from their camps in the neighboring Arab states but acted similarly toward internal refugees. Even people who were promised to be allowed back home in a few weeks (such as those from Iqrith and Kafr Ber'im) were prevented from doing so by the army. Furthermore, in 1951 the houses of these villages were destroyed in line with the Israeli policy of demolishing deserted villages. In some areas during the 1950s, many Arab villages were demolished, leaving the few remaining villages very far from one another. For example, in the upper eastern region of the Galilee, four villages near Safad (Zfat) remained: Jish (mostly Christian), Rihaneyye (populated by Circassians displaced centuries earlier by the Russian conquest of the Caucasus), Arab al-Heeb in Tuba-Zangariyya, and 'Akbara (settled by the present absentees from Qaditha and elsewhere). In the coastal area, only two villages survived: Furidees and Jisr al-Zarqa. And two remained in the Jerusalem hills: Abu-Gush and Beit Naqquba.

Demolishing Arab villages was another element of the fear-inducing policy conducted by the military regime. Present absentees and their neighbors were traumatized as they watched living villages being turned into ruins and empty landscapes. Israel opted to destroy small villages, particularly in the Wadi Ara area. Indeed, about 10 small Arab settlements were demolished by the army and new

Jewish Israeli settlements were established on their ruins while the case of the original inhabitants was litigated in the High Court of Justice (see, for example, the case of the Naddaf family from the village of Jalameh) (Cohen, 2000, p. 130; Manna, 2017, pp. 233–234). Such actions were a brazen abuse of the legal system and sent a clear message to the survivors that their formal citizenship did not secure their basic rights.

In addition to preventing the return of most Palestinian refugees, Israel expelled about 20,000 Palestinian citizens between 1949 and 1956 (Manna, 2017, pp. 194–195). However, about the same number of Palestinian refugees did succeed in returning to their homes during that same period. Some of the returnees came back under Israeli approval while others returned without it. The inhabitants of two villages that were expelled from their homes were allowed to officially but silently go back to their homes several months later. Those were the inhabitants of the Christian village of 'Elaboun, expelled to Lebanon, and the Muslim residents of 'Ilut, who had been living in a Christian monastery in Nazareth for a while.

A Change over Time

The Israel Border Police massacre of 49 innocent citizens of Kafr Qasim October 29, 1956, was a turning point in the history of the Arab minority in the Jewish state. The massacre took place in the evening of the first day of the Israeli war against Egypt (together with France and Britain). The people killed were residents of the village who returned to their homes from work after 5:00 p.m., unaware of the curfew imposed that same afternoon. About half of those killed were children aged 8–17. For the first time, many people in Israel perceived this assault as a war crime and demanded that the perpetrators be brought to justice. The government, led by Prime Minister David Ben-Gurion, initially tried to suppress the details of the massacre and spread disinformation for several weeks. However, political and public pressure forced the prime minister to change his mind. As a result, Israeli officers and soldiers who took part in the massacre were imprisoned—for the first time in Israeli history—for killing Palestinians (Rosenthal, 2000).

Conclusion

Much of the geopolitical environment in which Jewish and Palestinian citizens of Israel live took shape around 1948. Traumas of the Nakba continue to influence Palestinian citizens' perceptions of the conflict and will have an impact on its solution. This is particularly true in the case of the present absentees in the Galilee and the unrecognized Bedouin villages in the Negev. Past atrocities are still linger in present realities and should be addressed together with current inequalities. An end to the occupation of territories beyond the Green Line is the first step toward reaching a historical reconciliation between Jews and Arabs in the region. The Nakba of the Palestinians in 1948 was the beginning of their predicament, and each new assault exacerbates open wounds. Hence, healing the scars of the past is imperative for lasting peace and genuine reconciliation. The case of the Palestinian citizens in Israel, including the atrocities of the Nakba, should be part of the final settlement and historical reconciliation between peoples.

Painful memories of the Nakba, anticipation for a better future, and distress in the present have been constant elements of Palestinian citizens' experience in Israel since 1948. The dissolution of the military government at the end of 1966 raised hopes for a normal life for this trapped community. However, such wishful thinking did not last long. The Israeli occupation of the West Bank and Gaza Strip, the Golan Heights, and the Sinai Peninsula in June 1967 intensified the dialectics of the new realities. On the one hand, the survivors were able to meet their brethren in the West Bank and Gaza after a long period of separation. On the other hand, they met them as citizens of the occupying power. It took the Palestinians on both sides of the Green Line many years to reconcile the differences and rediscover their common ground as Palestinians.

Most Jewish and Palestinian citizens in Israel hold opposing and unreconciled narratives of the conflict. Both sides of the Palestinian/Jewish divide believe that they are the victims of the other's aggression. For the Jews, the war was an act of defense and part of the legitimate establishment of the Jewish state. For the Palestinians, the Nakba, often silenced and denied in Israel, is the history of a national trauma.

ADEL MANNA is a historian and Senior Research Fellow at the Van Leer Jerusalem Institute, Israel. He is author of *Nakba and Survival*.

References

Abbasi, M. (2014). *The cities of Galilee during the 1948 war: Four cities and four stories.* Saarbrücken, Germany: Lambert Academic.

Al-Zu'bi, S. a. D. (1987). *Shahid 'ayan* [in Arabic]. Shefa 'Amr: Dar al-Mashriq.

Ben-Gurion, D. (1948). *Protocol of the cabinet meeting* [in Hebrew]. Jerusalem.

Cohen, H. (2000). *The present absentees: The Palestinian refugees in Israel since 1948* [in Hebrew]. Jerusalem: Center for the Study of Arab Society in Israel.

Firro, K. (1999). *The Druzes in the Jewish state: A brief history* (Vol. 64). Leiden: Brill.

Jiryis, Ṣ. (1966). *The Arabs in Israel* [in Arabic]. Haifa: El Etehad.

Jiryis, Ṣ. (1976). *The Arabs in Israel.* New York: Monthly Review.

Kretzmer, D. (1990). *The legal status of the Arabs in Israel.* Boulder, CO: Westview.

Manna, A. (2017). *Nakba and survival:The story of Palestinians who stayed in Haifa and the Galilee 1948–1956* [in Hebrew]. Jerusalem: Van Leer Jerusalem Institute and Hakibbutz Hameuchad.

Masalha, N. (1997). *Maximum land and minimum Arabs: Israel, transfer and Palestinians, 1949–1996* [in Arabic]. Beirut: Mu'assasat al-Dirāsāt al-Filasṭīnīyah.

Masalha, N. (2005). *Catastrophe remembered: Palestine, Israel and the internal refugees*. London and New York: Zed Books.

Monterescu, D., & Rabinowitz, D. (2007). *Mixed towns, trapped communities*. Burlington, VT: Ashgate.

Morris, B. (1996). *Israel's border wars 1949–1956* [in Hebrew]. Tel Aviv: Am Oved.

Rabin, Y. (1979). *Pinkas sherut* [in Hebrew]. Tel Aviv: Maariv.

Rabinowitz, D. (2001). The Palestinian citizens of Israel, the concept of trapped minority and the discourse of transnationalism in anthropology. *Ethnic and Racial Studies, 24*(1), 64–85.

Rosenthal, R. (2000). *Kafr Kassem: Myth and history* [in Hebrew]. Tel Aviv: Ha-Kibbbutz ha-Meuchad.

4

COLLECTIVE IDENTITY AND MENTAL HEALTH AMONG PALESTINIAN CITIZENS IN ISRAEL

Mahmoud Mi'ari and Nazeh Natur

Collective Identity

Miller (1963, 1983), among other scholars, defines identity as a set of observable and inferable attributes that identifies a person to him- or herself and to others. Miller differentiates between objective public identity (how the person is seen by others), subjective public identity (how the person perceives how others see him or her), and self-identity (how the person sees him- or herself).

Social psychologists (e.g., Deschamps & Devos, 1998; Stephan & Stephan, 1996) distinguish between two main types of identity: social and personal. Social identity refers to a feeling of similarity to (some) others, while personal identity refers to a feeling of difference in relation to the same others. Deschamps and Devos (1998) have argued that every individual is characterized both by social features, which show his or her membership in a group or a category, and by personal features or individual characteristics that are more specific. Stephan and Stephan (1996) proposed that a negative relationship exists between personal and social identities. If people emphasize themselves as unique individuals, they do not usually stress their group affiliation, and vice versa.

The concept of "identity" or "collective identity" used in this chapter is equivalent to the concept of "social identity" just described. It is defined as a sense of belonging to a group or number of groups. Accordingly, collective identity is a subjective state and can exist at many different levels from family unit to professional organization, political party, ethnic group, nation, state, or grouping of states, such as the European Union and the Arab nation. Although identity is a subjective state, it is generally affected by objective features such as territory, language, history, and culture (Smith, 1991).

In most contemporary societies, collective identity is formed by a number of components (or subidentities) representing several group memberships. The importance given to these components may vary from one period to another depending on social and historical factors, such as state policy, social change, wars, and interracial contact. Collective identity, as such, is multidimensional and socially constructed and varies from time to time (Bostock & Smith, 2001; Mi'ari, 1998). Accordingly, the collective identity of Palestinian citizens in Israel is formed by at least four important components representing several group memberships: (1) Palestinian, being an integral part of the Palestinian people; (2) Arab, sharing a common language, history, and culture with the Arab world; (3) Israeli, as a result of holding Israeli citizenship and thus Israeli passports; and (4) predominantly Muslim, with two other distinct minorities, Christians and Druze. As noted, the importance given to these components may vary from one period to another (Mi'ari, 1998, 2011).

Identity before the Oslo Accords

During the first two decades of the establishment of the Jewish state, Palestinian citizens in Israel formed an isolated national minority, separated physically, socially, and culturally from the surrounding Arab world and from the sectors of the Palestinian people scattered in other countries. They lived in Israel without any real national leadership because all the social, political, economic, educational, and religious elites, who had been concentrated in the cities, had left the country during the 1948 Arab-Israeli War.

To control this minority effectively, the Israeli government initially imposed a military regime system. Willing to improve their socioeconomic status through their work in the Israeli labor market, Palestinian citizens in Israel accepted the new political reality and defined themselves in Israeli terms. In their study on the identity of Palestinian citizens in Israel before and after the Six-Day War of 1967, Peres and Yuval-Davis (1969) found that the order of identities (from strong to weak) before the war was Israeli, Israeli Arab, Arab, and lastly, Palestinian.

After the war of 1967, a new period in the collective identity of Palestinian citizens in Israel began as a result of two main factors: abolition of the military regime in 1966 and the outbreak of the Six-Day War. The former increased social interaction and integration among Palestinian citizens in Israel within their various regions (the Galilee, the Triangle, and the Negev), and the latter increased social interaction and solidarity between them and their brothers in the newly occupied West Bank and Gaza Strip. As a result, their Israeli identity weakened, their Arab identity intensified, and their Palestinian identity awakened (Mi'ari, 1992). Thus, Peres and Yuval-Davis (1969) also found that the order of identities among Palestinians after the war (from strong to weak) became Arab, Israeli Arab, Palestinian, and finally, Israeli.

Palestinian identity became more intensified and Israeli identity declined further during the 1970s and 1980s as a result of external and internal changes.

Two major developments took place on the external front. The first was the broad international recognition of the Palestinian Liberation Organization (PLO) as the sole legitimate representative of the Palestinian people. The second development was prompted by several massacres against Palestinians committed by Arab regimes and parties, the ugliest of which was the 1982 Sabra and Shatila massacre in Lebanon. The massacre of Sabra and Shatila was carried out in the Sabra and Shatila refugee camps in Beirut on September 16, 1982, where hundreds of civilian Palestinians and Lebanese were killed. The massacre was carried out by the Lebanese isolationist groups of the Lebanese Phalange Party and the South Lebanese Army. The Israeli commission investigating the events of Sabra and Shatila found "the Minister of Defense (Sharon) bears personal responsibility." It also recommended that "the Minister of Defense draw the appropriate personal conclusions arising out of the defects revealed with regard to the manner in which he discharged the duties of his office—and if necessary, that the Prime Minister consider whether he should exercise his authority under Section 21-A(a) of the Basic Law: the Government, according to which 'the Prime Minister may, after informing the Cabinet of his intention to do so, remove a minister from office'" (Malone, 1985, p. 374).

On the internal front, there were also two major developments: the rapid social transformation of agrarian Palestinian peasants into wage laborers working primarily in construction in Jewish cities and the broadening of a Palestinian educated stratum formed primarily of university graduates and students (Mi'ari, 2008).

Several studies have confirmed the intensification of the Palestinian identity in the 1970s and 1980s (Mi'ari, 1992; Rouhana, 1984; Smooha, 1984; Tessler, 1977). The activities of Palestinian citizens on Land Day reflected this upswing in the 1970s. The Land Day protest was rooted in a March 30, 1976 incident in which 6 Arab citizens were killed by the police in a clash over government confiscation of privately owned Arab land in the Galilee, Israel (Wolfsfeld, Avraham, & Aburaiya, 2000).

Palestinians participated in a general strike and mass marches to protest the Israeli government's plan to expropriate thousands of acres of land in the Galilee. During the confrontations with the army and police, six Palestinian citizens were killed, about 100 were wounded, and hundreds were arrested. In the 1980s, the deepening of Palestinian identity was reflected by the solidarity of Palestinian citizens with the first intifada, which erupted in the West Bank and Gaza Strip in December 1987. They expressed this sense of unity with demonstrations; strikes; and donations of money, food, and medications for the people in the West Bank and Gaza Strip.

Identity after the Oslo Accords: Four Perspectives

A review of the literature after Israel and the PLO signed the Declaration of Principles on Interim Self-Government Arrangements in 1993 (the Oslo Accords) identifies four distinct and important perspectives in relation to this topic: non-Palestinian

Israeli identity, Israeli Palestinian identity, localization of the national struggle, and incomplete Palestinian and Israeli identities.

Non-Palestinian Israeli Identity

This perspective, submitted by Israeli sociologist Sammy Smooha (1998), is based on a survey conducted in 1995 that sharpened his thesis about the Israelization of the Palestinian minority after the Oslo Accords with regard to identity and politics. Smooha hypothesizes that Israelization means increased integration in Israeli identity and politics, on the one hand, and estrangement from Palestinian identity and politics on the other (p. 41); thus, he argued that "Israelization overcame Palestinization" (Smooha, 1998, p. 44). His surveys, Smooha claimed, showed that the "non-Palestinian Israeli" identity became the strongest among most of the Arabs in Israel, the "non-Israeli Palestinian" identity declined, and the "Palestinian Israeli" identity remained accepted by only a third of the respondents. Unexpectedly, the latter had ceased to develop and spread from the late 1980s. Based on a later survey, Smooha (2005) argued that the non-Palestinian Israeli identity (45.1%) and the Palestinian Israeli identity (45.0%) were the most common and most attractive identities during and after the second (Al-Aqsa) intifada that began in September 2000, while the non-Israeli Palestinian identity remained marginal (8.6%). According to Smooha, these figures showed that the Israeli dimension in the identity of the Arabs in Israel was most central.

We may agree with Smooha that in the early years after the Oslo Accords the Palestinian identity was as described, but we disagree with his argument that "Israelization overcame Palestinization." In our opinion, he committed two main methodological errors in his classification of identities. In his 1976–1995 surveys, the identity of Palestinian citizens was measured by a closed questionnaire, requiring each respondent to choose one of the following seven identities: Israeli, Arab, Israeli Arab, Palestinian in Israel, Israeli Palestinian, Palestinian, and Palestinian Arab. Later, Smooha (2005) added two identities: Arab in Israel and Palestinian Arab in Israel. In his analysis, Smooha classified these identities into three categories: (1) "non-Palestinian Israeli," including Israeli, Arab, Arab in Israel, and Israeli Arab identities; (2) "Israeli Palestinian," including Israeli Palestinian, Palestinian in Israel, and Palestinian Arab in Israel; and (3) "non-Israeli Palestinian," including Palestinian and Palestinian Arab. Comparison of these categories in the two surveys shows that the "non-Palestinian Israeli" identity increased from 33% in 1988 to 54% in 1995, while the "non-Israeli Palestinian" identity declined from 27% to 10%, and the "Israeli Palestinian" identity dropped slightly from 40% to 36% (Smooha, 1998, p. 43).

We have found two errors in this classification: (1) The classification of "Arab" within the first category, "non-Palestinian Israeli" identity, errs because in most surveys Arab identity has been positively correlated with Palestinian identity and not significantly correlated with Israeli identity (Diab & Mi'ari, 2007). (2) The classification of "Palestinian in Israel" and "Palestinian Arab in Israel" within the second category, "Israeli Palestinian" identity, errs because, we argue, the word "Israel" in this category indicates place (or country) of residence and does not necessarily indicate Israeli identity (Mi'ari, 1992).

Israeli Palestinian Identity

Al-Haj (2004) proposed the second perspective we are examining here. He argued that the Oslo Accords, by neglecting the Palestinian citizens in Israel, intensified their status of double marginality—placing them at the margins of both Israeli and Palestinian societies. As a result, Palestinian citizens in Israel began to emphasize the issues of citizenship and civil rights in Israeli society in their struggle. Although still disturbed by the national issue, primarily the solution of the Palestinian-Israeli conflict, they are even more preoccupied by the problem of civil rights because this issue affects their everyday lives. This is also the case because, in their view, the fate of the Palestinian citizens in Israel is still linked to that of the state of Israel, even after the establishment of a Palestinian state (Al-Haj, 2004).

Al-Haj (2004) suggests that the feeling of double marginality has led Palestinian citizens in Israel to develop two central components in their identity. The civic component is reflected by Palestinian citizens who have linked their fate to the state of Israel, which they perceive as their homeland and in which they struggle for full equality in civil rights. The national component is reflected by the perception of Palestinian citizens that they are an integral part of the Palestinian people and by their support of Palestinian rights for self-determination, including the establishment of a Palestinian state alongside Israel. Al-Haj (2004) concluded that the sense of double marginality has led Palestinian citizens in Israel to develop a unique Palestinian Israeli identity in which commitment to the national component takes the civic one into consideration.

We have some reservations about Al-Haj's thesis. His thesis is not based on empirical data, and it presumes that the two components of the identity are harmonious and equal in strength. Our empirical data show that Palestinian and Israeli identities are negatively correlated and that the former is much stronger than the latter (Diab & Mi'ari, 2007).

Localization of the National Struggle

The third perspective is that of Rekhess (2002), who refers to "the localization of the national struggle." (p. 2). His view is based on a distinction between the identification and solidarity of Palestinian citizens with the external Palestinian issue, especially with the Palestinian Authority (PA) and the Palestine Liberation Organization (PLO), and the consolidation of particularistic national Palestinian patterns within Israel itself. Rekhess argued that external affinities were weakened in the Palestinization process as a result of two main factors. The first factor involved the recognition by Israel of the PLO and of the legitimate rights of the Palestinian people to self-determination, the return of the PLO leadership to the Palestinian territories, and the establishment of the PA. These actions constituted a partial or full realization of the Palestinian national platform and that of Israel's Palestinians (Rekhess, 2002). As a result, the Arabs in Israel felt they had done their share in supporting the Palestinian cause. Second, the Palestinian leadership (PLO and PA) maintained the traditional approach of ignoring the Palestinian population of Israel, or even harbored a discriminatory attitude toward Israeli Palestinians. As a result, the PLO and PA did not incorporate local Israeli Palestinian political leadership as a partner in the political process.

While the Palestinization process of Arabs in Israel was weakening in its external dimension, it gained strength in its internal one, the roots of which lay within the Green Line. This has been explored on three levels. The first is the opposition to the characterization of Israel as a Jewish and democratic state and proposed alternative models such as a state of all its citizens and a binational state. The second examines the ways in which Palestinian citizens can be recognized as a national minority and proposals for their collective rights. And the third looks at signs of a national awakening anchored within the Israeli context, such as proposals to reopen the question of land ownership and the right of return of uprooted residents and the desire to commemorate the Nakba. Rekhess (2002) indicated that despite the weakening of Palestinization in its external dimension, the peace process led to a significant reinforcement of the Israeli Palestinian's identity. A new era of national awakening had begun with distinctive characteristics. The establishment of the PA and the international recognition it gained reinforced the national consciousness of the Arabs in Israel.

Incomplete Palestinian and Israeli Identities

Rouhana and Ghanem (1998) proposed a fourth important perspective. They argued that the Arab minority in Israel faces hardship (or distress) in three fields: the Israeli, the Palestinian, and the internal. In the Israeli field, the struggle stems from factors such as the policy of discrimination against Arab citizens, the exclusion of Arabs from centers of power, Israel's neglect of Arab culture and Arabic language, the role of security forces in determining the policy toward Arabs, and the Jewish-Zionist character of the state. These factors undermine the hopes of Arab citizens that equality is an achievable goal.

With regard to the Palestinian field, the hardship stems from factors such as the PA leadership's apathy about including Arab Israeli citizens at the negotiating table with Israel; the PA's interference in the affairs of Arab Israeli citizens, especially in Knesset elections; and the PA's nondemocratic practices in the Occupied Territories. Palestinian citizens of Israel feel that they are outside the Palestinian national movement and are excluded from the Palestinian political center represented by the PA in the West Bank and Gaza Strip (Rouhana & Ghanem, 1998).

In the internal field, the distress is represented in daily life by the limited influence of the Arab Palestinian minority on the decision-making processes of the state, even as elected members of the Knesset, and by the absence of an elected, unified national leadership of this minority and its weak economic development. This hardship is also represented by the collective identity of the Arabs in Israel. Rouhana and Ghanem (1998) argued that "neither the Israeli identity nor the Palestinian identity of Arab citizens is complete and full under the current circumstances" (p. 66). This, they claimed, "is the summary of the collective identity crisis of Arab citizens" (p. 66). Although the Palestinian component in the identity of Arab citizens is "firm, prominent and salient" (p. 66), it cannot be complete as long as the Palestinian national movement is establishing a Palestinian homeland elsewhere. They further argued that the Israeli component in that identity "is incomplete because it lacks the feeling of belonging and of emotional support" (p. 66). Rouhana and Ghanem repeated elsewhere the same argument that the Israeli and Palestinian identities among Arab citizens of Israel are both incomplete. In the words of Rouhana (2002), these citizens "are not fully Israelis and, in a sense, not fully Palestinians" (p. 62). For Ghanem (2005), these citizens "have a partial Israeli identity and a partial Palestinian identity" (p. 938).

Although we agree with Rouhana and Ghanem's analysis of the factors leading to hardship and distress among Palestinian citizens in Israel, we have some reservations about their use of the terms "incomplete" or "partial" Israeli and Palestinian identities. In addition to the fact that these two identities are not equal in strength (see the discussion that follows), the collective identity of a person, as we understand it, means the sense of belonging to a group or a number of groups, and this sense of belonging may be strong or weak. It is more acceptable, therefore, to say that a certain collective identity is strong or weak rather than complete or partial.

Restrengthening of the Palestinian Identity

As indicated earlier, the Palestinian identity weakened and the Israeli identity strengthened among Palestinian citizens in Israel in the first few years after the Oslo Accords (Ghanem & Ozacky-Lazer, 2003; Reiter, 2009; Smooha, 1998). This resulted from the feeling that they were being neglected by the Palestinian national movement. However, the failure of the Oslo Accords, followed by the Al-Aqsa intifada, which erupted on September 28, 2000, tipped the scale again toward a restrengthening of the Palestinian identity. A survey conducted in 2003 during the Al-Aqsa intifada among a representative sample of 167 Arab students in the David Yellin College of Education in Jerusalem, comprising about 48% of all Arab students in the college, showed that 91% of the respondents felt Arab to a great extent or to a very great extent, 76% felt Palestinian, and 18% felt Israeli. When asked about their most important identity, 31% of the students selected the Palestinian or Palestinian Arab identity; 28%, the Arab identity; 18%, the religious identity; 5%, the Israeli identity; and the remaining 18% mentioned primarily the *hamula* (clan or tribe) and local (place of residence) identities (Diab & Mi'ari, 2007; Mi'ari, 2011). These results clearly show that the Palestinian identity, which had slightly weakened in the first few years after the Oslo Accords, regained strength, especially with the explosion of the Al-Aqsa intifada, and became much stronger than the Israeli identity.

Other survey studies support our argument that after the Oslo Accords, especially in the last decade, the Palestinian identity of Arabs in Israel became stronger than the Israeli identity. A survey conducted by the Information and Research Center of the Knesset (Berda, 2002) asked, "To what extent does each one of the three definitions (Israeli, Arab and Palestinian) describe the identity of Palestinian citizens in Israel?" The Arab identity ranked the highest (average score of 9.3 on a scale ranging from 1 to 10), followed by the Palestinian identity (8.4), while the Israeli identity was the lowest (6.0). Another survey conducted by Arad and Alon (2006) on a random sample of 800 Israeli respondents, of whom 170 were Arabs, showed that 56% of the Arab respondents were not proud of their Israeli identity, and 73% were unwilling to fight to defend the state. In addition, 24% defined themselves to a great extent as Israeli patriots, while 48% identified themselves to a great extent as Palestinian patriots. In 2010 the Saban Center conducted the Israeli Arab/Palestinian Public Opinion survey (*N* = 600). This study showed that, in response to a question about the most important identity, 36% of the respondents selected Arab; 22%, Palestinian; 19%, religious; and 12%, Israeli (Telhami, 2010). The Democracy Index 2012 poll, conducted by the Israel Democracy Institute, also showed that only 28% of Arab respondents felt (to a great extent or to a very great extent) that they were part of the state of Israel and its problems, 45% felt proud of being Israeli, and 75% felt deprived compared to Jewish citizens (Hermann, Atmor, Heller, & Lebel, 2012). The Mada al-Carmel civil service survey, conducted in 2012 among a sample of 504 Arab youth aged 16–22 years, found that the large majority of Arab youth believed that Arab citizens should not be enrolled in the civil service. As for their identity, 42% defined themselves either as Palestinian Arab or Palestinian Arab citizens in Israel; 22%, as Israeli or Israeli Arab; and 7%, as Israeli Palestinian Arab (Mada al-Carmel: Arab Center for Applied Social Research [Mada al-Carmel], 2012).

Two main factors contributed to the restrengthening of the Palestinian identity (Mi'ari, 2011): the failure of the Oslo peace process and the escalation of the Israeli policy of exclusion against the Palestinian Arab minority. The failure of the Oslo peace process led to the eruption of the Al-Aqsa intifada in the West Bank and Gaza Strip. The Israeli government applied repressive measures against Palestinians in these territories during and after the fighting: mass arrests, shootings, house demolitions, military checkpoints, limitations on movement, elimination of leaders, and use of airplanes and tanks to reach their targets. We argue that these actions, together with exclusionary policies, strengthened the Palestinian identity among Arab citizens in Israel. With the establishment of the Netanyahu government in 1996, legislative policies to exclude the Palestinian Arab minority from full citizenship escalated. Since the late 1990s, the Knesset has passed many anti-Arab law amendments (Adalah: The Legal Center for Arab Minority Rights in Israel [Adalah], 2012; Sultany, 2003). These new laws, as Adalah (2012) indicated, had several major goals: to dispossess Palestinian Arab citizens of Israel and exclude them from the land, to turn their citizenship from a right into a conditional privilege, to limit the ability of Arab citizens and their parliamentary representatives to participate in the political life of the country, and to criminalize political acts or speech that question the Jewish or Zionist nature of the state that gives privilege to Jewish citizens in the allocation of state resources.

Traditional Identities and Their Relationships

Previous studies (Diab & Mi'ari, 2007; Mi'ari, 1990; Mi'ari & Diab, 2005) have shown that traditional, primarily religious and *hamula* identities have also strengthened since the first intifada. A survey conducted in 1988 among a sample of Arab high school students (grade 12) indicated that 70% of the respondents felt they belonged to a great extent or to a very great extent to a religious group (Muslim, Christian, or Druze), and 63% felt they belonged to a *hamula*. Another survey conducted in 2003, during the second intifada, on a sample of Arab students in the David Yellin College of Education in Jerusalem, found that 84% felt to a great extent or to a very great extent that they belonged to a religious group, while 84% also felt that they belonged to a *hamula*. Pearson's correlation coefficients among the various identities in these two surveys found that religious and *hamula* identities were not significantly correlated with Arab, Palestinian, and Israeli identities. This finding contradicts a conclusion that we found in a survey conducted in 1976 among a sample of 293 Arab university graduates. Religious and *hamula* identities in that survey were positively correlated with Israeli identity ($r = 0.69$ and 0.64, respectively) and negatively correlated with Palestinian identity ($r = -0.31$ and -0.33, respectively) (Mi'ari, 1990). This means that in the 1970s, traditional Arab citizens tended to identify themselves as Israeli, while nontraditional Arab citizens tended to identify themselves as Palestinian.

The strengthening of Palestinian identity in the first intifada and subsequently during and after the second intifada, and the disappearance of its negative relationship with traditional identities, reflects the spread of the Palestinian identity in the last two or three decades among traditional as well as among nontraditional Arabs in Israel. It seems that the emergence of the Islamic movement in Israel in the late 1980s contributed to the spread of the Palestinian identity among traditional Arab citizens. Besides strengthening Palestinian identity, it also appears that the Islamic movement has weakened the Israeli identity among these traditional Arabs.

Reflections of the Palestinian Identity

As mentioned earlier, the expression of solidarity with Palestinians in the Occupied Territories during and after the second intifada in 2000 was one indication of the strengthening of Palestinian identity among Palestinian Arab citizens. The activities of Palestinian Arab citizens, Arab parties, and the Higher Arab Monitoring Committee—an independent political organization whose aim is to coordinate and lead the political actions of various Israeli-Arab bodies and parties—are also reflections of that change. In the last two decades, these individuals and organizations have begun to make efforts to preserve the history and memory of destroyed Arab villages during the 1948 war, to criticize the characterization of Israel as a Jewish and democratic state, and to demand that the Arab minority be recognized as an indigenous national minority with collective rights. Palestinian citizens in Israel now mark the Nakba of 1948, the Land Day of 1976, and the events of the Al-Aqsa intifada in October 2000 with protest marches called by the Arab Higher Monitoring Committee.

The restrengthening of Palestinian identity is also reflected by the Arab vote in Knesset elections. The voting percentage of Palestinian citizens in Israel decreased from 79% in 1996 to 64% in 2015. Additionally, the voting percentage for Arab (or non-Zionist) parties increased from 67% in 1996 to 87% in 2015 (Atmor & Friedberg, 2015; Mada al-Carmel, 2015; Shihade, 2013).

The intensification of the Palestinian identity may provide Palestinian Arab citizens with a sense of social support and social solidarity and thus may improve their mental health.

Ethnic Identity and Mental Health

No clear theoretical model exists to examine how an achieved ethnic identity increases psychological health (Grindal, 2014). Generally, the relationship between a strong ethnic identity and psychological health has been theoretically framed within a risk-and-resilience framework (Hawkins, Catalano, & Miller, 1992; Zimmerman & Arunkumar, 1994). A strong ethnic identity has been theorized and found to generate a stable, secure, and positively defined self-concept that provides mechanisms of resiliency to face the harmful impact of ethnic/racial discrimination (Smith & Silva, 2011). Indeed, strong identity and self-respect significantly decrease symptoms of depression and anxiety (Chae & Yoshikawa, 2008; Greene, Way, & Pahl, 2006; Mandara, Gaylord-Harden, Richards, & Ragsdale, 2009) and contribute to higher self-esteem. Minority members (e.g., African American and US Hispanic adolescents) with strong ethnic identity tend to have better mental health overall (Greig, 2003). As this identity weakens their own perception of being discriminated against (Rowley, Sellers, Chavous, & Smith, 1998), it serves as a buffer against the negative influence of discrimination in health care (Sellers, Caldwell, Schmeelk-Cone, & Zimmerman, 2003).

Two major themes have emerged in the research on the relationship between ethnic identity and health. One theme claims that strong ethnic identity could jeopardize mental health because it highlights the existing minority/majority differences and magnifies the negative discriminatory practices against minorities, thus having an impact on the person's self-perception and mental health

(Phinney, 1991). In addition, it may actually intensify vulnerability to distress (e.g., Yip, Gee, & Takeuchi, 2008; Yoo & Lee, 2008). The second theme proposes that a strong ethnic minority could function as a moderating factor, minimizing stress and the negative effect on perception of the self, thus increasing resiliency with reference to discrimination (Sellers et al., 2003).

Health and Mental Health among Palestinian Citizens in Israel

Health care in Israel is universal and participation in a medical insurance plan is mandatory. All Israeli citizens are entitled to basic health care as a fundamental right, including Palestinian citizens. Yet, Palestinian citizens in Israel face barriers in accessing mental health care (Chernichovsky, Bisharat, Bowers, Brill, & Sharony, 2017). Indeed, access to mental health services is at 21% among Palestinians compared to 39% among Jewish Israelis (Elroy, Rosen, Elmakias, & Samuel, 2017).

Poverty is another barrier that Palestinians citizens of Israel face in accessing health and mental care services. In 2016, 53% of Arab families lived in poverty compared to 14% of Jewish families, and 66% of Arab children lived in poverty compared to 20% of Jewish children (National Insurance Institute of Israel [NII], 2016). Palestinian families constitute 38% of all poor families, far above their proportion of all Jewish Israeli families (13%) (NII, 2016). Furthermore, researchers have found that a third of Palestinian citizens in Israel do not purchase prescribed medications owing to financial difficulties (Chernichovsky et.al., 2017).

Other possible indicators of limited access to health care, such as health promotion, are observed in the data on life expectancy of Palestinians, which is lower when compared to the Jewish population. Among Palestinian women life expectancy is 78.1 compared to 82.7 for Jewish women; among Palestinian men it is 76.5 compared to 81.2 for Jewish men (Rosen, Waitzberg, & Merkur, 2015). Similar problems are observed in infant mortality rates: among Muslims it is 5.3 deaths per 1,000 live births compared to 2.4 per 1,000 among Jews (Israel Central Bureau of Statistics, 2017). Furthermore, the Palestinian population of Israel has fewer primary care clinics and fewer physicians per capita (1.4 per 1,000 Palestinians compared to 2.6 per 1,000 Jews).

Some of these disparities in medical and mental health, while higher in past years, are the consequence of institutionalized policies such as the disproportionate allocation of funds. For example, the average expenditure on welfare (including self-generated supplements allocated by the localities) in economically strong regions in the country is NIS 9,095 per client, while in Arab Israeli areas the expenditure is only NIS 3,387 per client (Gal, Madhala, & Bleikh, 2017).

The mental health status of a population can be measured by the presence or absence of mental health-related conditions (i.e., stress, depression, low self-esteem, or reduced well-being). The prevalence of common mental disorders is higher among Palestinians than among Israeli Jews. Palestinians have higher scores in emotional distress and lower self-appraisal of mental health (perception of one's own mental health), but they make fewer requests for psychiatric help (Levav, Ifrah, Geraisy, Grinshpoon, & Khwaled, 2007).

Relationship between Identity and Mental Health

Studies on the mental health of Palestinian citizens in Israel, as noted elsewhere in this book, are limited, and studies on the relationship between mental health and collective identity are even more scare. In this section, we review the relationship between collective identity and mental health, then attempt to formulate a research problem on the relationship between mental health and collective identity among Palestinian citizens in Israel.

Often, minority groups worldwide—and the Palestinian minority in Israel, the focus of this book—suffer from various forms of discrimination. Ferdinand, Paradies, and Kelaher (2015) reported that experiencing discrimination is associated with high psychological stress and experiencing racial discrimination is associated with worse mental health (Banks, 2012; DeGruy, 2009; Dovidio et al., 2008). For example, studies have shown higher rates of anxiety, depression, and substance abuse among African American, Latino, and Asian American women compared to European American women in the United States (McDonald, Keys, & Balcazar, 2007).

The psychological importance of ethnic identity among ethnic minority groups can be attributed to previous experiences of discrimination and disparities (Tajfel & Turner, 1986). Identifying with a minority can serve as a protective function against perceived environmental threats (Ashmore, Deaux, & McLaughlin-Volpe, 2004). It provides a sense of social connectedness, a positive sense of self, and a sense of purpose that can serve as psychological resources for youth when facing stressful life events (Costigan, Koryzma, Hua, & Chance, 2010; Stein, Kiang, Supple, & Gonzalez, 2014).

Ethnic exploration as well as ethnic belonging have been significantly correlated with higher self-esteem and lower depressive symptoms, while higher levels of perceived racial/ethnic discrimination and economic stress have been significantly correlated with more depressive symptoms and lower self-esteem (Stein et al., 2014). Strong ethnic identity helps individuals to recognize positive features about their own ethnic group, and it minimizes the effects of negative beliefs and stereotypes in society (Outten, Schmitt, Garcia, & Branscombe, 2009). Strong ethnic identity has been found to be associated with improved functioning among Asian American adolescents, increased self-esteem, decreased depressive symptoms, and better academic outcomes (Fuligni, Witkow, & Garcia, 2005; Iwamoto & Liu, 2010; Phinney & Ong, 2007). Other aspects of strong ethnic identity have also been found to be beneficial among the Navajo native population in the United States. Greater ethnic exploration among Navajo youth, for example, has protected them against substance abuse when facing ethnic/racial discrimination (Galliher, Jones, & Dahl, 2011). No studies have been carried out on Palestinian citizens in Israel to examine the impact of identity level on mental health, yet it is safe to assume that, as in other instances in the world, stronger identity improves mental health while weak identity hinders it.

The link between ethnic identity and self-esteem is statistically significant for ethnic minorities (Worrell, 2007). African American and Hispanic adolescents in the United States who achieve a secure sense of themselves as ethnic group members have a higher sense of self-esteem and tend to have better mental health overall (Greig, 2003). Similarly, a strong identification with an ethnic group is directly associated with fewer depressive symptoms among Filipino Americans (Mossakowski, 2003). Having a sense of ethnic pride, involvement in ethnic practices, and cultural commitment to one's racial/ethnic group may protect mental health and buffer the stress and depressive symptoms of racial/ethnic discrimination. Other studies (e.g., Cheryan & Tsai, 2007; Gray-Little & Hafdahl, 2000; Phinney, 1990) have reported that a strong ethnic identity is vital to the psychological well-being of ethnic minority group members. Numerous research studies have been consistent in their findings of positive relationships between ethnic identity and indicators of self-esteem and personal adjustment (Smith & Silva, 2011).

Significant positive correlations between ethnic identity and a variety of positive attributes, such as coping ability, mastery, self-esteem, and optimism have also been found in a large study ($N = 5,423$) of young adolescents from diverse ethnic groups in the United States (Roberts et al., 1999). Ponterotto and Park-Taylor (2007) suggested that these consistent correlations indicate that positive ethnic identity buffers against distress experienced by ethnic minority groups. Yet others have observed that in some cases stronger ethnic identity may actually intensify vulnerability to distress (e.g., Yip et al., 2008; Yoo & Lee, 2008). One explanation could be that stronger identity highlights the existing minority/majority difference perceived by minority members.

Interestingly, Hughes, Kiecolt, and Keith (2014) found that strong racial identity among African Americans buffers the deleterious effect of financial stress on depressive symptoms. Racial identity does not eliminate the effect of financial stress, but it does reduce it by protecting psychosocial resources that help lessen depressive symptoms. This finding strengthens the conclusion that the connection of positive group evaluation to self-esteem, emphasized in social identity theory (Tajfel & Turner, 1986), explains how racial identity helps to protect mental health.

The positive relationship between ethnic-national identity and mental health is supported by the findings of a recent qualitative study conducted among Palestinians from the West Bank who were injured by Israeli military forces during the second intifada (Abusoboh, 2014). This study concluded that collective-national identity was perceived as a motivating force to participate in the intifada activities against the Israeli occupation and, at the same time, as a mechanism of coping and psychological resilience. Palestinian identity was considered a factor in achieving psychological adjustment for individuals suffering trauma caused by confrontations with the Israeli military (Abusoboh, 2014).

A recent comparative survey on the relationship between reported discrimination and mental health was conducted among a sample of 900 Israeli residents, aged 30–65, of whom 400 were Jews born in Israel, 200 were Jewish immigrants from the former USSR, and 300 were Muslim Arabs (Shala'ata, 2014). The findings of this survey showed that the feeling of discrimination is negatively correlated to mental health among Jews born in Israel and among immigrant Jews but is not correlated to mental health among Muslim Arabs. It seems that the collective character of Palestinian society (coherence, solidarity, and social support) prevents the negative effects of discrimination. Referring to the relationship between ethnic-national identity and mental health, the survey showed that ethnic identity (measured by the feeling of belonging to an ethnic group; feeling glad about being a member of this group and proud of this membership, participating in cultural activities with other members of the group; having good relations with other members of the group; and feeling good in the group) is positively correlated to mental health among Jews born in Israel and among Muslim Arabs but is not correlated to mental health among immigrant Jews.

Previous findings about the relationship between ethnic-national identity and mental health and the lack of studies on the relationship between minority group members' type of identity (e.g., ethnic identity vs. civic or state identity) and their mental health lead us to raise three questions.

First, what is the relationship between each component of the collective identity (Palestinian, Israeli, and religious) and mental health among Palestinian citizens in Israel? In other words, is the relationship between Palestinian identity and mental health different from that between Israeli identity and mental health and that between religious identity and mental health?

Second, what is the relationship between the main collective identity and mental health among Palestinian citizens in Israel? That is, do mental health measures differ among Palestinian citizens in Israel who identify themselves primarily as Palestinian, those who identify themselves primarily as Israeli, and those who identify themselves primarily as Muslim or Christian or Druze?

Finally, what is the relationship between feelings of discrimination, collective identity, and mental health among Palestinian citizens in Israel? Do feelings of discrimination among this population affect its collective identity and mental health, and do they affect the relationship between these two variables?

Empirical studies are needed to answer these three questions.

Conclusion

This chapter focuses on collective identity and mental health among Palestinian citizens in Israel. We show that after the Oslo Accords, while Palestinian identity remained much stronger than Israeli identity, to some extent the former was weakened and the latter was strengthened. This shift primarily occurred because the 1993 Oslo Accords had totally ignored Palestinian citizens in Israel and thus affirmed that they would remain part of the state of Israel. These Palestinians felt that they had been marginalized not only in Israeli society but also in Palestinian society.

However, since the late 1990s, and particularly since the Al-Aqsa intifada, the Palestinian identity has become stronger and has spread among both traditional and nontraditional Palestinian citizens in Israel. The disappearance of its negative relationships with traditional—especially *hamula* and religious—identities confirms this change. Two main factors have contributed to the restrengthening of Palestinian identity: the failure of the Oslo peace process, leading to the eruption of the second intifada, and the escalation of the Israeli policy of discrimination and exclusion, reflected by many anti-Arab law amendments aimed at the Palestinian minority passed by the Knesset. As a result, in the past decade, Palestinian citizens have begun to make efforts to preserve their history and collective memory, to criticize the Jewish character of the state of Israel, and to demand state recognition as an indigenous national minority with collective rights.

The intensification of Palestinian identity among Palestinian citizens may provide them with a sense of social support and social solidarity and thus may improve their general mental health. Two approaches are recommended in the literature to investigate mental health: examination of social determinants such as poverty, housing, education, and access to resources; and examination of psychological functioning and dysfunction.

Mental health is a neglected area in Palestinian society in Israel. This society is characterized by a higher poverty rate, a lower employment rate, less access to education, and a high dropout rate; it also suffers from underdeveloped infrastructure. An examination of health measures (e.g., lower life expectancy, higher rates of mortality and infant mortality, and higher rates of diabetes) and mental disorders (higher common mental disorders, emotional distress, and less help-seeking practices), although improving over time, still show discrepancies with regard to the Jewish Israeli population. Corrective actions are needed.

Studies on the relationship between mental health and the types of collective identity of Palestinian citizens in Israel, as indicated in this chapter, are scant. But in our review of the research literature, in most studies, we have found a positive relationship between ethnic-national-religious identity and mental health. This positive relationship is also supported by a recent comparative study conducted in Israel (Shala'ata, 2014) that reports that ethnic identity is positively correlated to mental health among Jews born in Israel and among Muslim Arabs. Based on this literature, we end the chapter by raising questions about the relationship between the type of collective identity (Palestinian, Israeli, and religious) and mental health and call for further studies.

MAHMOUD MI'ARI is Professor of Sociology of Birzeit University, Palestine. He is editor of *Arab Teaching Curricula in Israel*

NAZEH NATUR is Dean of Students and Senior Lecturer in the Department of Psychology at Al-Qasemi Academic College of Education, Baqa, Israel.

References

Abusoboh, A. (2014). The role of social Palestinian identity in psychological adjustment following military violence [in Arabic]. *Pangaea Journal, 5*. Retrieved from http:// sites.stedwards.edu/pangaea/the-role-of-social-palestinian-identity-in-psychological -adjustment-following-military-violence/.

Adalah: The Legal Center for Arab Minority Rights in Israel [Adalah]. (2012). *Discriminatory laws in Israel*. Retrieved from https://www.adalah.org/uploads/2009-2012_Discrim inatory_laws_and_bills_English.pdf.

Al-Haj, M. (2004). Whither the green line? Trends in the encounter between and orientation of the Palestinians in Israel and the territories. [in Hebrew]. *State and Society, 4*(1), 825–844. Retrieved from https://www.jstor.org/stable/23637430?seq=1#metadata_info_tab_contents.

Arad, U., & Alon, G. (2006). *Patriotism and Israel's national security: Herzliya Patriotism Survey 2006*. Herzliya: Institute for Policy and Strategy. Retrieved from https://www.idc.ac.il/he /research/ips/documents/2006/2129patriotism_hebrew2006.pdf.

Ashmore, R. D., Deaux, K., & McLaughlin-Volpe, T. (2004). An organizing framework for collective identity: Articulation and significance of multidimensionality. *Psychological Bulletin, 130*(1), 80–114.

Atmor, N., & Friedberg, C. (2015). *Participation in elections 2015* [in Hebrew]. Jerusalem: Israel Democracy Institute. Retrieved from https://www.idi.org.il/articles/3458.

Banks, M. E. (2012). Multiple minority identity and mental health: Social and research implication of diversity within and between groups. In R. Nettles & R. Balter (Eds.), *Multiple minority identities: Applications for practice, research, and training* (pp 35–58). New York: Springer.

Berda, M. (2002). *Perception of identity and extent of loyalty among Israel's Arab citizens*. Jerusalem: Knesset Research and Information Center. Retrieved from https://fs.knesset .gov.il/globaldocs/MMM/f1c0577e-9332-e811-80de-00155d0a0235/2_f1c0577e-9332-e811 -80de-00155d0a0235_11_10174.pdf.

Bostock, W. W., & Smith, G. W. (2001). On measuring national identity. *Social Science Paper Publisher, 4*(1), 1–6.

Chae, D. H., & Yoshikawa, H. (2008). Perceived group devaluation, depression, and HIV-risk behavior among Asian gay men. *Health Psychology, 27*(2), 140–148.

Chernichovsky, D., Bisharat, B., Bowers, L., Brill, A., & Sharony, C. (2017). The health of the Arab Israeli population. Jerusalem: Taub Center for Social Policy Studies in Israel. Retrieved from http://taubcenter.org.il/wp-content/files_mf/healthofthearabisraelipopu lation.pdf.

Cheryan, S., & Tsai, J. L. (2007). Ethnic identity. In F. T. Leong, A. G. Inman, A. Ebreo, L. Yang, L. Kinoshita & M. Fu (Eds.), *Handbook of Asian American psychology* (2nd ed., pp. 125–139). Thousand Oaks, CA: Sage.

Costigan, C. L., Koryzma, C. M., Hua, J. M., & Chance, L. J. (2010). Ethnic identity, achievement, and psychological adjustment: Examining risk and resilience among youth from immigrant Chinese families in Canada. *Cultural Diversity and Ethnic Minority Psychology, 16*(2), 264–273.

DeGruy, J. A. (2009). Post-slavery syndrome: A multi-generational look at African American injury, healing and resilience. In A. Kalayjian & D. Eugene (Eds.), *Mass trauma and emotional healing around the world: Rituals and practices for resilience and meaning-making.* (Vol. 2). *Human made disasters* (pp. 227–250). Santa Barbara, CA: Breager.

Deschamps, J.-C., & Devos, T. (1998). Regarding the relationship between social identity and personal identity. In S. Worchel, J. F. Morales, D. Páez, & J.-C. Deschamps (Eds.), *Social identity: International perspectives* (pp. 1–12). London: Sage.

Diab, K., & Mi'ari, M. (2007). Collective identity and readiness for social relations with Jews among Palestinian Arab students at the David Yellin Teacher Training College in Israel. *Intercultural Education, 18*(5), 427–444.

Dovidio, J. F., Penner, L. A., Albrecht, T. L., Norton, W. E., Gaertner, S. L., & Shelton, J. N. (2008). Disparities and distrust: The implications of psychological processes for understanding racial disparities in health and health care. *Social Science & Medicine, 67*(3), 478–486.

Elroy, I., Rosen, B., Elmakias, I., & Samuel, H. (2017). *Mental health services in Israel: Needs, patterns of utilization and barriers. Survey of the general adult population.* Jerusalem: Myers-JDC-Brookdale Institute. Retrieved from https://brookdale.jdc.org.il/wp-content/uploads/2017/09/English_summary_749-17.pdf.

Ferdinand, A. S., Paradies, Y., & Kelaher, M. (2015). Mental health impacts of racial discrimination in Australian culturally and linguistically diverse communities: A cross-sectional survey. *BMC Public Health, 15*, 1–14.

Fuligni, A. J., Witkow, M., & Garcia, C. (2005). Ethnic identity and the academic adjustment of adolescents from Mexican, Chinese, and European backgrounds. *Developmental Psychology, 41*(5), 799–811.

Gal, J., Madhala, S., & Bleikh, H. (2017). Social service budgeting in Israeli local authorities. State of the nation report 2017. Jerusalem: Taub Center for Social Policy Studies in Israel. Retrieved from http://taubcenter.org.il/state-of-the-nation-report-2017-pr/.

Galliher, R. V., Jones, M. D., & Dahl, A. (2011). Concurrent and longitudinal effects of ethnic identity and experiences of discrimination on psychosocial adjustment of Navajo adolescents. *Developmental Psychology, 47*(2), 509–526.

Ghanem, A. (2005). On the situation of Palestinian-Arab minority in Israel, 2003 [in Hebrew]. *State and Society, 4*(1), 933–952.

Ghanem, A., & Ozacky-Lazer, S. (2003). The status of the Palestinians in Israel in an era of peace: Part of the problem but not part of the solution. In A. Bligh (Ed.), *The Israeli Palestinians: An Arab minority in the Jewish state* (pp. 258–283). London: Frank Cass.

Gray-Little, B., & Hafdahl, A. R. (2000). Factors influencing racial comparisons of self-esteem: A quantitative review. *Psychological Bulletin, 126*(1), 26–54.

Greene, M. L., Way, N., & Pahl, K. (2006). Trajectories of perceived adult and peer discrimination among black, Latino, and Asian American adolescents: Patterns and psychological correlates. *Developmental Psychology, 42*(2), 218–236.

Greig, R. (2003). Ethnic identity development: Implications for mental health in African-American and Hispanic adolescents. *Issues in Mental Health Nursing, 24*(3), 317–331.

Grindal, M. (2014). *A theoretical development of the relationship between ethnic identity and psychological health* (Unpublished doctoral dissertation). University of California, Riverside.

Hawkins, J. D., Catalano, R. F., & Miller, J. Y. (1992). Risk and protective factors for alcohol and other drug problems in adolescence and early adulthood: Implications for substance abuse prevention. *Psychological Bulletin, 112*(1), 64–105.

Hermann, T., Atmor, N., Heller, E., & Lebel, Y. (2012). *The Israeli democracy index 2012* [in Hebrew]. Jerusalem: Israel Democracy Institute. Retrieved from http://www .herzliyaconference.org/_Uploads/2129Patriotism_Hebrew.pdf.

Hughes, M., Kiecolt, K. J., & Keith, V. M. (2014). How racial identity moderates the impact of financial stress on mental health among African Americans. *Society and Mental Health,* 4(1), 38–54.

Israel Central Bureau of Statistics. (2016). *Statistical abstract of Israel* [in Hebrew]. Table3.1 Marriages, divorces, live births, deaths, natural increase, infant deaths and stillbirths, by region. Retrieved from https://www.cbs.gov.il/he/publications/DocLib/2018/3 .%20ShnatonVitalStatistics/st03_01.pdf.

Iwamoto, D. K., & Liu, W. M. (2010). The impact of racial identity, ethnic identity, Asian values, and race-related stress on Asian Americans and Asian international college students' psychological well-being. *Journal of Counseling Psychology, 57*(1), 79–91.

Levav, I., Ifrah, A., Geraisy, N., Grinshpoon, A., & Khwaled, R. (2007). Common mental disorders among Arab-Israelis: Findings from the Israel national health survey. *Israel Journal of Psychiatry and Related Sciences, 44*(2), 104–113.

Mada al-Carmel: Arab Center for Applied Social Research [Mada al-Carmel]. (2012). *Public opinion survey on civil service among Arab youth, age group 16–22 years* [in Arabic]. Retrieved from http://mada-research.org/wp-content/uploads/2013/02/Mada-al-Carmel -Civil-Service-Presentation.pdf.

Mada al-Carmel: Arab Center for Applied Social Research [Mada al-Carmel]. (2015). *Percentages of voting in Arab villages and towns in elections 2015* [in Arabic]. Retrieved from http://mada-research.org/blog/2015/03/.

Malone, Linda A. (1985). *The Kahan Report, Ariel Sharon and the Sabra-Shatilla massacres in Lebanon: Responsibility under international law for massacres of civilian populations.* Retrieved from https://core.ac.uk/download/pdf/73972805.pdf.

Mandara, J., Gaylord-Harden, N. K., Richards, M. H., & Ragsdale, B. L. (2009). The effects of changes in racial identity and self-esteem on changes in African American adolescents' mental health. *Child Development, 80*(6), 1660–1675.

McDonald, K. E., Keys, C. B., & Balcazar, F. E. (2007). Disability, race/ethnicity and gender: Themes of cultural oppression, acts of individual resistance. *American Journal of Community Psychology, 39*(1–2), 145–161.

Mi'ari, M. (1990). Religious identity and its relationship with other identities among Palestinians in Israel [in Arabic]. *al-Mustaqbal al-'Arabi, 137,* 65–74.

Mi'ari, M. (1992). Identity of Palestinians in Israel: Is it Israeli Palestinian? [in Arabic]. *Journal of Palestine Studies, 10,* 40–60.

Mi'ari, M. (1998). Self-identity and readiness for interethnic contact among young Palestinians in the West Bank. *Canadian Journal of Sociology, 23*(2), 47–70.

Mi'ari, M. (2008). Identity of Palestinians in the two sides of the green line [in Arabic]. *Journal of Palestine Studies, 74,* 41–61.

Mi'ari, M. (2011). Collective identity of Palestinians in Israel after Oslo. *International Journal of Humanities and Social Science, 1*(8), 223–231.

Mi'ari, M., & Diab, K. (2005). Social identity and readiness for social relations with Jews among Arab students in a teacher training college [in Hebrew]. In R. Boreshtien (Ed.), *Etai Zamran book* (pp. 533–564). Jerusalem: David Yellin College of Education.

Miller, D. R. (1963). The study of social relationships: Situation, identity and social interaction. In S. Koch (Ed.), *Psychology: A study of science* (pp. 639–737). New York: McGraw-Hill.

Miller, D. R. (1983). Self, symptom, and social control. In T. R. Sarbin & K. E. Scheibe (Eds.), *Studies in social identity* (pp. 319–338). New York: McGraw-Hill.

Mossakowski, K. N. (2003). Race, ethnicity, and mental health. *Journal of Health and Social Behavior, 44*(3), 318–331.

National Insurance Institute of Israel [NII]. (2016). *Poverty dimensions and social gaps annual report* [in Hebrew]. Retrieved from https://www.btl.gov.il/Publications/oni_report/Documents/oni2016-new.pdf.

Outten, H. R., Schmitt, M. T., Garcia, D. M., & Branscombe, N. R. (2009). Coping options: Missing links between minority group identification and psychological well-being. *Applied Psychology, 58*(1), 146–170.

Peres, Y., & Yuval-Davis, N. (1969). Some observations on the national identity of the Israeli Arab. *Human Relations, 22*(3), 219–233.

Phinney, J. S. (1990). Ethnic identity in adolescents and adults: Review of research. *Psychological Bulletin, 108*(3), 499–514.

Phinney, J. S. (1991). Ethnic identity and self-esteem: A review and integration. *Hispanic Journal of Behavioral Sciences, 13*(2), 193–208.

Phinney, J. S., & Ong, A. D. (2007). Conceptualization and measurement of ethnic identity: Current status and future directions. *Journal of Counseling Psychology, 54*(3), 271–281.

Ponterotto, J. G., & Park-Taylor, J. (2007). Racial and ethnic identity theory, measurement, and research in counseling psychology: Present status and future directions. *Journal of Counseling Psychology, 54*(3), 282–294.

Reiter, Y. (2009). *Israel and its Arab minority.* Jewish Virtual Library. Retrieved from http://www.jewishvirtuallibrary.org/jsource/isdf/text/reiter.html.

Rekhess, E. (2002). The Arabs of Israel after Oslo: Localization of the national struggle. *Israel Studies, 7*(3), 1–44.

Roberts, R. E., Phinney, J. S., Masse, L. C., Chen, Y. R., Roberts, C. R., & Romero, A. (1999). The structure of ethnic identity of young adolescents from diverse ethnocultural groups. *The Journal of Early Adolescence, 19*(3), 301–322.

Rosen, B., Waitzberg, R., Merkur, S. (2015). Israel: Health system review. *Health Systems in Transition, 17*(6), 1–212.

Rouhana, N. (1984). *The Arabs in Israel: Psychological, political and social dimensions of collective identity* (Unpublished doctoral dissertation). Wayne State University, Detroit, MI.

Rouhana, N. (2002). Outsiders' identity: Are the realities of "inside Palestinians" reconcilable? *Palestine-Israel Journal of Politics, Economics, and Culture, 8*(4), 61–70.

Rouhana, N., & Ghanem, A. (1998). Palestinian citizens in the state of Israel: The crisis of a national minority in an ethnic state [in Arabic]. *Journal of Palestine Studies, 25,* 49–75.

Rowley, S. J., Sellers, R. M., Chavous, T. M., & Smith, M. A. (1998). The relationship between racial identity and self-esteem in African American college and high school students. *Journal of Personality and Social Psychology, 74*(3), 715–724.

Sellers, R. M., Caldwell, C. H., Schmeelk-Cone, K. H., & Zimmerman, M. A. (2003). Racial identity, racial discrimination, perceived stress, and psychological distress among African American young adults. *Journal of Health and Social Behavior, 44*(3), 302–317.

Shala'ata, W. (2014). *Identification of personal and social factors which explain the relationship between reported discrimination and health among different groups in Israel* [in Hebrew] (Unpublished doctoral dissertation). Haifa University, Israel.

Shihade, M. (2013). *Readings in the results of the 19th Knesset elections held in 2013 in Israel* [in Arabic]. Haifa: Mada al-Carmel: Arab Center for Applied Social Research. Retrieved from http://mada-research.org/wp-content/uploads/2013/06/Elections.pdf

Smith, A. D. (1991). *National identity.* Harmondsworth, UK: Penguin.

Smith, T. B., & Silva, L. (2011). Ethnic identity and personal well-being of people of color: A meta-analysis. *Journal of Counseling Psychology, 58*(1), 42–60.

Smooha, S. (1984). *The orientation and politicization of the Arab minority in Israel.* Haifa: Institute of Middle East Studies, Haifa University.

Smooha, S. (1998). Israelization of collective identity and of political orientation of Palestinian citizens of Israel—Reexamination [in Hebrew]. In E. Rekhes (Ed.), *Arabs in Israeli politics: Dilemmas of identity* (pp. 41–53). Tel Aviv: Dayan Center, Tel Aviv University.

Smooha, S. (2005). *Index of Arab-Jewish relations in Israel 2004.* Haifa: Jewish-Arab Center, University of Haifa.

Stein, G. L., Kiang, L., Supple, A. J., & Gonzalez, L. M. (2014). Ethnic identity as a protective factor in the lives of Asian American adolescents. *Asian American Journal of Psychology, 5*(3), 206–213.

Stephan, W. G., & Stephan, C. W. (1996). *Intergroup relations.* Boulder, CO: Brown & Benchmark.

Sultany, N. (2003). *Citizens without citizenship: Mada's first annual political monitoring report.* Haifa: Mada al-Carmel: Arab Center for Applied Social Research.

Tajfel, H., & Turner, J. C. (1986). Social identity theory of intergroup behavior. In W. Austin & S. Worchel (Eds.), *Psychology of intergroup relations* (2nd ed., pp. 33–47). Chicago: Nelson-Hall.

Telhami, S. (2010). *Israeli Arab/Palestinian public opinion survey.* Washington, DC: Brookings Institution. Retrieved from https://www.brookings.edu/wp-content/uploads/2016/06/israeli_arab_powerpoint.pdf.

Tessler, M. A. (1977). Israel's Arabs and the Palestinian problem. *Middle East Journal, 31*(3), 313–329.

Wokfsfeld, G., Avraham, E., & Aburaiya, I. (2000). When prophesy always fails: Israeli press coverage of the Arab minority's Land Day protests. *Political Communication, 17,* 115–131.

Worrell, F. C. (2007). Ethnic identity, academic achievement, and global self-concept in four groups of academically talented adolescents. *Gifted Child Quarterly, 51*(1), 23–38.

Yip, T., Gee, G. C., & Takeuchi, D. T. (2008). Racial discrimination and psychological distress: The impact of ethnic identity and age among immigrant and United States-born Asian adults. *Developmental Psychology, 44*(3), 787–800.

Yoo, H. C., & Lee, R. M. (2008). Does ethnic identity buffer or exacerbate the effects of frequent racial discrimination on situational well-being of Asian Americans? *Journal of Counseling Psychology, 55*(1), 63–74.

Zimmerman, M. A., & Arunkumar, R. (1994). Resiliency research: Implications for schools and policy. *Social Policy Report, 8*(4), 1–18.

5

PALESTINIAN CITIZENS IN ISRAEL

A Sociological Portrait

Nohad 'Ali

Palestinian Citizens in Israel: Changes and Reversals

Palestinian society emphasizes harmony and the relationship between the person and the environment (Haj-Yahia, 1995). It places special value on interpersonal loyalty and mutual respect as the basis for human relations and on treating family elders with respect and esteem. Consequently, the importance of family and its interpersonal relationships outweighs the importance of the surrounding society. This perspective is expressed in, among other things, economic support and child care (Barakat, 1993).

Palestinian society in Israel has undergone many changes in all areas of life—for example, society, economy, education, women's status, family structure, and sociocultural changes (Haj-Yahia, 1995). The Palestinian family experienced its most significant change—the inversion of status—beginning in 1948. At that time, the Palestinian population, which until then had constituted a majority, suddenly became an ethno-national minority that was beaten, weakened, devoid of national and religious leadership, and suspected of hostility to the state of which it had just become a part ('Ali, 2007). This minority had fought against the establishment of Israel, the antagonistic entity that took Palestinian land and became a state in lieu of its own. Now it was forced to fight for its citizenship or, more accurately, the right to exist within the borders of this new state ('Ali, 2014).

As a result of the establishment of the state of Israel, the Palestinian political, cultural, social, and economic elite, as well as the educated and the middle class, fled or were expelled from their homeland. Most of those who stayed were rural, uneducated members of the lower class (Al-Haj, 1997, 2004; 'Ali, 1998, 2004). In addition, those who remained became a remote, weakened, and excluded minority. Today, the Palestinian minority in Israel comprises approximately 1,468,000 persons (not including East Jerusalem and the Golan Heights, which were occupied in 1967) (Israel Central Bureau of Statistics [Israel CBS], 2016).

The changes that the Palestinian minority underwent were, in part, unnatural and forced. Thus, for example, the modernization it experienced was coerced, and the transition from a traditional to a modern society was not coordinated with its leadership (Ghanem, 1996). A modern society is characterized in the literature as having transitioned into an urban society that is primarily based on different kinds of industry and services and includes cultural and consumer centers (Khattab & Miaari, 2013). It is also characterized by changes in patterns of political organization from the traditional, in which positions are generally filled on the basis of belonging to a particular *hamula* or ethnic background, to democratic patterns, characterized by elections that are open to all, and by a government that is based on elected officials (Mustafa, 2011). However, geographically, economically, and politically, the Palestinian society in Israel still lives on the margins of the Israeli-Jewish core (Mustafa, 2011).

Palestinian citizens of Israel have fought—and are still fighting—for rights equal to those of Jewish citizens—for example, the fair allocation of resources and allotment of land (the government's land-use policy is exclusively for the benefit of the Jewish majority) and the establishment of businesses and development of industrial zones in areas populated by Palestinians (in which the government virtually does not invest). Often, the government does not take the Palestinian minority and its needs into account. Thus, state budgets, particularly the education budget, is biased, and discrimination between Arab and Jewish schools is prominent. In addition, budget allocations to local authorities are unequal. Discrimination is deeply felt in every sphere, particularly, as already stated, in the establishment and investment in businesses in Palestinian villages in Israel. This dissonance has led to a situation in which a considerable part of the Palestinian minority in Israel lives on the verge of poverty, as unemployment is relatively high and the educational level is relatively low. The relationship between the Palestinian minority and the various governments of Israel has been punctuated by tension (Hasson, 2006). Accordingly, the Palestinian minority in Israel has developed many characteristics, some of which are sociodemographic, that have implications for its future, its integration patterns, and its relationship with the Jewish majority and with the state. Above all, these characteristics have an impact on the formation of a Palestinian community in Israel.

This chapter discusses some of those sociodemographic changes and assesses their influence on a number of levels, the most important of which are attempts by Palestinian citizens in Israel to establish an independent community in response to underdevelopment, exclusion, and discrimination on the part of the state. More specifically, I argue that the most meaningful response on the collective level is the attempt to build a distinctly separate community, independent of the majority group, that will manage the lives of its members. Its leaders call this community *al-mujtama al-asami*, a self-made community ('Ali, 2007).

Evolution of the Minority Status

The war of 1948—the War of Independence for the Jews and the Nakba for the Palestinians—caused the Palestinian community to undergo a complete transformation, including its status, shaped by the tragic circumstances of war, destruction, evacuation, and coercion. A Palestinian state, proposed by the United Nations in November 1947, was not established. From the Palestinians' perspective, their homeland was divided between Israel, Jordan, and Egypt, and their people were scattered throughout the Middle East. Many became refugees. The war had, has noted elsewhere in this book, caused death and loss of property; families were separated; the economy was harmed; and land was expropriated. In addition, the leadership and a large part of society, particularly the financially and politically robust, remained outside the borders of the state. Importantly, connections with the leadership were severed ('Ali, 2013; Ozacky-Lazar, 2001; Smooha, 1999, 2013).

As mentioned earlier, once the state of Israel became a reality, the features of Palestinian society changed drastically. From a majority in their homeland, they were reduced to a minority living in a country that was no longer theirs; once subjects of the British Mandate (1917–1948), they became residents of the Jewish state (Ozacky-Lazar, 1996), receiving citizenship in a country whose establishment they had actively opposed ('Ali, 2014).

The Basic Laws of Israel do not define the Palestinian minority that remained within the borders of Israel as a national minority. Israel's definition as the Jewish state or the nation-state of the Jewish people (Smooha, 2001) has turned inequality into a practical, political, and ideological reality from the perspective of Palestinian citizens of Israel. Often, the majority group perceives these citizens as a fifth column, a view that is supported by their Palestinian identity and their national, religious, ethnic, and cultural ties to their Palestinian brethren in the Occupied Territories and neighboring Arab countries (Adalah: The Legal Center for Arab Minority Rights in Israel [Adalah], 2011).

Generally speaking, Palestinian citizens in Israel comprise a separate ethnic, religious, linguistic, cultural, and national minority that does not want to assimilate into the majority group, nor does the majority group seek its assimilation (Smooha, 1989). It is both religiously and ethnically heterogeneous. Over 83% are Muslims, 8.7% are Christians, and 8.3% are Druze (a distinct population group). These people are geographically dispersed across four areas: most of Israel's Palestinian citizens live in the Galilee (approximately 55.5% of the Galilee population are Muslims, Christians, and Druze); 23.5%, most of them Muslims, inhabit the Triangle, the Palestinian towns adjacent to the Green Line; and 13%, also Muslims, live in the Negev. About half of the Bedouin population (Muslim residents of the Negev) live in villages, the municipal status of which is not recognized by the state. Consequently, the Bedouins receive no municipal, educational, or welfare support, nor any other services within their villages; these localities lack running water, electricity, communication, and road infrastructures. Finally, around 8% of Palestinian citizens in

Israel reside in mixed cities such as Haifa or Ramla, where most live on the margins of the Jewish city and in slums (Manna, 2008).

The sense of hostility and fear of disloyalty led Israel's first government to declare martial law against its Palestinian citizens from 1948 until 1966. This regime greatly limited the Palestinians' freedom of movement and their property rights. Some have described the military rule as a large "jail" for Palestinians—a ghetto and an economic and psychological siege (Ozacky-Lazar, 2001, p. 13). The regime took numerous actions without parliamentary approval, and rigorous measures were applied against Palestinian residents without having been brought to public knowledge (Ozacky-Lazar, 2001).

In 1963 the regulations were loosened, particularly those pertaining to freedom of movement, following demands to abolish military rule. Those demands were expressed in four bills brought before the Knesset. In 1966 then prime minister Levi Eshkol abolished the special military administration (however, the Defense [Emergency] Regulations, which were applied countrywide to all citizens, remained in force). Martial law did not restrict Palestinians' right to vote and to be elected to the Knesset, and Arabic was recognized as an official language along with Hebrew. Conversely, the state expropriated hundreds of thousands of dunams (1 dunam = about 900 square meters) of land from its Palestinian citizens and even took over supervision of *Al Waqf* (Islamic charitable endowments) land, which had served to finance Muslim religious activities. As a result, another 40% of the land held by Palestinian residents of Israel was transferred to the state (Ozacky-Lazar, 2001).

Formal Policy toward the Palestinian Minority in Israel

Lockard (as cited in Smooha, 1980) held that the term "policy" is not limited to decision making or to the definition of regulations by public bodies. It also encompasses operating norms and practices that have the force of official policy, even when no such policy has been formally decided on. This broad definition of policy recognizes at least three components when it pertains to minorities: there is a "manifest" component that includes declared policies, laws, regulations, and other official resolutions (e.g., apartheid legislation in South Africa or laws and regulations passed by the military administration in Israel); a "latent" component that refers to informal discrimination or double standards in implementing a policy of equality (such as making military service a condition for employment in the private and public sectors, when the job type is unrelated to security); and policy "by default"—that is, the unwillingness to alter a policy that is seemingly irrelevant to the minority but in practice is discriminatory (such as neglecting the problem of unemployment, although it mainly affects the minority) (Lockard, as cited in Smooha, 1980, p. 72). A comprehensive analysis of the policy toward minorities therefore requires an analysis of official and unofficial actions, as well as inaction (Smooha, 1980, 2013).

Accordingly, to gain an in-depth understanding of the Palestinians' collective behavior, the question of whether the governments of Israel have had a formal, clear policy, or if they have acted as dictated by resolutions adopted to deal with specific situations, needs to be addressed. Indeed, this issue is unclear in the literature, but it is an important consideration to understand the overall relationship between the Palestinians and the state, as well as the trials and tribulations of this minority.

After the establishment of the state, the military administration enforced regulations that subsequently remained part of Israeli policy toward the Palestinian community. The early imposition of military rule is considered by some as the expression of the manifest component of overt policy toward the minority. This assertion has met with criticism by some researchers. According to Ozacky-Lazar (2008) and Sandler (1995), it reflects the basic assumption that the government and other state institutions never had a definitive, formally declared policy with respect to Palestinian citizens of Israel. The military administration was also the result of natural developments after the 1948 war. Sandler has gone even further and attacked arguments of the existence of a crystallized policy of dominance and control (Lustick, 1980; Rekhess, 1998; Smooha, 1980). Bauml (2002) has noted that a clear, formal policy of exclusion and discrimination was in place via separate administrative treatment, control of the labor market, and noninclusion in development plans. In this context, Ozacky-Lazar (2008) has mentioned that even if there was no official declared policy, from a historical perspective, the aforementioned issues are significant.

The lifting of military rule gave rise to expectations among the Palestinian population that barriers would be removed and that the government would take action to narrow the differences between the two populations. However, little happened to justify those hopes (Abraham Foundation Initiatives, 2013).

After military rule was lifted and following the Six-Day War in 1967, government policy and relations between the state and its Palestinian citizens were affected by additional factors: the ongoing Israeli-Palestinian conflict; the Land Day demonstrations on March 30, 1976, when Palestinian citizens of Israel protested against the planned expropriation of land and six persons were killed by Israeli police; the first intifada, which broke out in December 1987; the international Madrid Peace Conference on October 30, 1991, that attempted to revive the Israeli-Palestinian peace process; and importantly, the visit to Al-Aqsa Mosque in Jerusalem by a Likud (right-wing) Knesset delegation led by then leader of the Israeli opposition Ariel Sharon (on September 28, 2000), leading to the outbreak of the second intifada, also known as the Al-Aqsa intifada. Palestinians saw this visit as a provocation, because the head of the opposition was perceived as provoking the Palestinians by entering their holiest place, against their will, to show that Israel is the sovereign in the Al-Aqsa mosque. During the demonstrations that October against the visit, 13 Palestinian citizens of Israel were killed by the Israeli police force ('Ali, 2014; Smooha, 2013).

Regional processes have also influenced relations between the state and Palestinian citizens in Israel. These include the First Gulf War, which broke out in late 1990, and the collapse of the former Soviet Union, a power that had supported the Palestinian position in the conflict.

In short, the 1970s and 1980s saw neither substantial change in the status of Palestinian citizens in Israel nor in attitudes toward them. The events of Land Day succeeded in generating a fundamental shift in the government's stance toward the Palestinians. Earlier that year, a document authored by the Northern District commissioner of the Israel Ministry of the Interior, which was presented to policy-making circles but never implemented, recommended that the rights of Palestinian citizens in Israel be curtailed, that their political and social movements be monitored, that Palestinian economic dependence on Jews be intensified, and that the emigration of Palestinians from Israel be encouraged ('Ali, 2006).

The promises of the governments to maintain complete equality between Palestinian and Jewish citizens went unrealized as a result of objective and subjective factors. Rapid population growth created new physical needs among the Palestinian public, but they were not appropriately addressed. The prime minister's senior consultant on Arab minority affairs recommended policies that referred to most of the important needs and rights of the Palestinian population but, however positive those policies were, they were not implemented. The senior consultant had no power to enforce or execute such recommendations, and government policy was characterized as "stopgap solutions" (Stendel, 1992, p. 30).

A turning point in the government's attitude to the Palestinian population occurred under the Rabin-Peres government (1992–1996). The change followed the government's more liberal attitudes as well as its political constraints. Yitzhak Rabin, elected prime minister in 1992, had trouble forming a coalition. To ensure a majority in the Knesset, he relied on the silent support of a blocking majority of Palestinian Knesset members. This alliance was fruitful in the eyes of the Arabs following an arrangement between the Labor Party, which formed the government, and the Hadash (Democratic Front for Peace and Equality) and the Madaa' (Arab Democratic List).

Benjamin Netanyahu's first government (1996–1999) did not prioritize issues relevant to the Palestinian population in Israel. On the contrary, there was a clear regression in terms of its willingness to address the subject. Palestinians received a single expression of interest—semantically—when the government reverted to making use of the anachronistic term "minorities" while displaying a patronizing attitude to the minorities that had joined their fate with that of the Jewish people, as formulated in the guidelines of the government. Most of the budget amendments introduced by the Rabin-Peres government were revoked, with the exception of continued affirmative budgetary action for education and for local authorities (municipalities or the like).

In 1999 Ehud Barak was elected prime minister, receiving genuine support (96%) from the Palestinian population (Abraham Foundation Initiatives, 2013).

The expectations for a change from the new government increased, yet its guidelines were similar to those of its predecessors. The report by the Or Commission, which, three years later examined the reasons for the October 2000 events, asserted:

> The government establishment in Israel has yet to prove itself in terms of the fitting attitude to the minority . . . the Arab citizens of the state live in a reality in which they are discriminated against, as Arabs. The lack of equality has been documented in a great number of professional surveys and studies, has been ratified in judgments and government resolutions, and has also received expression in the State Comptroller's Reports and other official documents. Although the level of awareness of this discrimination among the Jewish majority is often too low, it is central to the feelings and attitudes of the Arab citizens. In the opinion of many, both in and outside the Arab sector, including official parties, it forms a key factor of incitement. The same also applies to other levels, on which not enough has been done to address the unique difficulties and distress experienced by the Arab sector. (as cited in Bauml, 2007, p. 173)

Compared to the Netanyahu government that preceded it, Barak's government—despite its short term in office—tried to generate change by focusing on a single key issue: the investment of funds in developing the infrastructures and the educational system of the villages and towns populated by Israeli Palestinians. Yet, like its predecessor, it maintained a rigid enforcement policy with regard to unlicensed construction and refrained from devoting a government meeting to the issues of the Palestinian citizens.

The policies of governments in the decade after the events of October 2000, from 2001 to 2012 (the governments of Sharon, Ehud Olmert, and Netanyahu) reflected a certain backslide in the government's attitude to the Palestinian population (Abraham Foundation Initiatives, 2013). Since 2013, the government coalition has initiated numerous bills that are damaging to Israeli democracy and detrimental to the national and civil status of Israel's Palestinian citizens (e.g., the Nation-State Bill, the Nakba Law, the MK Suspension Bill) (Association for Civil Rights in Israel, 2016).

Despite the definition of the present Netanyahu government as the most right-wing in Israeli history, this same government initiated a five-year plan aimed at narrowing socioeconomic gaps between Jewish and Palestinian citizens in Israel, involving an allocation of approximately 15 billion shekels. This initiative has been developed to close structural gaps and erase the long years of institutional discrimination against Palestinian citizens. These steps were announced only in the wake of international pressure and the economic and social challenges Israel has been tackling following its 2010 accession to the Organization for Economic Cooperation and Development (OECD), and not as a result of a process of enlightenment by Israel and its leaders or by the Jewish majority. Meanwhile, the government has imposed obstacles for implementing this plan. These obstacles are mainly a result of the coalition structure, and because of internal disputes between the more radical faction and the less radical faction of the Likud party; nonetheless, the government recently began implementing it.

Sociodemographic Changes among Palestinian Citizens in Israel

Palestinians who remained on their land and in their cities after 1948 were neither a homogeneous nor united community. They comprised different religious groups and led different lifestyles—urban, rural, and semi-nomadic Bedouin. They included people who were religious, traditional, and secular; there were familial and political rifts. Most were farmers, and the Palestinian economy was not based on principles of capitalism and industry. The political and economic Palestinian leadership, as well as the middle classes, had been made to flee, been deported, or had opted to leave the country. The remaining population was therefore forced to become integrated within the Israeli economy from an inferior starting point. In addition to the underdevelopment and conservatism that characterized it, the minority that had been created overnight also suffered politically (Abraham Foundation Initiatives, 2013).

The Palestinian minority took a generation to rebuild itself. The process was influenced by the will of the state and the authorities. The character of Palestinian society was reshaped according to a desired policy founded on weakening the Palestinian national component and strengthening the Israeli component in its personal and collective identity ('Ali, 2014).

Importantly, the Palestinian citizens of Israel were severed from any Arab cultural, social, and political rear guard and had no reasonable chance of receiving any aid from Arab countries, a reality that strengthened the desired submissive identity that accepted the inversion of personal and collective status ('Ali, 2007). This was a doubly orphaned society: these people were maternally orphaned by the country of which they were citizens, discriminated against in all areas of life as they were not really wanted to begin with, and paternally orphaned by the Arab nation to which they belonged but that was unable to help, support, or protect in times of crisis ('Ali, 2014). This situation has led Palestinians in Israel to be more self-reliant in looking for their own solutions to collective hardships and identity problems. This shift began with the establishment of national representative institutions such as the High Follow-Up Committee for Arab Citizens of Israel in the early 1990s and culminated in attempts to establish an independent community.

A number of researchers have described and conceptualized the changes and sociopolitical behaviors experienced by Palestinian citizens in Israel. Peres and Davis (1968) pointed to compartmentalization in the identities and the lives of Palestinian citizens in Israel—the disconnect between national identification with the Arab world and practical adjustment to life in the state of Israel. These authors held that this compartmentalization made it easier for Palestinians to live in the country, albeit with a divided soul. Compartmentalization was possible in the 1960s because the Arab world did not demand that Palestinians in Israel identify on the practical or active level but rather ideologically, whereas Israel made practical demands of its Palestinian citizens, such as maintaining law and order, but did not require that they identify with the country ideologically or emotionally. At that time, compartmentalization was enabled because of the strong position held by the traditional *hamula* leadership, which on the one hand prevented any manifestation of national rebellion against the state that would have created a danger to the Palestinian minority and on the other hand condemned any act or statement that could be construed as denial of Arab nationalism or of belonging to the Arab world (Peres & Davis, 1968). Rouhana and Ghanem (1998) referred to such a social approach as normal development. This perspective holds that the 1948 war caused the trauma of the disintegration of the Palestinians' political and social system, but since then, the Palestinian minority has been on a normal development path in all areas of life. According to this approach, Palestinian citizens in Israel have begun to recognize their national minority status. Abu-Asbeh, Jayusi, and Sabar-Ben Yehoshua (2011) believe that after 1948 the Palestinian minority aspired to continue to live in Israel without demanding self-determination or disengagement from the state. It sought to be integrated and focused its efforts on democratic means that would bring about a change in the military administration's discriminatory policy (Abu-Asbeh et al., 2011). Smooha (2013) argued that the Palestinians accepted the status quo and that this acceptance of a Jewish state was grounded in the assumption that Israel was a democratic country in which Palestinians could live as a minority with equal rights. However, acceptance is not justification, as it is apparent that the Palestinians neither justify nor prefer the country's Jewish character. Clearly, the Palestinians prefer a binational state to a Jewish state. Acceptance attests to realism, to adjustment to the inevitable, to maturity that distinguishes between vision and the constraints of everyday life, and to realistic, practical considerations. However, contrary to the Palestinian population, most of which has accepted Israel as a Jewish state, the local leadership challenges Israel's Jewish character (Smooha, 2013).

The changes and reversals were not limited to the sociopolitical arena. Significant adjustments did not bypass the sociocultural and socioeconomic structures and were expressed in the process of modernization. This fundamentally transformed the face of Palestinian society, creating rapid social and occupational mobility. The educational level rose exponentially, and new social strata were created with the emergence of a middle class and an intelligentsia. The traditional clannish leadership was eroded and ethnic particularism weakened. As a result of the modernization process and Israel's expropriation of land, the Palestinian village became a source of labor but not a source of employment—a bedroom suburb without a job market. The village thus became an intimate refuge (Abraham Foundation Initiatives, 2013).

The villages, large and small, retained their traditional social structure. Despite the changes and economic upheavals that weakened the sense of *hamula* kinship, local elections neutralized these influences and led to the creation of new tools to preserve the family social structure and familial bond with it (Al-Haj, 1997; 'Ali, 2004; Mustafa, 2011). In fact, the modern election methods introduced by the state to the Palestinian villages strengthened the status of the extended family (*hamula*), contrary to the expectations of the advocates of modernization that it would contemporize the traditional social structure. An explanation of these contradictions and contrasts is provided by Ghanem (1996), who used terms and concepts such as partial modernization. The practical outcome of this process was that the traditional forces actually grew stronger (Abu-Asbeh et al., 2011).

Many researchers believe that the Palestinian population in Israel can be characterized as an ethnic minority that is internationally unique. This is expressed in the combination of a number of attributes:

1. It is a relatively large minority, accounting for about one-fifth of the country's total population (Smooha, 2013), whose (Arab) nation is in political conflict with its country (Israel). According to Landau (1993), most of this public is bound together by national, cultural, linguistic—and, to a great extent—religious ties. These bonds encourage identification with its people who live on the other side of Israel's borders.

2. This minority enjoys civil rights at the individual level but not collectively as an ethno-national group. In granting collective rights, the state makes distinctions between religious elements in the national minority ('Ali & Inbar, 2011). Thus, for example, Christians and Druze have a greater degree of autonomy in managing their religious affairs.

3. As pointed out, the Palestinian minority in Israel is heterogeneous. It includes groups that differ from each other in religion, way of life, political affiliations with parties and movements, and the degree of traditionalism and religiosity in the population (Ghanem, 1996; Manna, 2008).

4. The Palestinian minority in Israel did not consider itself as such in the first two decades after the founding of the state, mainly because of the suddenness in which it had become a minority. Today, most members of the population have not yet internalized this awareness. The feeling that they are a majority stems from their belonging to the Palestinian circle (Al-Haj, 1997; Rekhess, 2007). According to Lipschitz (1989), another reason for the lack of minority consciousness is that most members of the Jewish majority have not yet internalized that they are the majority, as for many years the Jews were a minority in their countries of residence. Israel's security situation, which is characterized by threats to its existence by Arab countries in the Middle East, strengthens this feeling (Abu-Asbeh et al., 2011).

As mentioned, Palestinian society has undergone changes in almost every sphere. I discuss a number of these changes next.

Demographic Changes

The most significant change among the Palestinian citizens in Israel is the demographic inversion of their status from majority to minority, a transformation that led to significant social changes. As noted earlier, those who remained within the borders of the new country wanted to be citizens of the country whose establishment they had opposed. It was their only option; otherwise, they would have risked deportation from their homeland. Most seeking citizenship received it: it was granted to them and their descendants. However, those among the uprooted, the deported, and the fugitives were prohibited from receiving citizenship. The Palestinian political leadership and intellectuals believe that Israeli citizenship was forced on the weakened group that continued to live within the borders of the new country (Ghaida, 2006).

Population

According to the Israel CBS (2016), approximately 8.522 million people live in Israel. The Jewish population makes up approximately 6.377 million (74.8% of the total population), the Palestinian population is approximately 1.432 million (less than 20%) (not including East Jerusalem and the Golan Heights, which were occupied in 1967), and those classified as "Other" makes up approximately 374,000 (4.4%) of the population.

About 53% of Palestinian citizens in Israel live in 71 local councils; 30% in 10 cities; 8% in mixed cities (Haifa, Acre, Tel Aviv–Jaffa, Lod, Ramla, Upper Nazareth, and Ma'alot-Tarshiha); 3% in 35 localities belonging to 14 regional councils, three of which include Palestinian-only settlements; and 4.6% in locations that are not recognized as settlements by the Israel Ministry of the Interior (unrecognized villages), most of them Bedouin communities in the Negev.

Religion

While the Palestinian population in Israel is heterogeneous, there is great variance in sociodemographic data between Muslims, Christians, and Druze. As reported by the Israel CBS, the growth rate of all Palestinian ethnic groups is on a consistent downward trend.

In terms of religious affiliation, 83.6% of the Palestinian population is Muslim (1.454 million), an increase from 70% in 1950; 8.4% is Christian (166,000), dropping from 21% in 1950; and 8% is Druze (138,000) (Israel CBS, 2016).

MUSLIMS

The growth rate of this population is on a downward trend, having dropped from 3.8% in 2000 to 2.0% in 2014. The fertility rate (the average number of children per family) of Muslim women is also decreasing: it was 3.4 children per woman in 2014 compared to 4.7 children in 2000. Approximately 37% of households headed by a Muslim comprises six or more persons compared to 9% of Jewish households (Israel Central Bureau of Statistics [CBS], 2016).

The labor force participation rate among Muslims aged 15 and over in 2014 was 44.3% (63.5%, men; 24.9%, women). The participation rate for Muslim women is significantly lower than the corresponding figures for Jewish, Christian, and Druze women (65.5%, 46.3%, and 32.2%, respectively) (Israel CBS, 2016).

In 2014 the rate of those entitled to matriculation certification in the Palestinian educational system reached 58% of twelfth graders compared to 62% in the Jewish educational system (Israel CBS, 2016; Weiss, 2016).

CHRISTIANS

On Christmas Eve 2015, more than 166,000 Christians lived in Israel, accounting for 2% of the population. At the end of 2014, 79.1% of Christians in Israel were Palestinian Christians, and the rest comprised Christians who had immigrated to Israel with their Jewish family members under the Law of Return (including their Israeli-born children). Most arrived as part of the large wave of former Soviet Union immigrants in the 1990s (Israel CBS, 2016).

The median age at first marriage for Christian bridegrooms in 2013 was 29.6, some two years older than Jewish bridegrooms and four years older than their Muslim counterparts. The median age of first-time Christian brides was 24.7, about one year younger than Jewish brides and three-and-a-half years older than Muslim brides. The average number of children up to age 17 in Christian families is 1.9, which is lower than Jewish families (2.3), and Muslim families (2.9) (Israel CBS, 2016).

The labor force participation rate in 2014 among Christians aged 15 and over was 68.0% (72.6%, men; 64.1%, women). In comparison, among Jews aged 15 and over, the participation rate was 67.9% (70.3%, men; 65.5%, women) (Israel CBS, 2016).

Matriculation exam records over the years indicate that Palestinian Christians enjoy high success rates in passing these exams compared to Muslims as well as to all students in the Hebrew educational system. Women accounted for 61.3% of all Palestinian Christian students studying toward a first degree compared to 57.5% of all undergraduate students in Israel.

The age composition of the Christian population differs from that of the Muslim population and is more similar to that of the Jewish population. The percentage of the population group up to age 19 is 28.6%, lower than the Jewish population (34.0%) and even lower compared to the Muslim population (47.5%). The percentage of people aged 65 and over among all Christians is 10.7% (compared to 12.7% of Jews and 3.7% among Muslims). The growth rate of the Christian population more closely resembles that of the Jewish population: 1.6% compared to 1.9% among Jews and 2.4% among Muslims (Israel CBS, 2016; Weiss, 2016).

DRUZE

At the end of 2015, the Druze population in Israel made up approximately 138,000 of the total population and 8.0% of the Palestinian population in the country. When the state was established, approximately 14.5 thousand Druze lived in Israel (1.2% of the total population). Over the years, the Druze population has grown, mainly as a result of natural increase (births less deaths). The total fertility rate in the Druze community has been on a downward trend since the mid-1960s (in 2014 the average birthrate was 2.2 per Druze woman). The peak rate, 7.9 births per woman, was recorded in 1964. In 1990 the rate had dropped to 4.1 births per woman; in 2000, to 3.1; and in 2010, to 2.5. This decrease has affected the size of the Druze household, which in 2015 comprised 4.1 members on average, higher than Jewish and Christian households at 3.1 and lower than Palestinian households at 4.8 (Israel CBS, 2016).

The male labor force participation rate among the Druze reached 68.0% in 2015 (equal to the Christians and 62.0% among Muslims). The Druze female labor force participation rate was 32.4% (compared to 24.6% for Muslim women and 45.2% for their Christian counterparts) (Israel CBS, 2016).

In the 2014/2015 academic year, 4.6 thousand Druze were students at all higher education institutions in Israel, an increase of 9.6% over the prior academic year. From a multiyear perspective, the number of Druze students has increased by 2.7 within a decade and a half (in the 1999/2000 academic year, Druze students amounted to 1.7 thousand) (Israel CBS, 2016).

Age Composition

As a result of the high fertility rate typical of the Palestinian population until some two decades ago, the median age of this population is low (21.7). The median age of the Jewish population is about 10 years older (31.5). Following the drop in the fertility rate in the Palestinian population in recent years, the percentage of children has decreased and the median age has risen (Israel CBS, 2016).

Education

HIGH SCHOOL EDUCATION

Recognition of the importance of education as a tool for competing in the political struggle and for advancing social factors, such as health status, among others, has risen among the Palestinian minority in Israel (Haj Yahia-Abu Ahmad, 2006). Since the mid-1970s, the educational level in Palestinian high schools has changed on both quantitative and qualitative levels: the quantitative difference has been more marked, expressed in a massive increase in the number of students, the number of teens completing high school, as well as the number of those entitled to a matriculation certificate. The qualitative change is expressed in the percentage of twelfth graders studying mandatory core subjects at the four-unit level and above. This advance is important for the students' future mobility because it improves their chances of being accepted into a university or other institution of higher education. Additional progress is evident in the number of Palestinian women in higher education, which has risen significantly in recent decades ('Ali, 2013). At the end of the 1980s, only 9% of the young people aged 15 years and over had studied for 13 years or more; in 2012 their share had risen to 23% ('Ali & Da'as, 2018).

The incidence of school dropouts in the Palestinian population in Israel has become marginal. In the 2011/2012 academic year and in the transition to the following year, 4.7 % of all seventh to twelfth graders had dropped out of school. The dropout rate for boys was 6.7% and for girls, 2.8%. In the Hebrew educational system, for comparison, the corresponding figures were 2.8%, 3.8%, and 1.7%, respectively (Israel CBS, 2016).

HIGHER EDUCATION

Representation of Palestinian citizens in Israel in the higher educational system is of great importance for many reasons, such as the creation of skilled professional human capital and new employment opportunities. Higher education is a key route to social and economic mobility (Dirasat: Arab Center for Law and Policy [Dirasat], 2011) and, in particular, to participation in decision-making bodies. This reflects the attempt to reshape the public space and create an equilibrium of power in the academic world ('Ali, 2013).

In the 2011/2012 academic year, there were approximately 24,000 Palestinian students working toward a first degree in Israel's higher education institutions and 4,600 graduate students and 500 doctoral students. Palestinian students accounted for 12.5% of all Israeli undergraduates (14.4% of university students, 6.7% of students at academic colleges, and 26.2% of students at teacher training colleges). Palestinian students comprised 9.0% of all students working toward a master's degree and 4.5% of doctoral students ('Ali, 2013).

In summary, although the level of education among Palestinian citizens in Israel rose in 2001–2010, it remains considerably lower than the level of education in the Jewish population. The percentage of Palestinian males aged 20–64 with 13 years of schooling or more rose from 20.6% in 2001 to 25.2% in 2010, and the corresponding figure for Palestinian females in this age group rose from 14.5% in 2001 to 26.5% in 2010. The number of women aged 20–64 with at least 13 years of schooling in 2001 was lower than the corresponding figure for men that year, and higher in 2010. In 2010 the percentage of Jewish students with at least 13 years of schooling in the 20- to 64-year-old age group was 53.2% for men and 59.4% for women (Israel CBS, 2016).

The level of education of Palestinian women is similar to that of their male counterparts. In 2010, 10.3% of men had studied for 16 years or more compared to 10.5% of women, 9.8% of men and women held an academic diploma, 33.7% of men had 12 years of schooling compared to 29.6% of women, and 21.7% of men had up to 8 years of schooling compared to 30.3% of women ('Ali, 2013; Israel CBS, 2013; Gharrah, 2013).

Health

According to Israeli law, the state is required to provide equal health services at a high standard to all residents of Israel. However, various barriers, including an inadequate number of clinics in Palestinian towns and villages and limitations on mobility, have led to a situation in which many Palestinian citizens are unable to fully exercise the right to receive the highest standard of health care within a short time frame. Because of this and other reasons (see, for example, chapter 13 on smoking), life expectancy of Palestinian citizens in Israel is approximately four years shorter than that of Jewish citizens. In 2012 the life expectancy of Palestinian males was 76.9 and Palestinian women, 80.7 (Israel CBS, 2013). In the past few decades, the increase in life expectancy among Palestinian women has been greater than among Palestinian men. Palestinian mortality rates are higher than among their Jewish counterparts, particularly after the age of 60. The infant mortality rate among Palestinian citizens, except for Christians, is almost double that among Jewish citizens. Among the Bedouin population in the Negev it is even higher, reaching 15 deaths per 1,000 live births (Adalah, 2011).

Between 1985 and 1989 and between 2008 and 2012, the life expectancy of Palestinian women increased by a total of 4.9 years, greater than among Palestinian men (3.7 years) and lower than among Jewish women (6.0 years). Between 2000 and 2004 and between 2008 and 2012, Palestinian women's life expectancy increased by 2.1 years, higher than the increase among Palestinian men (1.6 years) and Jewish women (1.8 years) (Israel CBS, 2013).

Life expectancy at birth among women is 3.8 years longer than among men. Among Jews, women's life expectancy is 3.4 years longer than men's, and among Palestinians, 4.4 years. In the past decade (2004–2014) life expectancy at birth among men rose by 2.5 years and among women by 2.1 years. The increase in life expectancy among men is greater for Jews than for Palestinians (2.6 and 1.3 years in the same decade, respectively). Among women, the increase in the decade is equal for Jews and Palestinians (2.1 years). These differences in the rate of change in life expectancy are expressed in the growing gap in the life expectancy of Jewish and Palestinian males, which increased from 3 years in 2004 to 4.3 years in 2014, with a stable difference of 3.3 years among females (Israel CBS, 2016).

Employment

Unemployment in the Palestinian population in Israel remains significantly higher than in the Jewish population. The labor force participation rate among female Palestinian citizens is around 20% and is among the lowest in the world (Yashiv & Kasir, 2013). Palestinian citizens of Israel in general, and Palestinian women in particular, remain grossly underrepresented in the civil service, Israel's largest employer (Palestinians account for a mere 6% of civil service employees). This occurs despite legislated affirmative action designed to increase representation of the Palestinian minority and women in civil service (Adalah, 2011). Seemingly, the main problem does not lie in the legislation but rather in its enforcement.

In 2010 the number of unemployed Palestinians rose by 5.9% compared with a decrease of 10.9% among unemployed Jews (Gharrah, 2013). The unemployment rate among Palestinian men dropped from 6.8% in 2009 to 6.7% in 2010, while the corresponding rate among Palestinian women remained stable at 10%. In contrast, unemployment among Jewish males dropped from 7.4% in 2009 to 6.6% in 2010 and among Jewish women, from 7.4% to 6.3%. Dismissals were the main cause of Palestinian unemployment in 2010; 75.5% of unemployed Palestinians who had jobs in the year preceding the survey were let go (Israel CBS, 2013).

In 2013 the general unemployment rate in Israel was 6.2% of the labor force, whereas the unemployment rate among Palestinian citizens in the same year was 9.4%. The unemployment rate in the Palestinian localities in the Negev is alarming, where the figure ranges between 32% and 37% (Gharrah, 2013).

There are differences between Jewish and Palestinian societies in the percentage of one-income families: in 2012, 35% of families in the general population had a single breadwinner compared to 41.7% of Palestinian families, and, accordingly, in the general population 44.4% of families had two incomes or more compared to 35.7% of Palestinian families. Employment of one of the members of the couple is more prevalent in Palestinian society than in society as a whole (Yashiv & Kasir, 2013). The gaps in labor force participation rates paint the same picture: in 2014 the participation rate of Palestinian women (aged 25–62) was 34.8%, which is lower compared to 77.9% for Palestinian men and 82.7% for Jewish women. Moreover, a high percentage of Palestinian women are employed, sometimes unwillingly, on a part-time basis. In 2009 about 44.8% of these women worked part-time compared to 29.6% of all women, and 32% of them were employed part-time against their will because they would prefer full-time jobs (Yashiv & Kasir, 2013). In addition, there are differences between Palestinian and Jewish society in the percentage of working families living in poverty. In 2012, among poor families in the general population (according to income before transfer payments and taxes), around 41.7% of families were single-income families and 10% had two incomes compared to 51.5% of poor families in Palestinian society with a single breadwinner and 10.7% with two incomes or more. Poor families in the Palestinian population include a greater percentage of working families. In this context, it is noted that the average wage in Palestinian society is lower compared to Jewish society, and this may be one of the causes of the high percentage of working families in Palestinian society living below the poverty line (Levi, 2015).

Poverty

Poverty in Israel has not received adequate attention by decision makers, most likely as it exists on the margins of society, far from the center of attention and mostly concentrated in the ultra-Orthodox Jewish and Palestinian populations. Even after the 2011 social protest demonstrations by the Israeli population and the subsequent report by the Trajtenberg Committee (convened to examine Israel's socioeconomic problems), no serious policy for narrowing the economic gap has been implemented. According to the National Insurance Institute's (NII) *Poverty and Social Gaps Report* published in early December 2015, the number of Palestinian families living in poverty rose from 51.7% in 2013 to 52.6% in 2014, and no less severe, the data indicated that 37.4% of the poor in Israel are Palestinians, while Palestinians account for less than 20% of the population. Notably, among Jewish families in Israel there was virtually no change in the poverty rate in 2014, while there was a relatively significant deterioration in the situation of Israel's Palestinian citizens. The argument that the birthrate among Palestinian citizens is higher than the rest of the population can no longer serve as an excuse, as the birthrate among Palestinian citizens in Israel has dropped significantly in the past two decades. A reliable indication of the severity of the situation was presented in the 2015 Israel Democracy Index poll, in which 66.5% of Israel's Palestinian citizens stated that they felt part of a weak or fairly weak group, in contrast to 28% of Jewish citizens (Miaari, 2015).

According to the NII report (2015), the poverty rate among the Palestinian population in Israel was 59.2% before payment of allowances and taxes and decreased only to 53.4% after such payouts, whereas among the Jewish population the poverty rate—after payment of allowances and taxes—was 14.1%. This indicates that poverty among Palestinian citizens is not only more extensive but deeper as well, as taxes and allowances succeed in raising about half of poor Jewish families above the poverty line compared to only 8% of poor Palestinian families. Moreover, Palestinian localities and villages are highly represented in the lowest socioeconomic levels of society, and the unrecognized Palestinian Bedouin villages in the Negev are the poorest localities in the country (Adalah, 2011). The Israeli government has consistently refrained from taking sufficient and effective action to deal with the phenomenon of relative and absolute poverty among the country's Palestinian minority. Even when initiatives for development plans to benefit the Palestinian minority are undertaken, such as the multiyear modernization plan, they are implemented partially, gradually, or not at all (Adalah, 2011; Gharrah, 2013).

Standard of Living

In 2010 the majority of Palestinian households (62.87%) were in the three lowest income deciles according to disposable income, and only 5.67% were in the top three deciles (Dirasat, 2011). The average gross and net income of the Palestinian household in 2010 grew in real terms by 11.7% and 11.3%, respectively, amounting to NIS 9,232 and NIS 8,160 (in 2010 values). However, these averages were still approximately 40% lower than the average incomes of Jewish households, which amounted to NIS 15,312 and NIS 12,708, respectively. In 2009 the average monthly wage of a Palestinian salaried employee was only about 67.0% of a Jewish counterpart's salary, and the average income of a self-employed Palestinian was only 70.0% of that of a self-employed Jewish Israeli.

A comparison of the income of salaried employees in the Jewish and Palestinian populations in 2013 revealed relatively large gaps in both monthly salaries and hourly wages: the average gross monthly salary of employees in the Jewish population was NIS 9,267 compared to NIS 5,930 in the Palestinian population, which constitutes 64.0% of the earnings of their Jewish counterparts. This gap remains identical when comparing the gross hourly wage in the Palestinian and Jewish population groups (NIS 34.8 vs. NIS 54.4 per hour, respectively) (Dirasat, 2011).

A comparison of hourly wages between Palestinians and Jews based on the number of years of education completed reveals more of the same: the income in the Jewish population is higher than the income in the Palestinian population. The wage differences between the two groups grow smaller among people with less than 12 years of schooling and increase among those with more than 13 years of education. The greatest difference (34.3%) was found in the group with 16 years of education or more, and the smallest (6.8%) in the 0–8 years of schooling group (Dirasat, 2011).

The Adva Center's *Social Report 2015* reveals that the salary gaps between Palestinians and Oriental Jews (native-born Israelis whose fathers were born in Asia or Africa) and Occidental Jews (native-born Israelis whose fathers were born in Europe or the Americas) are highly significant. The following figures refer to the years 2012–2014 and are taken from the Household Expenditure Survey performed by the Israel CBS. In 2014 the income of Palestinian salaried workers was the lowest, at 29% below the average. The monthly income of Occidental salaried employees was 38% above the average monthly salary of all salaried employees. The income of their Oriental counterparts was 12% above the average (Swirski, Konor-Atias, & Zelingher, 2015).

Discussion

As a minority, the Palestinian population in Israel suffers from underrepresentation across almost all indexes of achievement in the country—for example, development and welfare—while it is overrepresented in all indexes of poverty. This community is not only marginal in politics but also, in my opinion, in the economy, in society, in communications, in culture, and in virtually all spheres of life as well.

The figures published by the NII, the Israel Association of Social Workers, the Ministry of Welfare and Social Services, the state comptroller, and other organizations and ministries paint a picture that demonstrates an inverse relationship between the problematic situation, which is growing steadily worse, and the response, which is growing steadily deficient.

In the past five years, the number of new cases opened in the welfare departments of Palestinian local authorities has doubled (compared to a 30% national increase). A social worker in a Palestinian locality handles an average of 350 cases compared to 180 in the Jewish community, and the welfare budget of Palestinian local authorities is 8.0% of the ministry's total budget, although Palestinians account for around 20.0% of the Israeli population (Abu-Asbeh et al., 2011).

Data published by *Sikkuy* (Hebrew for "opportunity"), the Association for the Advancement of Civic Equality, a joint organization of Jewish and Palestinian citizens, also point to an ongoing inequality between Palestinian and Jewish citizens of Israel, according to the weighted equality index, as well as the values across the five aggregated indexes on which it is based (education, health, welfare, employment, and housing). All annual reports published by *Sikkuy* from 1999 through 2008 (http://www.sikkuy.org.il/publications/) demonstrate a continuous rising trend in inequality values between Palestinians and Jews in Israel.

A review of the changes and reversals experienced by the Palestinian minority leads to the conclusion that after years of deliberate discrimination, unequal citizenship, and having their political voice silenced, Palestinian citizens of Israel are left with feelings of vulnerability, exclusion, insecurity, lack of trust, and alienation from the state.

Palestinian citizens do not enjoy equal access to the circles of public life and decision making, and their participation in the legislature, government, and civil service is lower than that of Jewish citizens. As a result, their access to decision-making processes and centers of power is limited, and their ability to cope with inequality and discrimination is hampered; Israel's definition as a Jewish state makes inequality and discrimination against Palestinian citizens not only a reality but also a political project. The juxtaposition of "Jewish" and "democratic" in defining the state of Israel anchors discrimination in the law and precludes the realization of full equality (Adalah, 2011).

This chapter examines some of the sociodemographic changes that have taken place in the Palestinian population in Israel and assesses their impact on a number of levels. In parallel, it looks at the inequality between Jews and Palestinians and discusses the policy of discrimination and exclusion toward the Palestinian minority. The chapter also argues that the minority has not accepted this status quo and has tried to change it. The attempts by some Palestinian leaders to establish an independent community organization is one example.

Numerous research projects illustrate the desire of Palestinian citizens in Israel to be integrated into Israeli society as part of an adjustment strategy ('Ali & Inbar, 2011; Smooha, 2013). But there are two sides involved in implementing this strategy—the Palestinian citizens of Israel and Israel's policy toward this minority. The literature shows that despite its cultural, ethnic, and national pluralism, Israel is a country that defines itself ethno-nationally as a Jewish state. Government policy is defined via the nation and does not grant other groups in society the right to take part in social control, thus increasing its dominance (Abu El-Hija, 2005). The Jewish nation has laid claim to the country and is using its claim to prioritize the Jewish national group above others (Smooha, 2013). Jewish nationalism has created barriers in the path of its other minority group citizens. The outcome is that the Jewish majority group has retained its position of power by controlling the various governmental institutions. Not only does this control neutralize and exclude Israel's Palestinian citizens from any practical ability to influence the distribution of social resources, but it also uses legal, political, and budgetary means to limit the ability of different minority groups in Palestinian society to influence the public agenda of the institutional and decision-making establishments, and alternatively, to establish institutions that will represent various goals sought by the minority group (Abu El-Hija, 2005).

Recommendations for Change and Improvement

The Palestinian population in Israel is an extremely weakened population that has borne the brunt of ethno-national discrimination displayed by the governments of Israel since the founding of the state. By contrast, the data I present here indicate a population with encouraging potential for improvement, were conditions to change. Consequently, I suggest a number of actions for decision and policy makers that if taken would advance the integration of Palestinians into the economy and improve their socioeconomic status and standard of living. The change would be a positive one for both the Palestinian minority and the state. The following recommendations address a variety of spheres to which reference is made in this chapter:

- Antidiscrimination legislation and increased enforcement is needed. Developed countries have antidiscrimination laws in place as well as strategies for raising public awareness of discrimination, of antidiscrimination laws, and of the rights of individuals who are the victims of discrimination. On this basis, legislation on the issue of occupational discrimination against Palestinian citizens in Israel could be expanded and enforcement of antidiscrimination laws increased.
- There must be complete equality, while applying affirmative action, in the allocation of resources to close gaps in different areas such as housing, infrastructure, budgets, and labor.
- Palestinians need to be included among Israel's decision and policy makers.
- Educational programs and textbooks should be developed in Arabic to enable the Arab educational system to adapt content in textbooks and curricula to reflect the national-cultural identity, history, and heritage of Palestinian society.
- Subsidy of education, including higher education, needs to be addressed. The educational system is a major key to improving the economic status of Palestinian citizens in Israel. Education is indispensable in terms of the effect on labor market performance in defining participation, occupational status, and productivity.
- Extensive occupational unsuitability currently exists among Palestinian academics, and a policy that encourages greater alignment between the education of employees and their jobs is needed that will help increase employee productivity as well as job satisfaction. Additionally, the number of Palestinian lecturers in Israeli academia must be increased.
- Women's participation in the workforce should be encouraged. As mentioned, the participation of Palestinian women in the labor force and their employment are extremely small-scale. Various means for encouragement, could be implemented.

- To increase employment demand, create infrastructure for production sites in regions adjacent to Arab residential areas where there is a relevant labor supply, apply a more vigorous effort for the inclusion of Palestinian employees in the public sector, apply a negative income tax policy that encourages the employment of Palestinians rather than of foreign workers, and provide professional training and occupational guidance, among others.
- Improve physical workplace accessibility. A major problem experienced by Palestinian citizens in Israel is related to geographical concentration and transportation problems. Infrastructure in many Arab locations is undeveloped, particularly for public transportation.
- Establish health institutions in Arab locations according to the principle of equity, establish mother and child clinics, and budget for mobile clinics in the unrecognized villages in the Negev.

NOHAD 'ALI is Director of the Arabs-Jews-State Unit at Samuel Neaman Institute, Technion, Head of the Center of Multiculturalism Study, and Senior Lecturer in Sociology at Western Galilee Academic College and University of Haifa, Israel. He is author of *Between Ovadia and Abdallah: Jewish and Islamic Fundamentalism in Israel, 2013* (Hebrew); author with Muhamad Al-atawnah of *Islam in Israel: Muslim Communities in Non-Muslim States* (Cambridge: Cambridge University Press, 2018); and author with Rima'a Da'as of *Higher Education among the Arab Minority in Israel: Representation, Mapping, Barriers and Challenges* (2018).

References

Abraham Foundation Initiatives. (2013). *Arab society in Israel, information file* [in Hebrew]. Jerusalem: Abraham Foundation Initiatives.

Abu-Asbeh, K., Jayusi, W., & Sabar-Ben Yehoshua, N. (2011). The identity of teenage Palestinian citizens of Israel, their identification with the state and with Jewish culture, and implications on the educational system [in Hebrew]. *Dapim:Journal for Studies and Research in Education, 52,* 11–45.

Abu El-Hija, Y. (2005). Why has an Arab university not yet been established in Israel? [in Hebrew]. In I. Gur-Zeev (Ed.), *The End of Academia in Israel?* (pp. 303–304). Haifa University of Haifa.

Adalah: The Legal Center for Arab Minority Rights in Israel [Adalah]. (2011). *The inequality report. The Palestinian Arab minority in Israel.* Haifa: Adalah: The Legal Center for Arab Minority Rights in Israel.

Al-Haj, M. (1997). Identity and oriented among Arabs in Israel: Double periphery. *State, Government and Interational Relations, 41/42,* 103–122.

Al-Haj, M. (2004). The status of the Palestinians in Israel: A double periphery in an ethno-national state. In A. Dowty (Ed.), *Critical Issues in Israeli Society* (pp. 109–126). Westport, CT: Praeger.

'Ali, N. (1998). *The Islamic movement in Israel: Ideology, goals and unique characteristics* [in Hebrew]. Haifa: University of Haifa.

'Ali, N. (2004). Political Islam in an ethnic Jewish state: Historical evolution, contemporary challenges and future prospects. *Holy Land Studies, 3*(1), 69–92.

'Ali, N. (2007). The Islamic movement in Israel's concept of "Al-Mujtama Al-Asami" [in Hebrew]. In E. Rekhess (Ed.), *The Arab minority in Israel and 17th Knesset elections*. Tel Aviv: Tel Aviv University, Moshe Dayan Center for Middle Eastern and African Studies and the Konrad Adenauer Program for Jewish-Arab Cooperation.

'Ali, N. (2013). *Between Ovadia and Abdallah: Jewish and Islamic fundamentalism in Israel* [in Hebrew]. Tel Aviv: Resling.

'Ali, N. (2014). *Violence and crime in the Arab society in Israel: The establishment's conspiracy or cultural crime* [in Hebrew]. Haifa: University of Haifa, the Jewish-Arab Center and the Aman Center: The Arab Center for a Safe Society.

'Ali, N., & Inbar, S. (2011). *Who's in favor of equality? Equality between Arabs and Jews in Israel: Summary of an opinion survey* [in Hebrew]. Jerusalem: Sikkuy.

'Ali, N., & Da'as, R. (2018). *Higher education among the Arab minority in Israel: Representation, mapping, barriers and challenges* [in Hebrew]. Tel Aviv, Israel: Resling.

Association for Civil Rights in Israel. (2016). *Anti-democratic legislation in Israel: Status report* [in Hebrew]. Retrieved from http://www.acri.org.il/he/wp-content/uploads/2016/03/anti-democratic-legislation0316.pdf.

Barakat, H. (1993). *The Arab world: Society, culture, and state*. Los Angeles: University of California Press.

Bauml, Y. (2002). *The attitude of the Israeli establishment toward the Arabs in Israel: Policy, principles and activities: The second decade, 1958–1968* [in Hebrew] (Unpublished doctoral dissertation). University of Haifa, Israel.

Bauml, Y. (2007). *A blue and white shadow: The Israeli establishment's policy and actions among its Arab citizens: The formative years 1958–1968* [in Hebrew]. Haifa: Pardes.

Dirasat: Arab Center for Law and Policy [Dirasat]. (2011). *Obstacle course: Challenges and approaches for substantial integration of Arab citizens in the higher education system in Israel*. Nazareth: Dirasat: Arab Center for Law and Policy.

Ghaida, R. Z. (2006). *The national committee for the heads of the Arab local authorities in Israel: The future vision of the Palestinians in Israel* [in Arabic]. Nazareth: National Committee for Heads of Arab Local Authorities in Israel.

Ghanem, A. (1996). *Political participation among Arabs in Israel* [in Hebrew] (Unpublished doctoral dissertation). University of Haifa, Israel.

Gharrah, R. (2013). *Arab society in Israel*. Vol. 6: *Population, society, economy* [in Hebrew]. Jerusalem: Van Leer Jerusalem Institute and Hakibbutz Hameuchad.

Haj-Yahia, M. M. (1995). Toward culturally sensitive intervention with Arab families in Israel. *Contemporary Family Therapy, 17*(4), 429–447.

Haj Yahia-Abu Ahmad, N. (2006). *Couplehood and parenting in the Arab family in Israel: Processes of change and preservation in three generations* [in Hebrew] (Unpublished doctoral dissertation). University of Haifa, Israel.

Hasson, S. (2006). Barriers to development and equality between Arabs and Jews in Israel: A proposal for a framework of thought. In S. Hasson & M. Karayanni (Eds.), *Barriers to equality: The Arabs in Israel*. Jerusalem: Floersheimer Institute for Policy Studies.

Israel Central Bureau of Statistics [Israel CBS]. (2013). *Population*. Retrieved from http://www.cbs.gov.il/reader/cw_usr_view_SHTML?ID=629.

Israel Central Bureau of Statistics [Israel CBS]. (2016). *Table B/1, Population, by population group*. Retrieved from http://www.cbs.gov.il/publications16/yarhon0416/pdf/b1.pdf.

Khattab, N., & Miaari, S. (2013). *Palestinians in the Israeli labor market: A multi-disciplinary approach*. New York: Springer.

Landau, J. (1993). *Arab minority in Israel, political aspects 1967–1991* [in Hebrew]. Am Oved.

Levi, A. (2015). *Description and analysis of the dimensions of poverty and inequality in Israel and developed countries—Marking poverty day in the Knesset* [in Hebrew]. Paper presented at the the Knesset Labor, Welfare and Health Committee, Jerusalem, Israel.

Lipschitz, M. (1989). *The Arab-Israeli conflict 1882–1989* [in Hebrew]. Ramat Gan, Israel: Or-Am.

Lustick, I. (1980). *Arabs in the Jewish state: Israel's control of a national minority*. Austin: University of Texas Press.

Manna, A. (Ed.). (2008). *Arab society in Israel 2: Population, society, economy* [in Hebrew]. Jerusalem: Van Leer Jerusalem Institute and Hakibbutz Hameuchad.

Miaari, S. (2015). *Arab poverty report* [in Hebrew]. Jerusalem: Israel Democracy Institute. Retrieved from https://www.idi.org.il/articles/2784.

Mustafa, M. (2011). Political participation of the Islamic movement in Israel [in Hebrew]. In E. Rekhess & A. Rudnitzky (Eds.), *Muslim minorities in non-Muslim majority countries: The Islamic movement in Israel as a test case*. Tel Aviv: Moshe Dayan Center for Middle Eastern and African Studies and The Konrad Adenauer Program for Jewish-Arab Cooperation.

National Insurance Institute [NII]. (2015). *Poverty and social gaps report* [PowerPoint slides; in Hebrew]. Retrieved from https://www.btl.gov.il/publications/oni_report/documents /oni2015.pps.

Ozacky-Lazar, S. (1996). *Formation of reciprocal relations between Jews and Arabs in the state of Israel: The first decade 1948–1958* [in Hebrew] (Unpublished doctoral dissertation). University of Haifa, Israel.

Ozacky-Lazar, S. (2001). Representation of Jewish-Arab relations in the first decade [in Hebrew]. In A. Shapira (Ed.), *A State in the Making: Israeli Society in the First Decades*. Jerusalem: Zalman Shazar Center for Jewish History.

Ozacky-Lazar, S. (2008). Arab citizens of Israel: National unification and political change [in Hebrew]. In Z. Tzameret & C. Jablonka (Eds.), *The third decade 5728–5738*. Jerusalem: Yad Yitzhak Ben-Zvi Institute.

Peres, Y., & Davis, N. (1968). On the national identity of the Israeli Arab [in Hebrew]. *Hamizrah Hahadash, 18,* 106–111.

Rekhess, E. (1998). First steps in the formulation of Israeli policy toward Israeli Arabs [in Hebrew]. *Skira Hodshit Journal 35,* 33–37.

Rekhess, E. (2007). The evolvement of an Arab–Palestinian national minority in Israel. *Israel Studies, 12*(3), 1–28.

Rouhana, N., & Ghanem, A. (1998). The crisis of minorities in ethnic states: The case of Palestinian citizens in Israel. *International Journal of Middle East Studies, 30*(3), 321–346.

Sandler, S. (1995). Ethnonationalism and the foreign policy of nation-states. *Nationalism and Ethnic Politics, 1*(2), 250–269.

Smooha, S. (1980). Existing and alternative policy towards the Arabs in Israel [in Hebrew]. *Megamot Journal, 26,* 7–36.

Smooha, S. (1989). The Arab minority in Israel: Radicalization or politicization? In P. Y. Medding (Ed.), *Israel—State and society, 1948–1988: Studies in Contemporary Jewry* (Vol. 5, pp. 59–88). Jerusalem: Institute of Contemporary Jewry, Hebrew University of Jerusalem and Oxford University Press.

Smooha, S. (1999). *Autonomy for Arabs in Israel?* [in Hebrew]. Beit Berl: Institute for Israeli Arab Studies.

Smooha, S. (2001). The model of ethnic democracy, ECMI working papers, No. 13, Flensburg. Taagepera, Rein 1992, Ethnic Relations in Estonia 1991. *Journal of Baltic Studies, 23*(2), 121–132.

Smooha, S. (2013). *Still playing by the rules: The index of Arab-Jewish relations in Israel 2012.* Haifa: University of Haifa and the Israel Democratic Institute.

Stendel, O. (1992). *The Arabs in Israel: Between Hammer and Anvil* [in Hebrew]. Jerusalem: Academon.

Swirski, S., Konor-Atias, E., & Zelingher, R. (2015). *Social report 2015* [in Hebrew]. Tel Aviv: Adva Center.

Weiss, A. (Ed.). (2016). *A picture of the nation: Israel's society and economy in figures, 2016.* Jerusalem: Taub Center for Social Policy Studies in Israel. Retrieved from http://taubcenter.org.il/wp-content/files_mf/pon2016english.pdf.

Yashiv, E., & Kasir, N. (2013). Arab women in the Israeli labor market: Characteristics and policy proposals. *Israel Economic Review, 10*(2), 1–41.

PART II

MENTAL HEALTH ISSUES
RELATED TO FAMILY
AND GENDER

6

THE PALESTINIAN FAMILY IN ISRAEL

*Its Collectivist Nature, Structure, and Implications
for Mental Health Interventions*

Muhammad M. Haj-Yahia

THE FAMILY REMAINS ONE OF THE CENTRAL SYSTEMS in Palestinian society in Israel, as in other Arab societies. In recent decades, Palestinian society has experienced numerous economic, social, political, and educational changes accompanied by processes of globalization. Although these changes have apparently had a substantial impact on the family, the close family—sometimes including other relatives as well—remains the primary support system for Palestinian citizens in Israel (Abu-Baker, 2007; Abudabbeh, 2005; Abdul-Haq, 2008; Rinnawi, 2003). Essentially, despite the changes and attendant upheavals, formal and informal services have not totally replaced the close family as a system of protection and support for family members in many areas (Rinnawi, 2003). Notably, the Arabic term for family (*'aila* or *usra*) reflects the importance and significance of mutual commitment, interdependence, and reciprocity (Barakat, 1993).

Until five decades ago, the basic unit in Palestinian society in Israel was the extended family (*ahal, dar*), which included the father, wife (or wives), unmarried sons and daughters, and married sons and their respective wives and children. This social structure incorporated a common place of residence, where extended family members lived either in several dwellings in the same building or in several housing units in close proximity. Extended family members almost always managed a business together. The nuclear family (father, mother, and children who had not reached young adulthood) had almost no independent existence, and they lived as an integral part of the extended family (Abu-Baker, 2007; Avitzur, 1987; Haj-Yahia, 1995).

The extended family fulfilled important social and economic functions for its nuclear families and sometimes for other relatives. Until the 1960s, extended families often played a role in local politics (i.e., by voting in the local council elections and holding seats in those councils) as well as in national politics (i.e., by voting in elections to the Israeli parliament and supporting parties that form the government) and sometimes even in the national labor union (the *Histadrut*). They engaged in political activities together with several other extended families related by blood from the same *hamula*. However, the transitions in Palestinian society in Israel, mainly in the economic and employment domains, have considerably weakened the economic connection between the nuclear family and the extended family. These changes are reflected in the decline of agriculture, the extended family's main source of income in the past, both as a result of increasing land division among a growing number of nuclear families within the land-owning extended family and as a result of land expropriation by the Israeli government. In addition, the economic functions of the extended family have been affected by accelerated industrialization and wide-ranging dependence on the Israeli labor market (e.g., in various services and in construction), as well as by an increase in educational and academic achievements. These social and economic transitions and transformations have contributed to a great extent to weakening the power of the collective financial sources (e.g., land and agriculture) of the extended family, on one hand, and enhancing the individual financial sources and the economic independence of the nuclear family, on the other (Abu-Baker, 2007; Avitzur, 1987; Haj-Yahia, 1995). Urbanization in Palestinian localities in Israel (as reflected in an increase in the number of residents and expansion of locality size) has also intensified. However, growth in these areas has not been accompanied by an improvement in the standard of living and quality of life in urban localities. Moreover, there is evidence of increasing mobility among families within localities (i.e., nuclear families living far from the home of the head of the extended family). These processes have also apparently accelerated the nuclearization of Palestinian families (Haj-Yahia, 1995).

Nonetheless, the family is still the primary support system in Palestinian society (Abu-Baker, 2007; Haj-Yahia, 1995; Rinnawi, 2003). Emotional bonds, collective values, and loyalty to kin have remained important for preserving connections among members of the extended family (i.e., among nuclear families) and in certain cases even among the extended families in the same *hamula* (during elections to the local council and sometimes in disputes with people in other families) (Abdul-Haq, 2008; Sharifzadeh, 2011). Loyalty and mutual support have persisted even when families do not share living accommodations or reside close by (Abdul-Haq, 2008; Abu-Baker, 2007; Barakat, 1993; Rinnawi, 2003). Importantly, the intensity of these connections and underlying values can differ by area of residence and by religion. They are stronger among Bedouins and in rural areas than in urban areas and stronger among Muslims and Druze than among Christians (Abu-Baker, 2007; Avitzur, 1987; Haj-Yahia, 1995).

As previously noted, it is commonly agreed that family ties in Arab societies, including Palestinian society in Israel, are in the process of change—yet they remain more cohesive and extensive than family ties in Western postindustrial societies (Abdul-Haq, 2008; Abu-Baker, 2007; Abudabbeh, 2005; Barakat, 1993; Haj-Yahia, 1995; Sharifzadeh, 2011). The relationships with other nuclear families within the extended family and with relatives and family friends constitute a significant network and vital support system in situations of personal, marital, and familial distress and crisis (Abdul-Haq, 2008; Abudabbeh, 2005; Haj-Yahia, 1995; Sirhan, 2005).

Such relationships have long-term implications for the individual's value system as well as for intrapersonal and interpersonal processes and individual behavior. This support system is often the only natural source of assistance for family members. Hence, in professional interventions with Palestinian families in Israel, the network of family relationships and the family support systems could facilitate intervention success on both family and individual levels (Abdul-Haq, 2008; Abudabbeh, 2005; Haj-Yahia, 1995). Nonetheless, the network of family relationships may also hinder the progress of the family or its members in solving problems (Haj-Yahia, 1995; Haj-Yahia & Sadan, 2008). To understand the transformations in Palestinian society in Israel, particularly within the family, it is crucial to recognize the collectivistic nature of the Palestinian family as well as its structure and composition.

The Collectivistic Nature of the Palestinian Family in Israel

Definition of Collectivism

Collectivism is a cultural pattern, sometimes including economic and sociopolitical elements, that exists mainly in Middle Eastern, Asian, African, South American, and Pacific countries, and, to a certain extent, in some Eastern European countries (Matsumoto, 1996; Triandis, 1995). Collectivism is also often found in minority communities living alongside individualistic majority societies (e.g., Arabs in Western Europe, Asians in North America, indigenous people in Australia and New Zealand, and Palestinian citizens in Israel). The first, second, and third generations of these communities belong to collectivistic societies (Matsumoto, 1996). Triandis (1995) argued that there are many types of collectivism and that the main types attribute considerable importance to the family as well as to work groups, the tribe, the community, and the nation.

Family members in collectivistic communities maintain a primary sense of commitment to their family and often to all components of their collective, as described earlier, which is reflected in a strong desire to fulfill the basic human needs and desires of their family. This yields a sense of personal satisfaction and self-actualization, as well as a sense of living harmoniously with one's collective (Haj-Yahia & Sadan, 2008).

Because of the collectivistic nature of the Palestinian family, family members often tend to subordinate their personal needs and goals to those that promote the well-being of the entire family or of some family members. Members of Palestinian families believe that their own personal survival, growth, prosperity, and quality of life are closely linked with those of their families. Therefore, in many cases, they may believe that the good of their family takes precedence over their personal good, and that their personal well-being is an outcome of their family's well-being. In other cases, they give priority to the benefits, quality of life, prosperity, and well-being of their families (Abudabbeh, 2005; Dwairy, 1998, 2006; Haj-Yahia & Sadan, 2008; Sharifzadeh, 2011). Hence, unsurprisingly, Palestinian family members often act to promote the goals and well-being of the family as a whole rather than their own personal goals and well-being. As a rule, individuals may attempt to promote personal goals and well-being that do not conflict with the goals of their families (Haj-Yahia, 1995; Sirhan, 2005).

Against this background, this section deals with the significance of three dimensions: (1) the self, (2) attitudes and values, and (3) activities and behaviors of the Palestinian family in Israel. These dimensions and their manifestations are examined in light of the collectivistic nature of Palestinian society. Based on the conceptual framework of Triandis, Brislin, and Hui (1988) and Triandis (1995), I explain the relevance of each of the three dimensions to the reality and life conditions of the Palestinian family.

The Self

In Palestinian society, the self is attached to family identity—although in certain situations it is also an integral part of community, ethnic, and national identities. Accordingly, family identity in Palestinian society in Israel, as in virtually all other Arab societies, is a major component of the personal identity (Abdul-Haq, 2008; Abudabbeh, 2005; Barakat, 1993; Dwairy, 1998, 2006; Haj-Yahia, 1995, 2000, 2011; Haj-Yahia & Sadan, 2008).

In Palestinian society, self-esteem, self-image, and self-concept are mainly dependent on the family and, in some cases, on the ethnic and national image. Thus, one's self-image, self-esteem, merits, security, and personal identity are evaluated on the basis of relations with the family, whereas friends and other contacts are considered secondary to family needs and commitments (Haj-Yahia, 1995, 2011). The reputation and status of the family in Palestinian society are more significant for the individual than personal achievements and have a strong impact on one's self and identity. Accordingly, the success or failure of one member of the Palestinian family is the concern of the entire family, not merely the concern of that individual. Likewise, the reputation of the family depends on the behavior of its members. Thus, in the collectivistic context of the Palestinian family, there is often a mutual connection between the personal self and identity, on the one hand, and the familial collectivist self and identity, on the other. In most cases, each family member is viewed as responsible for the behavior and life conditions of every other family member (Abu-Baker, 2007; Abudabbeh, 2005; Dwairy, 1998, 2006;

Haj-Yahia, 1995, 1996, 2000; Haj-Yahia & Sadan, 2008). This commitment may potentially lead to denial of individual needs and aspirations and may cause people to subordinate their own needs and interests to those of the family—or at least to the needs and interests of some family members (Dwairy, 1998, 2006; Haj-Yahia, 1995, 1996, 2000; Matsumoto, 1996; Triandis, 1995). But this does not mean that the family expects all of its members to completely subordinate and deny their individual selves and identities. On the contrary, the Palestinian family is known for encouraging the growth of each member and even imbues them with individualistic traits, such as ambitiousness and success, especially at school and at work. The family also encourages people to advance their status in the community and nation, as long as these aspirations, growth, and achievements do not conflict with the interests, goals, and well-being of the family as a unit. In addition, while the Palestinian family encourages separation and individuation, at least as a means of achieving personal growth and healthy independence, it also encourages interdependence, mutual bonding, and attachment as a way of preserving the collectivistic self of the family and as another facet of family health (Haj-Yahia, 1995; Sharifzadeh, 2011).

Attitudes and Values

One of the collectivist features of the Palestinian family is the expectation that its members maintain positive attitudes toward their family. Because members of Palestinian families derive their selves and identities from the family, and often from their ethnic and national collective, there is a strong tendency to attribute considerable significance to family ties and to believe that the family's good name and status reflect on their own personal reputation (Crabtree, Husain, & Spalek, 2008; Haj-Yahia, 1995, 2000, 2011; Haj-Yahia & Sadan, 2008). Accordingly, the Palestinian family emphasizes preserving and strengthening family ties and interdependence within the nuclear family. In addition, emphasis is often placed on relationships with members of the extended family, who are expected to serve as a major source of cognitive, emotional, and social support in distress or crisis. In most cases, family is preferred over formal sources of support (Abdul-Haq, 2008; Abu-Baker, 2007 Dwairy, 1996, 2006; Haj-Yahia, 1995, 1996, 2005). Thus, denial of family support or threats to discontinue such support can damage the individual's self-confidence, cause anxiety about his or her ability to cope with life's demands, and arouse fear of ostracism by the family or at least by some of its members (Haj-Yahia, 1995, 1996, 2000).

Furthermore, Palestinian family members are usually expected to maintain positive attitudes about vertical family relationships. In Palestinian society, as in most collectivist societies, power hierarchy and vertical relationships in the family are determined according to gender and age. Hence, adult men have more economic, social, political, cultural, and religious power than women and children (Abdul-Haq, 2008; Abu-Baker, 2007; Barakat, 1993; Beitin & Aprahamian, 2004; Haj-Yahia, 1995, 1996, 2000, 2003; Haj-Yahia & Sadan, 2008; Sharifzadeh, 2011).

Despite the considerable improvement in the status of Palestinian women in Israel in recent decades in private as well as public spheres, they are still expected to submit to their families, their husbands, and, oftentimes, to their brothers. Children in Palestinian society, as in most other collectivistic societies, are expected to comply with the demands of older family members (Abdul-Haq, 2008; Abudabbeh, 2005; Barakat, 1993; Dwairy, 1998, 2006; Haj-Yahia, 1995). Furthermore, the Palestinian family maintains positive attitudes toward mutual support, cooperation, and reciprocity, on the one hand, and negative attitudes toward selfishness, competition, and confrontation among family members, on the other. Attempts to resolve conflicts among family members through confrontation may often generate lack of understanding, disgust, and even ostracism. In many cases, confrontations among family members are viewed as an indication of rebelliousness and lack of respect for mediators and facilitators—especially if they have the potential to undermine family cohesion and solidarity (Crabtree et al., 2008; Haj-Yahia, 1995, 2000; Haj-Yahia & Sadan, 2008; Matsumoto, 1996; Triandis, 1995).

Indeed, the major values that prevail in the Palestinian family in Israel are harmony; face-saving; commitment to the family of origin, to the family of procreation, and often to the extended family and relatives; cooperation; modesty; moderation; thriftiness; and subordination and sacrifice of the individual self to the collective self of the family (Barakat, 1993; Dwairy, 1998, 2006; Haj-Yahia, 1995, 1996, 2000; Haj-Yahia & Sadan, 2008). The Palestinian family cultivates these values, especially family harmony, and fosters them as a means of preserving family ties and maintaining the collectivistic behavior of families while condemning individualistic behavior that conflicts with the aims, aspirations, and well-being of the family as a cohesive unit (Crabtree et al., 2008; Haj-Yahia, 1995, 1996, 2000; Haj-Yahia & Sadan, 2008; Rinnawi, 2003).

In addition, the Palestinian family fosters the value of honor among its members. The concept of honor is much broader and more complex than the simple, stereotyped interpretation of honor that many people have about Arab societies, which focuses only on sexual behavior. Rather, in the Palestinian family, honor essentially encompasses vital values for the family, such as economic prosperity and growth, educational success and academic achievements, hard work, and conservatism, as well as refraining from antisocial behavior and from involvement in criminal activity or any other unacceptable behavior that might harm the family's reputation (Abudabbeh, 2005; Abudabbeh & Aseel, 1999).

Activities and Behaviors

In Palestinian society, people tend to organize communal activities to preserve and strengthen the collectivist domain. At wedding celebrations, festivities, feasts, condolence gatherings, and other social and religious occasions, nuclear and extended families and other relatives come together and support each other. At such gatherings, family members and relatives share experiences, exchange ideas, and update each other on personal, familial, and community developments and concerns. In this context, people engage in social behavior that connects them with each other. They support each other willingly, both as individuals and families (Abu-Baker, 2007; Al-Krenawi, 2002; Barakat, 1993; Dwairy, 1998, 2006; Haj-Yahia, 1996, 2000, 2011; Haj-Yahia & Sadan, 2008; Sharifzadeh, 2011).

The collectivist character of the Palestinian family leads to the expectation that members will exercise self-discipline, control their emotions, and remain patient. As such, family members are expected to refrain from publicly protesting at times of crisis and distress. Coping patiently with difficult situations is considered preferable to hasty complaints and impulsive behavior (Beitin & Aprahamian, 2014; Dwairy, 2006; Haj-Yahia, 1995, 1996, 2000, 2011; Haj-Yahia & Sadan, 2008; Sharifzadeh, 2011).

The Palestinian family in Israel does not view outside intervention favorably. This includes intercession from nonfamily members and those working in formal and informal organizations. Family members fear that outsiders will be insensitive and disrespectful toward the family and are apprehensive about sharing sensitive issues that might stigmatize and harm their reputation. In addition, in Palestinian society, as in most collectivist societies, outside parties that intervene in family affairs may likely be blamed for upsetting the harmony and cohesiveness of the family. Hence, intervention from outside of the family often arouses feelings of disappointment with the one who involved the external party and hostility toward the outsider (Al-Krenawi, 2002; Cohen & Savaya, 1997; Haj-Yahia, 1995, 1996, 2000, 2011; Haj-Yahia & Sadan, 2008; Savaya, 1997; Savaya & Cohen, 2003; Triandis, 1995).

Importantly as well, it should be noted that these families are a minority in a society with a Jewish Israeli majority. Recall here that the history of the Arab-Jewish conflict has been characterized by intense hostility, death, and destruction for over 100 years. In the shadow of the conflict, the Palestinian minority in Israel has experienced continuous national, political, economic, and sociocultural oppression, as well as exclusion, discrimination, and racism. Note, too, that there are high rates of unemployment and poverty in Palestinian society in Israel in addition to poor infrastructure in all services in Palestinian localities. These experiences and life conditions have generated a sense of helplessness and hopelessness among most of the Palestinian population in Israel, as well as distrust in and hostility toward state institutions. Unsurprisingly, therefore, the collectivist Palestinian minority in Israel is wary of the changes taking place as a result of the encounter with Israeli society, which is both individualist and perceived as oppressing Palestinians.

It is also not surprising that, when dealing with the problems in Palestinian society, one hears responses such as: Why should the state want to help us? Does the state really acknowledge the injustice and problems it has caused us, or is it belittling us, and just seeking to continue oppressing and excluding us? We've always been oppressed and deprived—suddenly they care about us? (Haj-Yahia & Sadan, 2008, pp. 8–9). Clearly, these reactions show a profound sense of distrust among a large share of Palestinians, which is sometimes reflected in reluctance to seek help from and disclose their problems to mental health and social services (Haj-Yahia, 1996, 2000; Savaya, 1997).

The Structure of the Palestinian Family in Israel

Research has shown that in collectivist societies that are in the process of change, such as the Palestinian society, family ties (within the nuclear family and among family members comprising the extended family) are expected to be more cohesive and extensive than in individualist societies (Beitin & Aprahamian, 2014; Haj-Yahia, 1995; Sharifzadeh, 2011; Stanton, 2006; Triandis, 1995, 2001). Therefore, these relationships can serve the function of providing essential support to the family, or at least to individual members who are in a situation of crisis or distress (Beitin & Aprahamian, 2014; Crabtree et al., 2008; Sharifzadeh, 2011). These relationships can also have ongoing implications for the perspectives, value systems, and behaviors of individuals. Moreover, it can be reasonably assumed that these relationships will affect the success of professional and informal interventions with the family. Although these networks are not always available to provide the necessary support, they are often the natural source of assistance to family members. However, they can also impede solutions or even lead to failure in solving the problems of the family as a whole or individual family members (Al-Krenawi, 2002; Haj-Yahia, 1995, 2000). This section explores the structure of the Palestinian family within the framework of mate selection and courtship, marital relations, parent/offspring relations, sibling relations, and divorce.

Mate Selection and Courtship

In Palestinian society in Israel, intimate relations between a man and a woman are only permissible in the bounds of marriage (Sherif-Trask, 2006). The marriage must be acknowledged in accordance with religious law, and it must be publicly announced by the families of both partners and registered in the Population Registry of the Israel Ministry of the Interior (Abu-Baker, 2007; Haj-Yahia, 1995). Therefore, extramarital intimate relations between a man and a woman are not accepted and can often seriously damage the family's reputation. In fact, extramarital sexual relations are referred to as *zina* (fornication) and can result in harsh social punishments (Sherif-Trask, 2006).

Nonetheless, the earlier tradition of matchmaking is almost nonexistent in Palestinian society today. Introductions between potential partners are made secretly (at school, work, and even through social media), with a view toward formalizing the relationship through engagement and marriage. Despite this change, the final choice of a partner is still to some extent mediated by the parents of the potential bride and groom. A young man who is interested in marrying is still expected to send his parents or parents' representatives to the potential bride's parents. The potential bride's mother is usually the first to be approached. She then shares the proposal with her husband and with the potential bride's brothers. It is also considered desirable for the father of the potential bride to involve his brothers and even his wife's brothers in deciding on the proposal (Haj-Yahia, 1995).

In some cases, mate selection and courtship do not begin without the mutual consent and blessing of both families (Abu-Baker, 2007; Barakat, 1993; Haj-Yahia, 1995; Sherif-Trask, 2006). As soon as both potential partners receive the consent and approval of their families, they announce the engagement together with their families. The announcement is usually celebrated at a festive event attended by the extended families of both couples and their friends. However, if both families oppose the engagement and the couple chooses to remain engaged despite their disapproval, both partners often suffer negative consequences, including social isolation and ostracism. Undoubtedly, such responses and consequences are sources of stress and concern. The harm to the families' reputation can be transmitted from one generation to another and can have a detrimental effect on the couple's offspring as long as their families have not forgiven them (Crabtree et al., 2008; Haj-Yahia, 1995; Sherif-Trask, 2006).

Before an engagement, as part of getting to know each other, the couple may meet in various settings within and outside of their own locality, but it is undesirable for the pair to be seen together in public. Nonetheless, it is commonly known that such encounters do occur outside the village or town where the couple has opportunities to meet—for example, at work, at college or university, or nowadays, via social media.

Once the couple has received the consent of the two families, plans for the nuptial ceremonies can proceed. Although the engagement ceremony is a religious confirmation that the partners will bear the status of a married couple, the prospective bride and groom continue to live with their own families until the marriage ceremony, usually held several months after the engagement or once the couple's economic situation allows them to live independently. Although both partners see each other during this period, at the end of each day they return to their own families.

Notably, the engagement ceremonies also provide an opportunity for both partners to receive social and financial support from their nuclear and extended families, as well as from friends of their families and from their own friends. Although most of the burden of expenses for the marriage ceremony and for setting up the new household is borne by the groom and his family, the bride's family usually covers some of those expenses (Haj-Yahia, 1995; Sherif-Trask, 2006).

Marital Relations

Notwithstanding major gains in the status of women in Palestinian society over the past fifty years, their status has always been lower than that of males (especially compared with their older brothers), and wives' status is lower than their husbands'. Moreover, despite improvement in the domains of education and employment outside of the home, and despite women's improved economic situation in Palestinian society, they are often still expected to be dependent on their partners in most matters relating to their marriage and to family affairs in general. They are expected to fulfill the needs of their husbands and children and to maintain the home (Abu-Baker, 2007; Haj-Yahia, 1995; Rinnawi, 2003; Sherif-Trask, 2006). The husband is usually expected to fulfill the dominant instrumental roles in the family as main provider and protector, whereas the wife is expected to fulfill expressive roles as intimate partner, mother, and housewife (Abu-Baker, 2007; Crabtree et al., 2008; Haj-Yahia, 1995; Sharifzadeh, 2011).

Haj-Yahia (1995) argued that the changes in the status of Palestinian women in Israel, both within and outside of the family, can be viewed as "quantitative" (p. 439) (i.e., more women are educated, more women work outside the home, and more women are socially and politically involved). However, it is difficult to view these as "qualitative" (p. 439), deep-rooted developments that have led to a serious substantive structural change in the status of women in the private sphere (i.e., in the family and in the marital relationship) as well as in the public sphere (at work places, in politics, and in the economy). Unsurprisingly, the role of Palestinian women in Israel has continued to be nonegalitarian, both as wives and as mothers (Abu-Baker, 2007; Haj-Yahia, 1995; Rinnawi, 2003). It is still not self-evident that husbands will take responsibility for household chores and child care, although they may be more involved in these matters than in the past. In certain parts of Palestinian society (mainly among Bedouins and among couples with low levels of education), it is a common perception that "the woman's place is in the home and the husband's place is outside of the home" (Abu-Baker, 2007; Haj-Yahia, 1995; Rinnawi, 2003; Sharifzadeh, 2011). This division of roles may probably enhance the power of women in the family (as partners and as mothers) behind the scenes, even though they show apparent support for their husbands' authority (Abudabbeh, 2005; Haj-Yahia, 1995; Rinnawi, 2003). Although Palestinian women do not tend to underestimate their role as marital partners, they are most likely to consider their role as mother more important than their role as partner. It may be argued that in the Palestinian family, children establish the marriage and cement the marital relationship. Yet it is also commonly argued that maternal love is considered more powerful than a wife's love for her husband (Barakat, 1993; Haj-Yahia, 1995; Sharifzadeh, 2011).

The Palestinian nuclear family has to reconcile two conflicting forces and values: those that encourage "modernization," and those that pull the family toward "traditionalism." This struggle is most likely to cause stress in the family and may generate conflicts between marital partners or even conflicts between the partners, both sets of the couple's parents, and the extended families (Cohen & Savaya, 2003a, 2003b; Haj-Yahia, 1995).

Some researchers have found that, in contrast to the past, and unlike relationships between older couples, most husbands in the younger generation consult with their wives about family matters (Haj-Yahia, 1995; Rinnawi, 2003). Furthermore, young Palestinian wives have been expanding their involvement, influence, and role in the family. This has been affected by sociocultural and sociopolitical developments and mainly by the wife's increasing contribution to the family income as a result of changes in the employment structure in Palestinian society in Israel since the 1960s (Avitzur, 1987; Haj-Yahia, 1995; Rinnawi, 2003; Shokeid, 1993). When the wife earns a salary and contributes to the family income, her status rises in the family and most likely in the public sphere as well. Even if some Palestinian husbands are not fully conscious of the need and importance of involving their wives in family decisions, most young couples are likely to find that the objective circumstances of modern life leave them no other choice (Avitzur, 1987; Haj-Yahia, 1995; Rinnawi, 2003; Shokeid, 1993).

Parent/Offspring Relations and Discipline

Parental functions in the Palestinian family in Israel are consistent with the sociocultural norms governing marital relations (Haj-Yahia, 1995; Sharifzadeh, 2011). Naturally, the three parenting patterns that prevail in families throughout the world (authoritative, permissive, and authoritarian) are also found in the Palestinian family (Beitin & Aprahamian, 2014; Sharifzadeh, 2011). Authoritative parenting is characterized by high demands and control of children based on clear rules and standards while parents express considerable warmth. Permissive parenting is characterized by low demands and low levels of control while parents express high levels of warmth. Authoritarian parenting is characterized by high demands, extensive control, and low levels of warmth (Sharifzadeh, 2011). However, it can also be argued that parent/offspring relations in Palestinian society do not fit these three styles of parenting in that Palestinian parenting is generally characterized by high demands, high levels of control, and high levels of warmth (Barakat, 1993; Beitin & Aprahamian, 2014; Haj-Yahia, 1995; Sharifzadeh, 2011).

Often, the father's main role is to demand obedience, provide discipline, and control or punish certain behaviors; whereas the mother's main role is to support, nurture, educate, and raise the children. Children in the Palestinian family are expected to obey their parents, submit to their demands and directions, and fulfill their expectations. Love, affection, and warmth are usually expressed openly when the child is small. The mother is typically expected to devote most of her time and energy to the children, whereas the father is expected to play with them and provide tangible and moral support. The father is most likely to be congenial toward young children and more strict and assertive (even aggressive, "if necessary") toward older offspring. Furthermore, in Palestinian society in Israel, as in all Arab societies, parents are not expected to befriend their children. Parents usually gain their children's respect through various complementary interactions between them and expect that children will be obedient and disciplined (Beitin & Aprahamian, 2014; Haj-Yahia, 1995; Sharifzadeh, 2011).

However, the expectations and rules that govern parent/offspring relations can vary depending on the child's age and gender and the parent's gender and education. The younger the child, the more permissive the parents. Parents are also more permissive with boys than with girls. The older the child is and the less educated the parents are, the more strict and demanding the parents are likely to be (Sharifzadeh, 2011).

Although the family gives children more room for independence as they grow older, they are still expected to continue consulting with their parents, and they are expected to refrain from placing too much emphasis on their independence in front of their parents. For example, despite the economic transformations in Palestinian society over the past five decades that have enabled young adults (mainly sons) in the family to be economically independent, in many cases they are not expected to be socially independent. It is not considered appropriate for young men to decide for themselves whether to study in Israel or abroad, where to buy a plot of land for their homes, or when and whom to marry. In these matters, they are expected to consult with their parents (mainly the father). If they fail to do so, or if they overemphasize their independence and make their own plans, their behavior is often considered disrespectful and even rebellious. This may arouse anger and discontent and can even lead to ongoing conflict (Haj-Yahia, 1995).

The expectation that daughters will be obedient and disciplined is even more rigid, despite the considerable improvement in their status, as mentioned earlier. There are areas in the family and public spheres in which women have not gained independence. For example, it is undesirable and often even unacceptable for an unmarried woman to live far away from her parents—unless she is studying at a university in a locality that is far from her parents' home or, in exceptional cases, if she is working in another city. As indicated, women in Palestinian society should not meet men openly for social purposes (e.g., dating, friendship). In extreme cases, secret meetings with men may be reluctantly accepted by the family, but by no means are they condoned (Crabtree et al., 2008; Haj-Yahia, 1995; Sharifzadeh, 2011).

In the Palestinian family, it is considered natural and even beneficial for members of the extended family to be involved in child rearing as well as in dealing with the problems of older children in the family. Extended family members usually help parents perform basic tasks such as disciplining and taking care of children, which gives the parents space to fulfill other obligations. For example, financial obligations often require the Palestinian father to work long hours outside the home, and more Palestinian women are also employed on the outside. Nonetheless, it can be assumed that this will not adversely affect supervision, care, and education of the children because other family members (e.g., uncles and aunts, older brothers and sisters, and grandparents) willingly and happily step in to help the biological parents. Although the use of babysitters and day care has been increasing in Palestinian society, it is still common for children to grow up around adults from the extended family throughout the day and in the late afternoon. Relatives are also involved in providing for the children's needs in times of crisis and distress (e.g., if one of the parents is hospitalized), and it is still customary for the relatives (mainly grandparents) to raise the children if the mother passes away (Haj-Yahia, 1995).

Sibling Relations

Gender and age are the main factors that determine the hierarchy of sibling relations. Older brothers are expected to be more dominant than their younger brothers and sisters, often irrespective of their age. Notwithstanding the changes in many domains in the Palestinian family, including family relations, many parents still believe that through their sons (particularly their older sons) they can maintain the family's reputation and perpetuate the memory of their ancestors. Hence, it is not surprising that many parents prefer to bear sons (Abu-Baker, 2007; Al-Krenawi, 2002; Haj-Yahia, 1995; Sharifzadeh, 2011). These parents tend to give older sons authority and delegate tasks such as supervision, care, consultation, and guidance of their younger siblings. In many Palestinian families, the older son is still expected to be a role model for his younger siblings and care for them as much as possible (Barakat, 1993; Haj-Yahia, 1995; Sharifzadeh, 2011).

At the same time, children in the Palestinian family are supposed to develop sibling relationships characterized by friendship, mutual support, solidarity, cooperation, and respect. Parents expect their children to develop these relationships from a young age and continue fostering them. In addition, parents discourage disputes, hostility, and negative competition among their children. The children are also supposed to develop such relationships with other members of the extended family such as grandparents, aunts and uncles, and cousins (Barakat, 1993; Beitin & Aprahamian, 2014; Haj-Yahia, 1995; Sharifzadeh, 2011). The conditions of poverty and unemployment that prevail among a large percentage of families in Palestinian society and the low quality of services and infrastructure in every domain (e.g., education, health, welfare, and employment) in Palestinian localities in Israel constitute a strong rationale for promoting such relationships among children in Palestinian families (Rinnawi, 2003).

Divorce

Divorce is permitted in Islamic religious law as well as in the Druze faith, but it is not permitted in most of the Christian denominations. Nonetheless, in all sectors, divorce is considered socially and culturally undesirable. Although divorce rates are increasing in Palestinian society in Israel, it is thought to symbolize the failure of the couple. Accordingly, divorce has harsh implications for the couple and their children and often for their entire families as well (Cohen & Savaya, 2003a, 2003b; Haj-Yahia, 1995, 2000, 2011; Sherif-Trask, 2006). The legalities of divorce in these religions are beyond the scope of this chapter, thus I focus on the familial, cultural, and social aspects of divorce. Just as marriage is considered a legal and religious union of two partners and as a social alliance between the two families, divorce represents the breakup of these relationships (Sherif-Trask, 2006).

In Palestinian society, divorce is considered an extreme process and often has long-term social implications beyond the tension and unhappiness of the divorced couple. Divorce usually bears a heavy social stigma, and therefore, unsurprisingly, the families of both partners make concerted efforts to achieve reconciliation between the partners in order to prevent divorce (Haj-Yahia, 2000; Sherif-Trask, 2006). Divorce can symbolize not only the failure of both partners and the discord and lack of harmony between them but may also symbolize the failure of their families to support the couple and resolve their conflicts. Divorce can also harm the woman's reputation as well as the reputation of her family (Cohen & Savaya, 2003a, 2003b; Haj-Yahia & Sadan, 2008).

For many couples, divorce proceedings are the last step in a long and debilitating process that is accompanied by tension and disputes between the partners and, in many cases, among members of their respective families. Therefore, family members try to intervene in the couple's problems early to prevent them from escalating to the point of divorce (Abu-Baker, 2003, 2007; Haj-Yahia, 2000, 2011; Sherif-Trask, 2006). In such situations, the woman usually tries to involve her father, brothers, and other men from her extended family. Although she also informs her mother and older sisters, they tend not to intercede as long as the male family members are intervening with the husband and his family (Sherif, 1996; Sherif-Trask, 2006).

Savaya and Cohen (1998) argued that emotional problems and incompatibility, which are major causes of divorce among couples in Western societies, play a minor role among Palestinian couples in Israel who divorce. In a study conducted among Palestinian Muslim women in Israel, the participants mentioned the following causes for their divorce: (1) sexual torment (e.g., "It's shameful to say; I haven't slept with my husband in 10 years," "He would ask me to do things that God and religion forbid," "He wanted to sleep with me with blows and force"); (2) husband's physical violence (e.g., "He drank, beat, and humiliated me. I went to his family; they sent me back"); (3) violence by a member of the extended family (e.g., "He said 'Your parents told me I have to beat you'"); (4) interference of extended family members (e.g., "My mother-in-law interferes in my marital life," "My father-in-law would tell him, 'Treat her like a servant'"); (5) communication problems (e.g., "He made my life miserable," "No understanding"); (6) husband's addiction (e.g., "[He's an] alcoholic. The children saw their father drinking all the time. He would walk along the street drunk. The children would be called 'the drunkard's kids,' and I would be called 'the drunkard's wife'"); and (7) husband's bizarre behavior (e.g., "Where is he? Sleeping in the garbage. So I suffered. And he goes and picks up all the garbage and brings it home. And I had a beautiful home, beautiful," "I was ashamed to go out with him. I'd go only with the children and my friends, not with him") (Savaya & Cohen, 1998, pp. 172–173).

Studies conducted in Western societies have shown that adjustment to divorce is affected by numerous factors, including demographic and sociodemographic variables (e.g., age, gender, educational level, economic status, employment, presence of young children), the characteristics of the divorce process (e.g., who asked for the divorce, current life strains and stressors, satisfaction with the divorce procedures), changes in life circumstances after the divorce (e.g., economic situation, housing conditions), social conditions (e.g., social ties, social support, participation in social activities), and personal variables (e.g., self-confidence, sense of coherence, coping patterns and skills) (Cohen & Savaya, 2003a, 2003b). However, Cohen and Savaya (2003b) claimed that although these factors can be related to the way Palestinian women cope with and adjust to divorce, other social and cultural factors can also strongly influence their coping. Al-Krenawi and Graham (1998) found that divorced Palestinian women experience various psychosocial problems as a result of restricted liberty and social censure imposed on them, mainly by their families and relatives, in addition to the decline in their social status. Cohen and Savaya (1997) found that divorced Palestinian women cope with a stigma, and they are treated as socially and sexually wanton. So they try to adjust by proving to their suspicious neighbors and relatives that they can maintain their chastity, keep a clean house, and care for their children.

Some Implications for Intervention

The topics discussed in the previous sections are highly significant for mental health practitioners working with Palestinian families in Israel—including practitioners working in public welfare and mental health services as well as those working in private clinics. Segregation exists between Jewish and Palestinian service users in most of the services in Israel (mainly in education and welfare services, and in most local community health and mental health services). Therefore, most practitioners working with Palestinian families in Israel are presumably Palestinian themselves and conduct therapeutic meetings in Arabic (although in some organizations, such as hospitals, Palestinian families meet with Jewish therapists). However, because both Jewish Israeli and Palestinian mental health practitioners have been educated according to individualistic ideals and ideologies, their knowledge and intervention skills are characterized by an individualist orientation. Therefore, it can be assumed that many of them lack awareness of the essence and significance of the structure and collectivist nature of the Palestinian family. Their ignorance of the differences between these dimensions in Palestinian families in contrast to families in individualist societies, as well as their basic assumption that their knowledge and skills are universal rather than dependent on sociopolitical and sociocultural contexts, can lead to difficulties and conflicts in their work with Palestinian families.

I do not claim that this analysis can be generalized to all Palestinian families in Israel nor that they are totally homogeneous. Undoubtedly, differences may be found among Palestinian families with regard to some aspects (in terms of their intensity but not in terms of their nature). The differences depend on several variables, including the couple's levels of education and sometimes the educational level of the couple's parents, the family's place of residence (urban localities, mixed Jewish-Arab localities, rural areas, and Bedouin areas), the family's income, religion (Muslim, Druze, Christian), gender, age, unemployment and women's employment outside of the home, political attitudes, number of children in the family, proximity of the family's residence to the rest of the nuclear families that compose the extended family and other relatives, and some personal variables (Abu-Baker, 2007; Haj-Yahia, 1995, 2000; Rinnawi, 2003; Savaya, 1997, 1998). At the same time, it seems clear that any intervention with Palestinian families must be sensitive to their sociocultural and sociopolitical contexts.

A full intervention model for work with Palestinian families in Israel is clearly beyond the scope of this chapter. However, I offer synoptic insights and challenges to be taken into account when intervening with these families. One major insight derives from the nature of professional socialization for practitioners working with Palestinian families in Israel. As mentioned earlier, most Israeli mental health practitioners are trained at universities and professional institutes in Israel and/or other Western countries, where academic programs are heavily influenced by Western individualistic value systems that are likely to contradict the collectivist nature of Palestinian society. According to the Westernized individualistic approach, "it is possible to control nature" (Haj-Yahia, 1995, p. 433), no problem is beyond solution, and although equilibrium and harmony are preferred solutions, conflicts are still an integral and legitimate part of daily life. Notably, practitioners working with Palestinian families in Israel may find this approach in conflict with the collectivistic attitudes and values discussed previously. They must acknowledge these differences and try to find a middle-of-the-road approach to deal with the conflicting values, attitudes, orientations, and behaviors while also considering and respecting those of the family as a unit and those of the family members as individuals to the extent that this is professionally, ethically, and legally possible (Haj-Yahia, 1995, 1996, 1997, 2000).

Another important insight relates to the assumption that Palestinian families are more likely to prefer solutions that are oriented to the present reality and that they are most likely to cooperate with practitioners who help them achieve such solutions. Accordingly, solutions that overemphasize the historical development of the family and individual family members may be rejected, and the family may not willingly cooperate in achieving such solutions (Haj-Yahia, 1995, 1997). The preferred approaches should acknowledge the importance of reinforcing pride in the family and its history, as well as the importance of maintaining and enhancing positive aspects of the family heritage and the ability to learn from them. Similarly, even though emphasis has been placed on the here and now in interventions with Palestinian families, it is assumed that future-oriented interventions will not always be rejected as long as they remain concrete and task oriented. Hence, the aims of such interventions with the Palestinian family should be practical, operational, and attainable while remaining consistent with the goals, values, and attitudes of the family in particular and Palestinian society in general (Al-Krenawi, 2002; Haj-Yahia, 1995, 1997).

Another major challenge for practitioners relates to the importance of family focused interventions in Palestinian society in Israel. Considering the collectivist nature of the Palestinian family and the preference given to the collective self over the individual self, it seems logical that Palestinian families will welcome their involvement in dealing with individual, marital, and family problems and that in certain cases they might even prefer family oriented interventions over individual-focused and/or marital-focused interventions. I do not argue that Palestinian families will oppose interventions that are not family focused. Although I highlight the collective notion of self in the Palestinian family, I also emphasize that in the Palestinian family and in Palestinian society there is respect for the desire of individual family members "to build and establish themselves," "to progress on their own," and "to be independent as long as the individual's desires do not conflict with goals, values, desires, and aspirations of the family." Hence, individual-focused and marital-focused interventions might be welcomed by the family as long as they maintain family unity and emphasize the goals, desires, plans, aspirations, and interests of the family unit as opposed to those of individual family members. Any help or support rendered to individuals in the Palestinian family is also welcomed as long as it does not conflict with the needs and goals of the family. Nonetheless, practitioners who intervene with Palestinian families often have difficulty coping with situations of conflict between the interests of the family and the interests of individual family members (Al-Krenawi, 2002; Haj-Yahia, 1995, 1997).

Irrespective of the intervention method (i.e., family focused, marital focused, or individual focused), members of the nuclear family and nuclear families in the extended family as well as other relatives might want to be involved in the therapeutic process. It is thus essential to exercise caution and remain sensitive to ethical, professional, sociocultural, human rights, and sociopolitical issues when involving family members and relatives in this process. Three examples of issues that should be taken into account throughout intervention with individuals, couples, and families in Palestinian society follow.

First, apparently, the involvement of the family can be a source of support, protection, and resilience and may promote fulfillment of needs and aspirations for individual family members (Beitin & Aprahamian, 2014; Haj-Yahia, 1995, 1996, 2000). Nonetheless, it can also be a barrier to self-actualization for some family members whose needs and aspirations contradict the attitudes, beliefs, values, and aspirations of the family from a social, cultural, religious, and political point of view (Haj-Yahia, 1997, 2000, 2011).

Second, although practitioners are expected to promote harmony in the family, enhance family cohesiveness, promote cooperation among family members, and help the family maintain its good reputation, the family or some of its members may be reluctant to share their problems. In such cases, family members might fear that the professional perspective as well as the ethical and legal obligations of the practitioners will lead to the removal of some family members from the home (e.g., children who are victims of abuse and neglect, a violent husband) or to the breakup of the family (e.g., divorce). They might also fear that the family will be stigmatized because of undesirable social behavior (e.g., harming elderly persons, certain sexual tendencies) or because of problems considered a source of shame (e.g., mental illness among family members).

A third example relates to the barriers to involving family members in interventions. Some family members may ask practitioners to keep certain information confidential from other family members. However, practitioners might believe that they have an ethical, professional, and legal obligation to convey the information to the rest of the family. They may also feel ethically bound to involve legal, health, and/or welfare services.

In addition to the general insights already discussed, several specific challenges derive from some of the components of the structure of the Palestinian family. One component is courtship and marriage, which usually occurs at a relatively young age in Palestinian society (about the mid-20s on average for men and women) (Haj-Yahia, 1995). Both partners may need some advice, guidance, and orientation about intrapersonal, interpersonal, marital, parental, familial, and socioeconomic aspects of marital life and general family dynamics (Haj-Yahia, 1995; Sherif-Trask, 2006). Practitioners can play a particularly important role during engagement by organizing and offering relevant enrichment programs on different aspects of premarital, marital, and family life. Such programs could be run in cooperation with clergy who are involved in the engagement process and are officially responsible for carrying out the engagement in accordance with religious law and sociocultural customs (Haj-Yahia, 1995).

Regarding marital relations, one challenge that should be considered by practitioners is the inequality in marital relations. In light of the extensive and ongoing transitions taking place in Palestinian society in Israel and given the implications of those processes for marital relations, one main challenge for practitioners is to encourage egalitarianism and delegitimize the notion of male supremacy (Crabtree et al., 2008; Daneshpour, 2017; Haj-Yahia, 1995). These attempts might be accompanied by resistance and conflicts because of the patriarchal nature of Palestinian society. As such, some Palestinian men might be unwilling to accept the introduction of these concepts into the therapeutic process (Haj-Yahia, 1995).

Another challenge practitioners face today relates to the extent to which they should encourage women to work outside of the home (especially in poor families and when both partners have middle-to-low levels of education) and the extent to which women should be encouraged to develop careers in nontraditional domains, such as politics. Working wives might not only contribute to the financial well-being of their families, but employment might also promote self-fulfillment and psychological well-being among the women (e.g., positive implications for marital relations and parenting). However, women's employment outside of the home and development of a career can also lead to marital conflicts (Haj-Yahia, 1995). As mentioned, marital conflicts are not viewed favorably in Palestinian society and have the potential to undermine family harmony and cohesiveness that, in turn, might negatively affect the family's reputation. When such conflicts arise, the wife is often expected to submit to her husband's demands and subordinate her own needs and aspirations to those of her husband (Haj-Yahia, 1995, 2000, 2011). Therefore, practitioners must convey the message that spousal conflicts are integral parts of marriage and family life and can be resolved on a mutual basis (e.g., by win-win solutions in which both partners feel satisfied, rather than win-lose solutions, with the wife submitting to her husband's demands) (Haj-Yahia, 1995).

Another challenge relates to the role of both partners' extended families and the impact of their involvement on marital relations and family life in general. Despite the increased cohesiveness of the nuclear family in Palestinian society in Israel, practitioners must be aware of the couple's relationships with their families of origin; the families' resources and availability; the families' expectations from the couple; and pressure exerted by the families to conform to these expectations, often at the expense of the couple's personal and/or interpersonal needs. In this context, practitioners face the challenge of helping young people achieve a balance between maintaining self-respect and pursuing their own needs, goals, and aspirations and satisfying the needs and expectations of their families.

In addition, practitioners should take several challenges into consideration when they intervene in issues related to parent/offspring relations. For example, when they work with parents and children in Palestinian families, practitioners face a dilemma: on the one hand, they seek to develop and promote egalitarian relations within the family and discourage blind obedience and rigid discipline; on the other hand, the expectation that one's parents must be obeyed is an integral part of Palestinian society and culture. However, this expectation contradicts the principle of egalitarian and horizontal communication, as it emphasizes the rigid boundaries between the roles of parent and child (Abudabbeh, 2005; Dwairy, 1998, 2006; Haj-Yahia, 1995; Sharifzadeh, 2011). It is vital to acknowledge this issue in planning the stages and content of interventions with Palestinian parents and offspring. Thus, when practitioners seek to create a violence-free family environment for raising children, in which discipline is enforced without fear or blind obedience, special care should be taken not to harm the therapeutic relationship with the family. In particular, it is important to be sensitive to the parents' need to supervise and control the family and enforce discipline. Yet the practitioner should not express approval of these and other patriarchal dimensions of family life (Haj-Yahia, 1995; Sharifzadeh, 2011).

Regarding interventions in sibling relations, one major insight that should be highlighted is that the intervention plan must consider the significance of gender, age, and position of siblings in the Palestinian family (Dwairy, 1998, 2006; Haj-Yahia, 1995). Factors affecting the boundaries of relations in the Palestinian family in general and relationships among adult siblings in particular include the economic situation and educational level of each sibling (particularly sons and parents) as well as the other relatives residing in the household (particularly parents and grandparents, uncles and aunts). They are also influenced by the geographic proximity of each sibling's home and the extent to which the siblings legitimize the involvement of other siblings in various aspects of their lives and in processes that occur in the family (Dwairy, 1998, 2006; Haj-Yahia, 1995; Sharifzadeh, 2011).

Accordingly, while practitioners should encourage egalitarian relationships among siblings and discourage dominance and blind obedience, they should be careful not to undermine the importance of respect for older siblings. Although these relationships are traditionally hierarchical, they constitute an effective way of maintaining harmony in the Palestinian family without creating unnecessary conflicts. For example, if the practitioner collaborates with one or more siblings in designing interventions to encourage independence and fulfillment of personal aspirations and needs, efforts should be made to ensure that these goals do not weaken or blatantly challenge the importance of interdependence, cooperation, and support among siblings. Considering the collectivistic nature of the Palestinian family, exclusive emphasis on individualistic-oriented goals may endanger the intervention and its outcomes as well as the relationships with siblings who have individualistic aspirations. Because siblings constitute a source of different types of tangible and intangible resources, the importance of this source of support in the intervention cannot be underestimated or ignored (Abudabbeh, 2005; Barakat, 1993; Haj-Yahia, 1995; Sharifzadeh, 2011).

Regarding interventions in cases of divorce, some challenges should be highlighted. First, both of the divorcing partners (but mainly the woman) cope with the social stigma of failing to build a cohesive, harmonious, and conflict-free family. Because Palestinian society views the family as a major institution that is considered sacred, harmony and cohesiveness are fostered among family members, especially among couples. Thus, divorced couples are believed to have failed in this sacred and essential task. The social stigma, the internal sense of failure, and the stressful process of divorce itself (including the legal, economic, financial, religious, sociocultural, familial, and emotional aspects) adversely affect each partner's psychological well-being and impede adjustment to the separation and divorce (Cohen & Savaya, 2003a, 2003b). Thus, practitioners face a complex challenge in interventions with each of the two partners. First, they can play a significant role in alleviating the adverse effects of divorce and in helping the couple cope with the situation by providing support and establishing self-help groups, as well as by enhancing the couple's self-esteem and sense of personal coherence (Cohen & Savaya, 2003a, 2003b). Practitioners should also focus on educating the couple to accept the divorce not as a failure but rather as an option for dealing with spousal problems and even as a potential opportunity for personal growth and for building a new family. In so doing, however, they should be cautious not to appear to be encouraging divorce and undermining the sanctity of the family.

Second, practitioners should work with the families of both partners. Because spousal disputes often have a negative impact on relationships between families, these disputes and tensions also effect the partners' ability to cope with separation and divorce and adjust to it. The tensions also make it difficult for both families to provide the support that the couple needs during this process. In these situations, practitioners can play significant roles by educating the families of origin about the adverse intrapersonal, interpersonal, and familial effects of the divorce. They can also enhance the families' awareness of the vital need to support the couple rather than causing escalation, and they can educate them about helping the partners grow from the conflict and the separation instead of limiting the woman's movements through superfluous investigations and control. Practitioners can try to reconcile and achieve a compromise between the families of origin and help them alleviate tensions and conflicts. In that way, the families can work together to help both partners cope with the separation and its difficult consequences.

Conclusion

In this chapter, I discuss the collectivist nature of the Palestinian family in Israel as reflected in the family identity, in the attitudes and values of the family, and in the daily activities and behavior of family members. I also discuss the structure of the Palestinian family and provide a selective presentation of several insights that mental health practitioners should take into account in their work with Palestinian families in Israel.

The discussion of insights and challenges for practitioners' interventions is based on the analysis of the collectivist nature of the Palestinian family and its structure. My major assumption is that although most aspects of family focused intervention models have been developed and practiced in Western and individualistic societies, they can also be applicable to interventions with Palestinian families. However, in some cases, these models may not be appropriate for intervention with Palestinian families, and they may even harm the families and adversely affect the intervention process (Al-Krenawi, 2002; Dwairy, 1998, 2006; Haj-Yahia, 1995, 2000). The effectiveness of mental health practitioners is, to a large extent, enhanced by their awareness of the sociocultural and sociopolitical contexts of Palestinian society in Israel, as well as by their sensitivity to and active incorporation of these contexts into all phases of the intervention process. Undoubtedly, the practitioners' personal background as well as their professional qualifications and experience can also affect the intervention and play an influential role in determining its effectiveness. For example, in some cases differences between the practitioner and the family (or some family members) in gender and age as well as in sociopolitical and sociocultural attitudes might arouse conflicts, resistance, and opposition to the intervention or to some of its components. Consequently, the entire family or some of its members may feel that the practitioner is insensitive and is not cognizant of their unique values, attitudes, help-seeking behaviors, and patterns of coping with different types of problems or crisis situations (Haj-Yahia, 1995).

Most Palestinian and Jewish mental health practitioners in Israel who work with Palestinian families have been trained at Israeli universities, where the curriculum is based on material developed and practiced in Western individualistic and postindustrial societies. Hence, the sociocultural and sociopolitical differences between Palestinian society and the prevailing Western-oriented content may pose additional conflicts that might be reflected negatively in work with Palestinian families. Practitioners must vitally enhance their awareness of and sensitivity to these differences and to their ramifications for work with Palestinian families. In particular, it is highly important to increase the Palestinian practitioners' awareness of personal changes that they themselves have experienced following their exposure to Western individualistic scientific and professional content and how these changes affect their professional relationships with Palestinian families. Accordingly, these practitioners should have the tools to develop additional socioculturally and sociopolitically sensitive theoretical and practical content appropriate for intervention with Palestinian families. Moreover, these practitioners should be equipped with skills to develop interventions that are sensitive to the significance of the family in Palestinian society and its collectivistic nature and structure.

Rather than presenting a comprehensive intervention model, I offer several insights and challenges based on issues discussed in the chapter that relate to the nature and structure of the Palestinian family. I do not discuss political and sociopolitical issues in Israel, their relevance to the structure and problems of the Palestinian family, and their implications for intervention processes. Therefore, the challenges for intervention proposed here do not include insights that are sensitive to the political and sociopolitical contexts of daily life in Palestinian society and Palestinian families in Israel that may have crucial ramifications for intervention. Although these issues are highly significant, they are beyond the scope of this chapter.

The Arab-Israeli conflict, persisting from the end of the nineteenth century to the present, continues to affect the relationships between the two nations in the region as well as the quality of their lives. For both nations, this violent conflict has been accompanied throughout history by death, loss, and many traumatic experiences. For many Palestinian citizens in Israel, the conflict is particularly distressing in light of the difficulties they have experienced since the establishment of the state. As other chapters in this book show, the founding of the state following the Nakba was accompanied by the destruction of over 430 Palestinian localities and the mass exodus of about seven hundreds of thousands of Palestinian refugees. As an ethnic and national minority, Palestinian citizens in Israel have experienced exclusion, discrimination in all domains of life, rejection, and racism, and they are prevented from involvement in decision making and allocation of resources. In addition, they have experienced traumatic events perpetrated by their state, such as the expropriation of lands and the destruction of homes, besides having poor infrastructure in many areas. The conflict has also caused unemployment, poverty, and other distressing experiences that have undoubtedly affected the quality of life and emotional well-being of Palestinian families. Although this chapter does not deal with the conflict and its implications for Palestinian society or for the Palestinian family in particular, mental health practitioners working with Palestinian families must be aware of and sensitive to the nature of the conflict. They should also be aware of its implications for the quality of life of Palestinian families as well as for the therapeutic encounter, expectations from the therapeutic process, and the quality and nature of their relationship with Palestinian families. As mentioned, more comprehensive exploration of these issues and their impact on the well-being of Palestinian families is necessary and even crucial.

MUHAMMAD M. HAJ-YAHIA is Gordon Brown Chair and Professor of Social Work, Paul Baerwald School of Social Work and Social Welfare, the Hebrew University of Jerusalem, Israel. He is author of *Violence against Women in the Palestinian Society.*

References

Abdul-Haq, A. (2008). The Arab family: Formation, function and dysfunction. In L. S. Nasir & A. K. Abdul-Haq (Eds.), *Caring for Arab patients* (pp. 77–88). Oxford, UK: Radcliffe.

Abu-Baker, K. (2003). Marital problems among Arab families: Between cultural and family therapy interventions. *Arab Studies Quarterly, 25*(4), 53–74.

Abu-Baker, K. (2007). *The Palestinian family in Israel* [in Hebrew]. Ra'anana, Israel: Open University Press.

Abudabbeh, N. (2005). Arab families: An overview. In M. McGoldrick, J. Giordano, & N. Garcia-Preto (Eds.), *Ethnicity and family therapy* (pp. 423–436). New York: Guilford.

Abudabbeh, N., & Aseel, H. A. (1999). Transcultural counseling of Arab Americans. In J. McFadden (Ed.), *Transcultural counseling* (2nd ed., pp. 283–296). Alexandria, VA: American Counseling Association.

Al-Krenawi, A. (2002). Social work with Arab clients in mental health systems [in Hebrew]. *Society and Welfare, 22*, 75–97.

Al-Krenawi, A., & Graham, J. R. (1998). Divorce among Muslim Arab women in Israel. *Journal of Divorce and Remarriage, 29*, 103–119.

Avitzur, M. (1987). The Arab family: Tradition and change [in Hebrew]. In H. Granot (Ed.), *The family in Israel* (pp. 99–115). Jerusalem: Council of Schools of Social Work in Israel.

Barakat, H. (1993). *The Arab world*. Berkeley: University of California Press.

Beitin, B. K., & Aprahamian, M. (2014). Family values and traditions. In S. C. Nassar-McMillan, K. H. Ajrouch, & J. Hakim-Larson (Eds.), *Biopsychosocial perspectives on Arab Americans* (pp. 67–88). New York: Springer.

Cohen, O., & Savaya, R. (1997). "Broken glass": The divorced woman in Moslem Arab society in Israel. *Family Process, 36*(3), 225–245.

Cohen, O., & Savaya, R. (2003a). Adjustment to divorce: A preliminary study among Muslim Arab citizens of Israel. *Family Process, 42*(2), 269–290.

Cohen, O., & Savaya, R. (2003b). Lifestyle differences in traditionalism and modernity and reasons for divorce among Muslim Palestinian citizens of Israel. *Journal of Comparative Family Studies, 34*(2), 283–302.

Crabtree, S. A., Husain, F., & Spalek, B. (2008). *Islam and social work: Debating values, transforming practice*. Bristol, UK: Policy Press.

Daneshpour, M. (2017). *Family therapy with Muslims*. New York: Routledge.

Dwairy, M. A. (1998). *Cross-cultural counseling: The Arab Palestinian case*. New York: Haworth.

Dwairy, M. (2006). *Counseling and psychotherapy with Arabs and Muslims: A culturally sensitive approach*. New York: Teachers College Press.

Haj-Yahia, M. M. (1995). Toward culturally sensitive intervention with Arab families. *Contemporary Family Therapy, 17*(4), 429–447.

Haj-Yahia, M. M. (1996). Wife abuse in the Arab society in Israel: Challenges for future change. In J. L. Edleson & Z. C. Eisikovits (Eds.), *Future interventions with battered women and their families* (pp. 87–101). Thousand Oaks, CA: Sage.

Haj-Yahia, M. M. (1997). Culturally sensitive supervision of Arab social work students in Western universities. *Social Work, 42*(2), 166–174.

Haj-Yahia, M. M. (2000). Wife abuse and battering in the sociocultural context of Arab society. *Family Process, 39*(2), 237–255.

Haj-Yahia, M. M. (2005). On the characteristics of patriarchal societies, gender inequality, and wife abuse: The case of Palestinian society. *Adalah's Newsletter, 20,* 1–6.

Haj-Yahia, M. M. (2011). Contextualizing interventions with battered women in collectivist societies: Issues and controversies. *Aggression and Violent Behavior, 16,* 331–339.

Haj-Yahia, M. M., & Sadan, E. (2008). Issues in intervention with battered women in collectivist societies. *Journal of Marital and Family Therapy, 34*(1), 1–13.

Matsumoto, D. (1996). *Culture and psychology.* Pacific Grove, CA: Brooks/Cole.

Rinnawi, K. (2003). *The Palestinian society in Israel: An ambivalent agenda.* Tel Aviv: The Academic Track, College of Administration.

Sirhan, B. (2005). *Transformations of the Palestinian family in the diaspora: A comparative sociological study.* Beirut: Institute for Palestine Studies.

Savaya, R. (1997). Political attitudes, economic distress, and the utilization of welfare services by Arab women in Israel. *Journal of Applied Social Sciences, 21*(2), 111–121.

Savaya, R. (1998). Associations among economic need, self-esteem, and Israeli-Arab women's attitudes toward and use of professional services. *Social Work, 43*(5), 445–454.

Savaya, R., & Cohen, O. (1998). A qualitative cum quantitative approach to construct definition in a minority population: Reasons for divorce among Israeli Arab women. *Journal of Sociology and Social Welfare, 25,* 125–179.

Savaya, R., & Cohen, O. (2003). Divorce among Moslem Arabs living in Israel: Comparison of reasons before and after the actualization of the marriage. *Journal of Family Issues, 24*(3), 338–351.

Sharifzadeh, V. S. (2011). Families with Middle Eastern roots. In E. W. Lynch & M. J. Hanson (Eds.), *Developing cross-cultural competence* (4th ed., pp. 392–436). Baltimore: Paul H. Brookes.

Sherif, B. (1996). *Unveiling the Islamic family: Concepts of family and gender among upper-middle class Muslim Egyptians* (Unpublished doctoral dissertation). University of Pennsylvania, Philadelphia, PA.

Sherif-Trask, B. (2006). Families in the Islamic Middle East. In B. B. Ingoldsby & S. D. Smith (Eds.), *Families in global and multicultural perspective* (2nd ed., pp. 231–246). Thousand Oaks, CA: Sage.

Shokeid, M. (1993). Ethnic identity and the position of women among Arabs in an Israeli town. In Y. Azmon & D. N. Izraeli (Eds.), *Women in Israel* (pp. 423–441). New Brunswick, NJ: Transaction.

Stanton, M. E. (2006). Patterns of kinship and residence. In B. B. Ingoldsby & S. D. Smith (Eds.), *Families in global and multicultural perspective* (2nd ed., pp. 79–98). Thousand Oaks, CA: Sage.

Triandis, H. C. (1995). *Individualism and collectivism.* Boulder, CO: Westview.

Triandis, H. C. (2001). Individualism-collectivism and personality. *Journal of Personality, 69*(6), 907–924.

Triandis, H. C., Brislin, R., & Hui, C. H. (1988). Cross-cultural training across the individualism-collectivism divide. *International Journal of Intercultural Relations, 12,* 269–289.

7

MENTAL HEALTH ISSUES AMONG PALESTINIAN WOMEN IN ISRAEL

Sarah Abu-Kaf

THIS CHAPTER ADDRESSES MAJOR DETERMINANTS OF MENTAL HEALTH issues among Palestinian women in Israel, including political, social, cultural, and economic factors. Poverty, harsh living conditions, violence, disrupted family relations, polygamy, discrimination and stigma, and employment and working conditions, among other factors, are discussed in the contexts of negative mental health outcomes (e.g., depression, somatization, and anxiety) and positive mental health outcomes (e.g., marital quality, family functioning, life satisfaction, and well-being). The effects of these different determinants are examined with regard to coping resources, coping behaviors, and help-seeking behaviors. This chapter relates to the general Palestinian society in Israel. However, significant differences among subgroups within this society (based on religion and place of residence) also are addressed.

The WHO's *World Health Report 1998* noted that "women's mental health is inextricably linked to their status in society; it benefits from equality and suffers from discrimination" (World Health Organization [WHO], 1998). Women comprise 49.5% of Palestinian citizens in Israel (Israel Central Bureau of Statistics [Israel CBS], 2015). This population is young, and the majority of these women are married. This sector has a lower level of employment (compared to Jewish women and Palestinian men) and faces a difficult economic situation (Israel CBS, 2015; Galilee Society: The Arab National Society for Health, Research and Services [Galilee Society], 2013). Furthermore, Palestinian society in Israel is highly collectivistic and patriarchal, although it is currently undergoing a rapid process of transition (Al-Haj, 1988; Azaiza, 2013; Haj-Yahia-Abu Ahmad, 2006). In this context, inequalities based on gender and age (and, in recent years, also on education) are very common (Al-Haj, 2000; Hofstede & Hofstede, 2005).

It has been stated that investment in the mental health of women is important for the improvement of the mental health of entire populations (Desjarlais, Eisenberg, Good, & Kleinman, 1995). This holds doubly true for Palestinian society, in which women play a crucial role in the mental and physical development of their family members. In this chapter, I provide several recommendations regarding how this population should be approached. I also discuss major issues that should be prioritized in intervention and prevention programs and principles of culturally competent intervention programs. The first section presents the demographic characteristics of Palestinian women in Israel.

The Demography

At the end of 2014, 550,500 Palestinian women aged 15 and over lived in Israel, representing 49.5% of the Palestinian society in Israel (Israel CBS, 2015). Importantly, the Palestinian population in Israel is heterogeneous with regard to religion—comprising Muslims (83%), Christians (9%), and Druze (8%) (Israel CBS, 2015; Gharrah, 2012)—as well as in terms of residential areas, including the northern region of Israel, Haifa, and the central and southern regions. The Palestinian population of the southern region is mainly composed of Palestinian Bedouins (a subgroup of Muslim Palestinians who live in the Negev). The Palestinian population is young, with a median age of 22.6. About 64.0% of the population is 15 years of age or over. This percentage is lower in Palestinian society in the south, where it is 50.9%, and it decreases further to 43.0% among the Palestinian Bedouins who reside in the unrecognized villages in the Negev and increases to 71.3% in ethnically mixed localities (Israel CBS, 2015; Galilee Society, 2013).

The percentage of married women (aged 15 years and over) in Palestinian society in Israel is 62.4%. In 2014 about half of all Palestinian women were mothers of children younger than 17 (compared to 35% of Jewish Israeli women). About 7% of these mothers were heads of single-parent families (Israel CBS, 2015).

With regard to the level of education among Palestinian women, 24.1% have at least some post-high school education compared to 50% of Jewish Israeli women. And 26.7% of Palestinian women have had no more than eight years of schooling, in contrast to 8.5% of Jewish women and 19.5% of Palestinian men in Israel (Israel CBS, 2015).

Epidemiological Studies of Mental Health Problems among Palestinian Women in Israel

In this section, I present three common mental health problems (depression, somatization, and anxiety) at the community level and among women in particular (Gater et al., 1998; Goldberg & Huxley, 1992; Patel, Kirkwood, Pednekar, Weiss, & Mabey, 2006; Piccinelli & Wilkinson, 2000; WHO, 2001). The first large-scale national health survey, conducted in 2003–2004, revealed no significant differences in the 12-month prevalence rates of any anxiety or affective disorder among Palestinians compared to Jewish Israelis. However, the survey indicated significant differences in relation to emotional distress and self-appraisal of mental health. Palestinians reported higher levels of emotional distress and lower self-appraisal of mental health (Levav, Ifrah, Geraisy, Grinshpoon, & Khwaled, 2007).

In 2007–2010, the Israeli Ministry of Health conducted a second large-scale national health survey that included 1,189 Palestinian women. That survey found that 2.2% of Palestinian women suffered from depression and/or anxiety disorders. The prevalence rate of these mental health problems among Palestinian women was lower than that estimated among Jewish women.

It is important to note that the population samples for those surveys were based on telephone lines, and survey data were collected in calls to landline telephones. Thus, the survey sample did not include populations that have no basic infrastructure (such as telephone lines) (Amara & Yiftachel, 2014; Association for Civil Rights in Israel, 2014). As a result, this survey did not include any women who live in unrecognized Bedouin villages or Bedouin villages in the process of becoming recognized (about 50% of the Bedouin Palestinian population) (Amara & Yiftachel, 2014).

Research on the Bedouin Palestinian population indicates a relatively high incidence of mental health problems among this group. For instance, a 2008 report of Physicians for Human Rights in Israel found that Bedouin Palestinian women in the Negev, especially those living in unrecognized villages, suffer from high levels of emotional distress, most of which is manifested as depression and anxiety. That report identified a prevalence rate of depression of 31%; anxiety, 30%; and low self-esteem, 27% (Physicians for Human Rights, 2008).

Kaplan et al. (2010) conducted another study that included Palestinian women from the Hadera area (in central Israel) and found that depression rates were 2.5 times greater among Muslim women participants in that study than among Jewish women. Interestingly, depression rates increased as a function of age, with Muslim women suffering substantially more than Jewish women later in life. Higher education and reported professional prestige acted as buffers against the negative association of ethnicity on depression.

In addition, the second national health survey showed a high rate of use of primary health services (46.1%) among Palestinian women compared to Jewish women and Palestinian men (38.2% and 37.7%, respectively). This finding may be related to the tendency to somaticize (instead of psychologize) distress, which is commonly observed in non-Western collectivistic cultures, such as the Palestinian culture (Abu-Kaf & Shahar, 2017; Hamdi, Amin, & Abou-Saleh, 1997; Kleinman, 2004; Sethi, 1986). Symptoms such as back pain, headache, gastrointestinal disturbances, musculoskeletal pain, fatigue, dizziness, and other physical complaints are the leading reasons for outpatient visits and are associated with substantial disability and health-care utilization (Spitzer et al., 1994). Cwikel, Lev-Wiesel, and Al-Krenawi (2003) found more support for this pattern of primary health service use among Palestinian Bedouin women. They examined health-care use of 202 Palestinian Bedouin women aged 22–75. These women had visited a doctor 10.2 times on average in the last year for health-care needs (range of visits was 0–50). This is a relatively high number of visits. As the socioeconomic level decreased, so did the percentage of women who did not turn to medical care for attention when needed. In addition, the more children a woman had, the more she visited the doctor. Women living in recognized villages visited the doctor more often than women living in unrecognized villages (11.8 visits vs. 8.6 visits, respectively) (Cwikel et al., 2003).

Determinants of Mental Health Issues among Palestinian Women in Israel

Major determinants of mental health issues among Palestinian women in Israel include political, economic, social, and cultural factors. Clearly, these factors are associated with and affected by one another. For instance, the political status of the Palestinian minority in Israel affects its economic status (participation in the workforce, lower income, and lower educational attainment) (Knesset Research and Information Center [Knesset RIC], 2016; Okun & Friedlander, 2005). This is also true of social factors (inferior social position, social exclusion, and intense conflictual relationship with the Jewish majority) (Ben-Ari, 2004; Ghanem, 2001; Keshet & Popper-Giveon, 2016).

Sociopolitical Determinants

The involuntary sociopolitical minority status experienced by Palestinians, which began with the establishment of the state of Israel in 1948, is believed to affect most aspects of their lives and, to a large extent, their health. As a minority group in Israel, Palestinians have experienced oppression, social exclusion, and related socioeconomic and political problems (Ghanem, 2001; Okun & Friedlander, 2005; Pinson, 2007; Yiftachel, 2009). This population is significantly disadvantaged compared to the Jewish population in terms of quality and quantity of educational and social services as well as in the development and industrialization of the Palestinian communities (Ben-Ari, 2004). Two different examples illustrate how discriminatory policies can have strong negative effects on different resources and protective factors among Palestinians in general, and Palestinian women in particular. The first refers to basic infrastructure and public transportation in Palestinian villages and cities in Israel, which are significantly inferior to those found in Jewish communities (Knesset RIC, 2016). Public transportation is essential for the day-to-day needs of a population—for example, work, education, commerce, and leisure. Different reports have shown that the limited availability or complete lack of public transportation in Palestinian communities is one of the barriers facing Palestinian women who want to enter the workforce (Keinan & Bar, 2007; Knesset RIC, 2016).

According to data from the Israel Ministry of Finance, in 2015 a large gap existed in the budgets directed to the Palestinian population compared to the Jewish population. For instance, only 7% of the annual budget for subsidies was directed to public transportation lines that serve the populations of Palestinian cities (Israel Ministry of Finance, 2015).

The second example concerns the large inequalities in early childhood education in Palestinian society compared to Jewish society. In 2003, 1,700 day-care centers functioned under the supervision of the Israel Ministry of Labor and Welfare, but only 36 of those centers were located in Palestinian communities. These day-care centers offer full-day programs for children whose mothers work and for children who have been referred to the centers by social services. A recent report of the State Comptroller of Israel (2015) points to a serious lack of preschools in Palestinian communities in general and in Palestinian Bedouin communities in particular. The physical condition of the facilities used by the existing programs in these communities is inferior and inappropriate for the children's developmental activities (State Comptroller of Israel, 2015). The lack of programs and solutions for preschool education is a significant issue that may discourage Palestinian women from pursuing further education and seeking employment. This fact is all the more significant as the majority of Palestinian women marry and become mothers at a relatively young age (in their early twenties) (Israel CBS, 2015).

Sociopolitical minority status may have a direct impact on health. Subjective and objective experiences of discrimination and racism may increase levels of stress experienced by members of minority groups, which can adversely affect their health (Williams, 1999). The continuing Palestinian-Israeli conflict has left the Palestinian minority under considerable stress and subject to expressions of discrimination that have adverse effects on their health (Ben-Ari, 2004; Epel, Kaplan, & Moran, 2010; Keshet & Popper-Giveon, 2016; Levav et al., 2007).

One of the most discriminatory practices experienced by the Palestinian population in general, and particularly among the Bedouins in the south, is that of house demolitions. In 2014, 859 houses, deemed illegal by the Israeli government, were demolished in Bedouin communities (Ziadna, 2013). For women, this practice is particularly depressing as the home is considered the woman's private and social space. Gottlieb and Feder-Bubis (2014) conducted 12 interviews with women and families from unrecognized Bedouin villages. The home is often the source of identity for women in collectivist societies, and they reported personal and collective trauma as a result of potential home demolitions. House demolitions elicited fear, feelings of helplessness, and, at times, included physical violence. Women are more affected by these processes because of their role in the family as the mother and their practice of staying at home and nurturing the home most of the day (Gottlieb & Feder-Bubis, 2014). Daoud and Jabareen (2014) examined depressive symptoms among Bedouin women following house demolitions in the Negev. In that study, 27% of 464 participants were under threat of house demolition. The findings indicate that the threat of house demolition is a stronger predictor of depressive symptoms than women's socioeconomic position (i.e., education level or income).

Economic Determinants

Compared to Israeli Jews, Palestinians are disadvantaged in terms of almost every socioeconomic indicator. They have lower incomes, higher levels of unemployment, and lower educational attainment (Okun & Friedlander, 2005). In 2015 the rate of workforce participation among Palestinian women aged 25–64 (31.5%) was significantly lower than the rates observed for Palestinian men and Jewish women of the same age (74.2% and 79.7%, respectively) (Knesset RIC, 2016).

Importantly, although there is a high rate of part-time employment among women who are in the workforce, that is not by choice and they desire full-time jobs. In 2015 the number of Palestinian women working part-time not by choice was 35.2% compared to 11.6% among Jewish women (Israel CBS, 2016; Knesset RIC, 2015). According to figures from the Israel CBS (2015), in 2014 the average gross monthly salary for Jewish women aged 25–64 was 45% higher than that of Palestinian women (7,633 shekels vs. 5,271 shekels, respectively).

With regard to employment, Palestinian women encounter mixed obstacles— that is, they face barriers because of their gender as well as barriers related to their Palestinian membership. Different reports and studies mention a lack of sufficient transportation to the areas in which jobs are located, as well as the low number of jobs present inside Palestinian localities, informal and structural discrimination (rules, norms, attitudes) by employers, and the need to care for relatively large numbers of children (young children in particular). These women also face a lack of day-care centers. Other barriers to the employment of Palestinian women include low salaries; lack of professional consultation and direction, education, and professional skills; limited knowledge of Hebrew; and different social conceptions regarding the role of women in the family (Keinan & Bar, 2007; Knesset RIC, 2015).

The lower level of education among this population and the difficulty of finding employment have severe implications for the economic situation of Palestinian women. In one survey, 25% of women reported being in a difficult or very difficult economic situation (Galilee Society, 2013). In addition, women become financially dependent on social welfare services, national insurance, and/or other family members.

Social and Cultural Determinants

Different social and cultural factors affect the mental health and well-being of Palestinian women. These include characteristics and values of Arab culture and social factors such as consanguineous marriages, polygamy, and violence. Palestinian society demonstrates a large degree of power distance. Palestinians accept a hierarchical order in which everybody has a set place that needs no further justification (Hofstede & Hofstede, 2005). Inequalities are common, based on gender and age: male over female and the older over the younger (Backer, 1983; Barakat, 1993; Haj-Yahia-Abu Ahmad, 2006; Patai & DeAtkine, 1973). However, in recent years, an additional variable related to educational level has been added to these inequalities—educated individuals now have more power over less-educated individuals. These values may affect the sense of power and levels of stress experienced by young people and female individuals. Moreover, Palestinian society endorses collectivism, with particular concern for relationships and their maintenance (Al-Haj, 1988, 2000; Haj-Yahia, 2000; Haj-Yahia-Abu Ahmad, 2006). Individuals are interdependent within their respective in-group, mainly the family, and they do what their in-group expects of them.

People in collectivistic cultures generally prefer methods of conflict resolution that do not dismantle relationships, even at the expense of their needs or personal interests (Triandis, 2001). In these societies, child-rearing practices stress security, conformity, and reliability (Hofstede & Hofstede, 2005). In terms of family structure, social roles in Palestinian families are still influenced by the patriarchal power structure: men have more power in relation to their wives, sisters, and daughters (Haj-Yahia, 2000). Furthermore, Haj-Yahia (2000) mentioned that despite women becoming stronger in terms of employment outside the home and their increased financial independence, it is still commonly accepted that women are caregivers and should look after family members, particularly those who suffer from physical or mental illnesses. Additionally, women's health is a lower priority than the health of other family members (Douki, Zineb, Nacef, & Halbreich, 2007; WHO, 2000). Palestinian women play active roles in their households. They are expected to be good daughters, good wives, and good mothers. Women are likely to lose the conditional support of their family if they do not meet the aforementioned expectations (Haj-Yahia, 2000). However, in the public sector and the broad social domain, their role is quite limited (Abu-Baker, 1998).

In Palestinian society, marriage is considered a family and social issue, with marriage connecting not only two individuals but two families (Barakat, 1993). Thus, the family plays a major part in the choice of spouse, the wedding arrangements, and even in family planning decisions (Lev-Wiesel & Al-Krenawi, 1999).

CONSANGUINEOUS MARRIAGES

The rate of marriages between relatives has decreased, but as of 2010, about one-third (31%) of marriages were consanguineous—that is, between relatives (Israel Center for Disease Control [ICDC], 2010; RHA Center for Bedouin Studies and Development, 2010). The factors that have been found to be related to this marriage pattern are living in rural communities, low socioeconomic status, low level of education, younger age, and the existence of family ties between the parents of the couple (ICDC, 2010). This marriage pattern shows the strong influence of parents and the extended family over young couples. Moreover, this pattern of marriage is related to health problems and hereditary illnesses (ICDC, 2010; Jaber & Halpern, 2006), presenting a particular burden for mothers and daughters, who are the main caregivers for the extended and nuclear family. However, consanguineous marriages may also provide protection and support from the husband's family because of familiarity with the future spouse before the marriage (Alfayumi-Zeadna, Kaufman-Shriqui, Zeadna, Lauden, & Shoham-Vardi, 2015; Sandridge, Takeddin, Al-Kaabi, & Frances, 2010).

POLYGAMY

Another practice that exists among Palestinian families, particularly Bedouin Palestinian families, is polygamy. Among Bedouin women of the Negev, the transition from monogamous to polygamous family structure can be a traumatic change for the senior wife, eliciting reactions similar to those that follow divorce, with mourning and low self-esteem being common (Al-Krenawi, 1999; Slonim-Nevo & Al-Krenawi, 2006). Polygamy may contribute to mental health adversities through the family environment. Polygamous marriage has been associated with increased family stress because of greater stressors in the lives of those involved that may be relational (jealousy and acrimony between the families) (Al-Krenawi, 1999) or economic, as polygamous marriages contain greater numbers of children but not necessarily an increase in income (Al-Krenawi, 1998; Al-Krenawi & Graham, 1999a, 1999b, 2006). Furthermore, women in a polygamous relationship reported greater psychological distress, anxiety, depression, hostility, paranoid ideations, somatic complaints, experiences of loneliness, and lower self-esteem (Al-Krenawi, 2001; Al-Krenawi & Graham, 2006; Daoud, Braun-Lewensohn, Eriksson, & Sagy, 2014); increased domestic violence (Al-Krenawi & Lev-Wiesel, 2002; Maziak & Asfar, 2003) and emotional abuse (Hassouneh-Phillips, 2001); as well as lower levels of family functioning and marital satisfaction (Al-Krenawi & Graham, 2006, 2011). Polygamy may contribute to poor family functioning, which in turn leads to mental health symptoms among women (Al-Krenawi & Slonim-Nevo, 2008). Palestinian Bedouin women in polygamous marriages reported poor health (Daoud, Shoham-Vardi, Urquia, & O'Campo, 2014) and greater use of health services (Al-Krenawi, 2004).

On the positive side, social support and the development of good relations between co-wives have been found to be protective factors against the negative effects of this type of marriage. Since the stresses in polygamous marriages are often relational (i.e., feuds between husband and wife, different children, and/or co-wives), the presence of social support and good relations between co-wives may substantially minimize stressors and, as a result, improve outcomes (Daoud, Shoham-Vardi, et al., 2014).

VIOLENCE

In a national survey conducted in 2001 that included 2,544 women, the prevalence of different forms of intimate partner violence (IPV) among Palestinian women in

Israel was found to be higher than that among Jewish women (Eisikovits, Winstok, & Fishman, 2004). A survey conducted during 2016 provided additional support for this finding. This latter research was based on a representative sample of 1,401 women aged 16–48 who were surveyed during their visits to 72 well-baby clinics in five districts in Israel. The research found that IPV is a common phenomenon in all sectors of society, although low-income families reported a higher rate of incidents. Among Palestinian women, the instances of violence were higher in families with a greater degree of religiosity and in families living in urban rather than rural localities. Furthermore, this research found that Palestinian women reported more IPV of all types compared to their Jewish counterparts. Among the surveyed Palestinian women, 11% reported physical violence, 50% reported psychological or verbal violence, and 50% reported social violence (isolating the woman from her support networks) or economic violence(restricting the women's access to economic resources). Among the surveyed Jewish women, the respective results were 2%, 19%, and 16% (Daoud & Shoham-Vardi, 2016).

IPV was linked to higher rates of postpartum depression (PPD), symptoms of depression and anxiety, and other health problems, such as miscarriages and premature births, among both Palestinian and Jewish women. The association between IPV and health problems was stronger among the Palestinian women (Daoud & Shoham-Vardi, 2016). Explanations for the higher prevalence rate of this phenomenon include social factors such as gender roles within the patriarchal culture, a cultural context that underscores the values of family integrity and superiority in the national group over the well-being and physical security of the individual, social exclusion, and higher rates of poverty and violence in the community (Haj-Yahia, 2001; Haj-Yahia & Peled, 2013; Levinson, 1989; Malley-Morrison & Hines, 2004).

Mental Health Issues among Palestinian Women across Different Age Groups

The prevalence of mental health challenges and problems varies across age groups. This section discusses mental health issues among Palestinian women during three important stages of development: in adolescence, as young adults in higher education settings, and during the period of fertility. Each age group may be affected by different risk and protective factors that may contribute to different levels of mental health problems.

Palestinian Female Adolescents

About 16% of Palestinian women are adolescents (15–19 years) (Israel CBS, 2016). Few studies of mental health issues have been done among this population (Azaiza, 2006; Daeem et al., 2016; Grinstein-Weiss, Fishman, & Eisikovits, 2005; Guterman, Haj-Yahia, Vorhies, Ismayilova, & Leshem, 2010; Mansbach-Kleinfeld et al., 2010; Shechory-Bitton & Kamel, 2014).

One preliminary study (Azaiza, 2006) explored perceptions of the concept of adolescent girls in distress among Palestinian female adolescents aged 13–18. In terms of their understanding of the concept, two main themes emerged from the data. First, for survey participants, the term "adolescent girls in distress" refers to (a) girls who have a problem, mainly familial but also social, personal or emotional, and abusive (physically or sexually); and (b) girls who have no one to turn to when in need. About 12% of the respondents identified themselves as adolescent girls in distress. Risk factors found to be related to the subjective experience of being a girl in distress derived from a large family (a family with more than seven children) and a home atmosphere rife with tension, conflict, and fighting (Azaiza, 2006).

When those female adolescents were asked to whom they would turn in case of need, more than half (57.4%) chose family members, particularly their mothers (48.9%). A 12% reported that they would turn to a friend, and 8% cited professionals. Surprisingly, the second most frequent category was "I don't turn to anyone when I am in need" (21.2%) (Azaiza, 2006, p. 195).

Shechory-Bitton and Kamel (2014) conducted a study among 120 Palestinian female adolescents living in Israel that included those defined as at-risk by the Israeli welfare authorities and normative adolescent females studying at regular schools. That study examined sociodemographic variables and levels of traditionalism, self-control, and aggression. The results showed that at-risk female adolescents tended to come from larger families with less-educated parents and harsh economic circumstances. A higher school dropout rate and more contact with delinquent peer groups were found among these teens compared to those in the comparison group. Twenty-five percent of the participants in the at-risk group had been exposed to violence and drug use (mainly of family members), and about 12% of those girls had run away from home, while none of the girls in the comparison group had done so. Moreover, levels of self-control and traditionalism were found to be lower among the at-risk girls compared to participants in the other group. In contrast, levels of aggression were higher among the at-risk participants. Furthermore, aggression levels among daughters of less-educated fathers were higher, whereas daughters of more educated fathers showed higher levels of self-control and traditionalism. No relationships were found between religiosity and the research variables of aggression, self-control, and traditionalism (Shechory-Bitton & Kamel, 2014).

A limited number of studies have been conducted to examine the willingness of Palestinian adolescents to seek help in times of distress. These studies have found ethnic differences and gender similarities (particularly among Palestinians). Grinstein-Weiss et al. (2005) examined the willingness to seek formal versus informal help among 6,017 Palestinian and Jewish adolescents who were living in a very stressful environment with a constant threat of terror. They found that the Palestinian adolescents were more likely to seek formal help (from social workers, psychologists, family doctors, and school teachers) and help from the family (parents, siblings, and relatives) compared to Jewish adolescents. However, the Palestinians were less likely to look for help from friends. In this research, gender differences related to the willingness to seek help were found only among the Jewish group (Jewish males were less likely to seek help) (Grinstein-Weiss et al., 2005).

More support for the pattern of results related to the greater willingness of Palestinian adolescents to seek help was found in a study conducted by Guterman et al. (2010). These researchers examined prevalence of help seeking as well as internal barriers to help seeking in the wake of exposure to community violence, adolescents' personal victimization, and witnessing of community violence in the past year. The 1,835 participants in the study included 858 Palestinian and 977 Jewish adolescents, with a female majority in both samples. The findings indicated more exposure to community violence among the Palestinian youth. The researchers also found a tendency among adolescents not to seek help in the wake of exposure to community violence. However, this tendency was stronger among the Jewish youths than among the Palestinian youths. (Only one in three Palestinian and one in four Jewish adolescents reported seeking help from anyone following their exposure to violence.) With regard to internal obstacles, Palestinian adolescents endorsed internal obstacles more frequently than Jewish adolescents did, with over half responding "yes" to seven different obstacles (in contrast to only two items endorsed by more than half of the Jewish respondents). For example, Palestinian adolescents most frequently noted that they "thought their feelings would go away" if they did not turn to someone for help or that they "did not want others to know what happened." In contrast, Jewish adolescents most frequently noted that they felt they "did not need help from anyone else" and they "did not think what happened was very important." (Guterman et al., 2010, p. 692). The authors suggested that the more frequent and severe exposure to violence among the Palestinian adolescents might partially explain their significantly higher rates of help seeking (Guterman et al., 2010). Together, these studies suggest that help from formal and informal sources may have been more commonly sought when adolescents were in distress.

Palestinian Women in Higher Education Settings

The percentage of Palestinian university students in Israel has risen significantly in recent years. According to an Israel CBS report (2016), in the 2015–2016 academic year, 37,800 Palestinian students were enrolled in institutions of higher education, and a majority of those Palestinian students were female (67.3%). Increased numbers of Palestinian women were observed among those studying for both undergraduate and advanced degrees. Previous research has shown that minority groups in multinational and multicultural societies will often attribute great importance to the pursuit of higher education, believing that it will help them to lift their status from the margins of society and avoid unemployment (Branch, 2001; David, 2007). Accordingly, Palestinian citizens in Israel consider education, and higher education in particular, to be a key element for personal and collective development, as well as a significant tool for political empowerment (Al-Haj, 2003; Arar & Abu-Asbah, 2010).

Adapting to new educational and social environments may be even more stressful for students who have different cultural values, language, academic preparation, and study habits (Mori, 2000; Zwingmann, Gunn, & WHO, 1983). Research indicates that 15.5% of Palestinian students in Israeli universities fail to finish their first academic year, and the percentage of Palestinian graduates is lower than the percentage of Jewish graduates. Researchers claim that political, economic, social, cultural, and psychological factors underlie these dropout statistics (Arar & Mustafa, 2011). Palestinian citizens in Israel have a separate K–12 educational system that endeavors to preserve Arabic language, traditions, and culture. In this school system, Hebrew is taught as a second language starting in third grade, and English is taught as a third language starting in fourth grade (Geiger, 2013). Palestinian students come from a different culture and speak a different language, and this might cause them to feel socially isolated and discriminated against when they reach university (Ben-Ari, 2004). A comparison study has found that Palestinian university students experience stress more acutely than their Jewish counterparts and consider some aspects of their academic life to be challenging, stressful, and even threatening (Zeidner, 1992). In addition to the fact that Palestinian students are less academically prepared than their Jewish Israeli peers (Ben-Ari & Azaiza, 1996; Haj-Yahia, 1997; Manzar, 1999), they also experience nonacademic personal, social, and cultural stress during their time at university (Ben-Ari, 2004). Palestinian students in Israel may face more difficulties than other foreign groups as they belong to an ethnic and racial minority, often experience marginalization as a result of culture and politics, and may find themselves, perhaps for the first time, in a cultural context different from their own (Jackson, 1998; Nishimura, 1998; Renn, 2000). Despite limited studies on the acculturation stress of Palestinian students in Israel, an attempt to examine this topic was offered by Geiger (2013), who found that female Palestinian students lack self-confidence and have poor mastery of the Hebrew language, which makes them feel marginalized by Jewish students. Furthermore, Palestinian women (particularly Muslims and Druze) usually wear distinctive clothing and have clear social boundaries and attitudes (Joseph, 1994). These women may experience additional adversity. Their distinctive clothing, which is often negatively stereotyped (Janson, 2011), can be a daily challenge that emphasizes their foreignness and limits their mobility. As a result, they may face social isolation (Benbenishty & Astor, 2005). Consequently, female Palestinian students may experience emotional distress and suffer negative adjustment to academic life.

Support for this claim is found in a recent study that examined relationships between depressive symptoms and somatic complaints among Palestinian Bedouin students in institutions of higher education in southern Israel. Of the 190 individuals who participated in that study, 89 were Palestinian Bedouin students and 101 were Jewish students. Two assessment waves, one year apart, were applied. At both Time 1 and Time 2, the Palestinian Bedouin participants' mean score on the Center for Epidemiological Studies Depression Scale (CES-D) was close to the stricter diagnostic cutoff point of 23 (in the total score) among both males and females.

A high prevalence of depressive symptoms was found among the Palestinian Bedouin group, particularly among Palestinian Bedouin women. At Time 1, 50% of the male Palestinian Bedouin participants and 60% of the female Palestinian Bedouin participants reported severe levels of depressive symptoms. Among the Jewish group, at Time 1, 16.7% of the male participants and 17% of the female participants reported severe levels of depressive symptoms. One year later, a decrease in the prevalence of depressive symptoms was observed only among the female Palestinian students (47%), but even at that time, about half of those students still reported severe levels of depressive symptoms (Abu-Kaf & Shahar, 2017). These results can be partially attributed to greater use of avoidant strategies for coping with stress (Abu-Kaf & Braun-Lewensohn, 2015; Abu-Kaf & Priel, 2008). Depressive symptoms have been found to affect learning and memory processes, leading to lower levels of academic achievement (Hysenbegasi, Hass, & Rowland, 2005), poor school attendance, failure to complete the academic degree (Hammen, Rudolph, Weisz, Rao, & Burge, 1999), dropping out of the academic institution (King & Bernstein, 2001), and even suicidal ideation (Garlow et al., 2008).

Coping Resources and Strategies among Female Palestinian Students

SOCIAL SUPPORT

Stress theory suggests that social and emotional support may serve as a major resource for coping with stressful situations (Lazarus & Folkman, 1984). Previous research has been conducted to examine social support among Palestinian students in Israeli universities. However, the majority of these studies included small samples of Palestinian students and did not pay any special attention to gender differences related to this resource (Ben-Ari, 2004; Ben-Ari & Gil, 2004; Ben-Ari & Pines, 2002; Pines, Ben-Ari, Utasi, & Larson, 2002). These studies have yielded three main findings: (a) higher levels of different types of social support are reported by Palestinian students compared to Jewish students, (b) Palestinian students tend to turn to family members in time of need (spouse, mother, father, and siblings), and (c) Palestinians reported significantly more often than Jews that they would turn to "no one" for support (Kaplan et al., 2010; Pines & Zaidman, 2003, p. 473). The tendency of Palestinians to turn to their nuclear families when facing a range of problems (from mild depression, to a need for advice about a job or other life change, to the need for a loan) was interpreted as reflective of a collectivist cultural orientation, with its ideals of familial solidarity and support (Haj-Yahia, 1997). However, the finding related to the Palestinians' greater tendency to turn to no one reflects the strong cultural interdiction among Palestinians against the "shameful" disclosure of personal affairs (Al-Haj, 1987; Barakat, 1985; Savaya, 1997, 1998, p. 205). Requesting assistance from others may involve exposing one's vulnerability and/or incompetence and risking rejection (Taylor et al., 2004). More support for the third finding is found in two studies carried out by Abu-Kaf and colleagues (Abu-Kaf & Braun-Lewensohn, 2015; Abu-Kaf & Priel, 2012), which showed that Palestinian Bedouin female students experience significantly lower levels of social support than their Jewish counterparts. This finding may be explained by the strong tendency among Palestinians not to disclose their personal problems and difficulties to others and by the fact that these Bedouin students are the first generation of their families to get a higher education. Thus, their nuclear families do not have the tools and knowledge to help them cope with academic stress. The availability of social support as a coping strategy in times of stress is greatly affected by a lack of enthusiasm for using it (Abu-Kaf & Braun-Lewensohn, 2015).

COPING STRATEGIES

Coping includes regulatory processes that can reduce the negative feelings that result from stressful events. Active coping strategies are behavioral or psychological responses designed to change the nature of the stressor itself or how one thinks about it, whereas avoidant coping strategies lead people into activities (such as alcohol use) or mental states (such as withdrawal) that keep them from directly addressing stressful events (Holahan & Moos, 1987). Active coping strategies are more effective in reducing negative psychological well-being (Braun-Lewensohn et al., 2009), and avoidant coping strategies tend to be associated with psychological distress (Braun-Lewensohn, Sagy, & Roth, 2010; Lambert, Lambert, & Ito, 2004).

Gender differences have been found in both active and avoidant coping, as females scored higher in both active and avoidant coping compared to their male counterparts (Abu-Kaf & Braun-Lewensohn, 2015). This is consistent with previous literature that has noted that coping mechanisms may be gender-specific (Folkman & Lazarus, 1980) and that females tend to face higher levels of stress that are associated with the use of more coping resources than males (Tamres, Janicki, & Helgeson, 2002). Abu-Kaf and Braun-Lewensohn (2015) confirmed that female students report higher levels of active coping than male students. They found that female students tend to use social support, emotional regulation, affective release, and emotion-focused strategies to a greater extent than males. Taylor et al. (2000) also noted that females tend to cope using social support—"the-tend-and-befriend response"(p. 423) to stress—emotion-focused strategies, affective release, and emotional regulation, whereas male coping efforts tend to be directed toward gaining control over the situation and disengagement.

Abu-Kaf and Braun-Lewensohn (2015) observed a higher level of avoidant coping among female Bedouin students compared to male Bedouin students. Understanding that females suffer disproportionately from life stressors is essential to highlighting gender differences in personal methods of coping and/ or efforts to overcome stressful situations (Lazarus & Folkman, 1984). In other words, the greater number of life stressors that females experience can be associated with the use of more coping mechanisms, whether avoidant or active (Tamres et al., 2002). Furthermore, avoidant coping strategies were found to play an important role in the development of mental health problems such as depressive symptoms.

Abu-Kaf and Braun-Lewensohn (2015) were interested in examining the potential pathways between vulnerability factors and depression among Palestinian Bedouin and Jewish students. Among Bedouin students, the effect of self-criticism is amplified through the indirect effects of avoidant coping. The self-critical Palestinian Bedouins tend to be more depressed because they tend to use avoidant coping strategies more often—that is, they attempt to reduce tension by avoiding dealing with problems (i.e., behavioral disengagement, self-distraction, denial, and self-blame) (Abu-Kaf & Braun-Lewensohn, 2015). More support for the important role of avoidant coping strategies, particularly among female Palestinian students, is found in the research of Khalaf and Abu-Kaf (2016). Khalaf and Abu-Kaf (2016) wanted to investigate the relationships between acculturation stress and depression among Palestinian students at institutions of higher education in northern and central Israel. Furthermore, they were interested in testing the roles of sense of coherence (SOC), social support, and different types of coping strategies (active and avoidant) in these relationships. They found that among female Palestinian students, avoidant coping and SOC each mediate the relationship between acculturation stress and depression.

Palestinian Women and Fertility

The fertility of Palestinian women (i.e., the average number of children a woman is expected to have during her lifetime) is experiencing a declining trend and varies across different religious groups and areas of residence. In 2014 the fertility rate of Muslim women, 3.4, was higher than that of other religious groups: Christians, 2.3; and Druze, 2.2. The highest fertility rate among Muslim women, 5.5 children per woman, was recorded among those living in the southern region, and the lowest, 2.8 children per woman, was recorded among those in the northern, Haifa, and central regions (Israel CBS, 2015).

Several studies have attempted to assess the scope of postpartum depressive symptoms (PPDS) among postnatal Palestinian women from different subpopulations. The rate of postnatal depression among Palestinian women in Israel is higher than that seen among Jewish Israeli women (Alfayumi-Zeadna et al., 2015; Eilat-Tsanani et al., 2006; Glasser, Stoski, Kneler, & Magnezi, 2011; Glasser et al., 2012). Differences between Palestinian subgroups have been found by area of residence and religion. The highest rates of PPDS were found among Palestinian Bedouin women in the south (range 32%–43%) (Alfayumi-Zeadna et al., 2015; Glasser et al., 2011). A moderate rate was found among Palestinian women in the central region (24.7%), and the lowest rates among Palestinian women were in the north (range 12.2%–16.3%,) (Glasser, 2010; Glasser et al., 2012). Moreover, the rate of PPDS was significantly higher among women living in Muslim versus Druze communities

(Edinburgh Postnatal Depression Scale [EPDS] ≥ 10: 19.0% vs. 13.4%, respectively) (Glasser et al., 2012).

Alfayumi-Zeadna et al. (2015) examined risk factors for the development of PPDS among Palestinian Bedouin women in the Negev. Over one year, they recruited 564 women, four weeks to seven months postdelivery, in eight maternal and child-health clinics in the Negev. The women were interviewed at the clinics.

Higher levels of PPDS were associated with chronic illness of the infant (four times more likely), history of emotional problems, low spousal social support, below-average income, a low level of education, unplanned pregnancy, marital conflict, and being unemployed or spouse being unemployed. Among women living in consanguineous marriages, the prevalence of PPDS was lower. This is consistent with studies showing that marriage within the family is a source of support and protection against depressive symptoms, partially a result of support from the husband's family and familiarity of the spouses (Alfayumi-Zeadna et al., 2015; Sandridge et al., 2010). Among women living in polygamous marriages, the prevalence of PPDS was higher, but there was no significant difference between the prevalence of PPDS among new mothers in polygamous versus monogamous marriages. These findings highlight the need to monitor emotional symptoms in this population to reduce chances of the development of postnatal depression.

CHILDBIRTH EXPERIENCES AMONG PALESTINIAN WOMEN

Halperin, Sarid, and Cwikel (2014) examined Palestinian and Jewish women's perceptions of their birth experiences. They were interested in assessing the extent to which aspects of childbirth and perceptions predict satisfaction with the birth experience and how traumatic women find the childbirth experience. This study was conducted in postpartum units of two major public hospitals in northern Israel. The sample included 171 respondents comprising 115 Jewish Israeli and 56 Palestinian women from Israel. The Palestinian women were much less likely to have attended childbirth preparation classes than the Jewish women (5% vs. 24%). The rate of self-reported traumatic birth was significantly higher among the Palestinian women than among the Jewish women (32% vs. 14%). A higher percentage of Palestinian women reported being afraid during labor, expressed fear for their newborn's safety, and reported that the level of medical intervention was excessive in their opinion compared to the Jewish women (Halperin et al., 2014).

To investigate the childbirth experiences of Jewish and Palestinian Bedouin women in terms of self-reported pain compared to exhibited pain, as interpreted by the attending obstetrician and midwife, Sheiner et al. (1999) approached 447 Palestinian Bedouin and Jewish women who gave birth during a six-month period and were interviewed by an obstetrician. Most of the Bedouin women defined themselves as religious or traditional, and about two-thirds of the Jewish women were secular. The Bedouin women were younger, had more children, had less formal education, had not attended childbirth preparation classes, and usually had no spouse present during birth. The practitioners perceived the Bedouin mothers as experiencing less pain, and practitioners were less prepared to offer epidural anesthesia to these service users. Epidural anesthesia was offered more often to Jewish mothers. The authors explained these biases in terms of the difficulty of recognizing pain in a member of a different, stigmatized cultural and ethnic group. The number of previous childbirths a mother has had could be another factor influencing the practitioners' pain perceptions. The level of pain experienced may decrease with more deliveries (Sheiner et al., 1999).

To sum up, a higher prevalence of PPDS is well documented among Palestinian women, particularly among Muslims in the south (Bedouins). Palestinian patients are younger, less educated, and less prepared for delivery. Their experiences during labor are characterized by higher levels of anxiety and fear. In addition, during their labor, they are often subject to biases and discriminating attitudes from Jewish obstetricians and midwives. Risk factors for PPDS are chronic illness of the infant, history of emotional problems, low spousal social support, below-average income, a low level of education, unplanned pregnancy, and marital conflicts. Protective factors include higher levels of education, social support, and consanguineous marriages.

PPD has a negative effect on the health and the quality of life of the mother and her newborn and has been found to affect the mother's attitude toward and care of her baby (Righetti-Veltema, Conne-Perréard, Bousquet, & Manzano, 2002). PPD may have a long-term effect on the development of the child that lasts until late childhood (Cogill, Caplan, Alexandra, Robson, & Kumar, 1986). Treatment for PPD improves the mother's ability to function and has a beneficial effect on the baby and the family (Wickberg & Hwang, 1996).

COPING WITH PPD AMONG PALESTINIAN WOMEN

Despite the relatively high interest in PPD among Palestinian women and the high prevalence rate of this mental health problem among these women, only one study has examined how Palestinian women cope with PPD. Eilat-Tsanani et al. (2006) conducted a study among 438 Jewish women and 89 Palestinian women who gave birth at HaEmek Medical Center in Afula (northern Israel). The main goal of this study was to compare the frequency of and reasons for consultations with physicians between women with and without PPD. The results of that work revealed an association between PPD and multiple consultations with family physicians and pediatricians. The authors found women with PPD may be characterized in terms of their consultation patterns.

Many of the somatic complaints cited by the women in that study—such as headache, abdominal pain, and joint pain—may be related to somatization, which is considered an acceptable idiom for emotional distress among women, particularly among women from collectivistic non-Western cultures (Abu-Kaf & Shahar, 2017; Eilat-Tsanani et al., 2006). Furthermore, Eilat-Tsanani et al. (2006) also considered nonspecific baby-related complaints—such as feeding problems, irritability, cry-ing, and lack of weight gain—which may actually reflect maternal distress (a kind of baby-related somatization). Participants in this research study did not agree to visit a psychiatry clinic, underscoring the importance of diagnosing and treating PPD at the primary care level. To that end, these researchers noted that screen-ing for depression and taking careful note of the woman's health condition during pregnancy and frequent visits and somatic complaints following delivery can aid the health-care team in the primary care setting to diagnose PPD. It is important to note that this research did not compare the frequency of and reasons for con-sultations with physicians between Palestinian and Jewish women. Moreover, this research was conducted 10 years ago and awareness of mental health services may have improved since then.

The Use of Formal and Informal Mental Health Services among Palestinian Women

A few studies have examined the use of formal mental health services among Pales-tinian women and found underuse of these services (Al-Krenawi & Graham, 2011; Ayalon, Karkabi, Bleichman, Fleischmann, & Goldfracht, 2015; Levav et al., 2007; Savaya, 1998). The reasons for this may be related to the stigma associated with mental illness and the use of mental health services (Al-Krenawi & Graham, 2011), the tendency to rely on the informal support of family members, the interdiction against discussing family and personal problems with outsiders (Savaya, 1998), and the scarcity of culturally sensitive services (Levav et al., 2007). Palestinian women, in particular, were more likely to adhere to traditional beliefs concerning the nature of mental illness rather than to the biopsychosocial model (Al-Krenawi & Graham, 1999a; Bener & Ghuloum, 2011).

Whereas the aforementioned studies focused on the use of informal mental health services among Palestinian females, Ayalon et al. (2015) conducted focus groups with primary care Palestinian female service users and providers to as-sess their attitudes toward informal mental health services. Three main informal help-seeking behaviors were identified: (a) social support, (b) religious support, and (c) self-help. Nuclear family and friends were considered potential sources of sup-port. However, disclosure of personal information about mental health problems may be seen as having negative emotional ramifications on other family members, as well as being a potential source of aggravation of mental health distress. The Palestinian women (i.e., patients) identified religiosity (belief in God and praying to God) as a coping resource, whereas none of the interviewed physicians identi-fied religiosity as potentially helpful. However, those women were more ambivalent toward religious figures as a potential source of informal help. In terms of informal help, the women also identified self-help strategies (i.e., active strategies such as en-gagement in activities and avoidant strategies such as disengagement from stressful life events) as potentially effective coping mechanisms (Ayalon et al., 2015).

Limitations and Directions for Future Studies

The preceding literature review shows that Palestinian women have not received much research attention. The lower social status of women in Israeli and Palestinian contexts is reflected in their mental health. There is also a dire shortage of research on Palestinian women in menopause transition and at older ages (aged 50 and over), despite the fact that women aged 50 and over represent 23% of the entire population of Palestinian women in Israel. To the best of my knowledge, no research has focused on mental health issues among these age groups and the transition periods women experience as they grow older. There is also a dearth of research on mental health issues among Palestinian female youths, particularly with regard to their lives outside of academic settings (uneducated adolescents and young females). Moreover, the majority of the previous research addressing mental health issues among this population (e.g., social support) was conducted about 10 years ago and has not been updated, thus these findings may be irrelevant given the rapid social transition Palestinians in Israel are experiencing. For this reason, more updated research should be conducted on the different mental health issues affecting this population. Furthermore, most of the previous research among this population has focused mainly on reproductive health—for example, childbirth and emotional experiences of mothers. More research is needed on reproductive processes, functions, and systems at all stages of life from adolescence through old age, and that work should include a wider range of reproductive health topics such as infertility issues, birth control, and appropriate health-care services that will enable women to go safely through pregnancy and childbirth and provide couples with the best chance of having a healthy infant.

Clinical Implications and Recommendations

Investment in the mental health of women is important for the improvement of the mental health of entire populations (Desjarlais et al., 1995). This holds doubly true for Palestinian society, in which women play a crucial role in the mental and physical development of the members of their families (Haj-Yahia, 1995, 2000).

I offer several recommendations to address the obstacles that may prevent Palestinian woman from seeking and using formal mental health services. First, it is important to address the accessibility and availability of mental health services for Palestinian women and the stigma related to mental problems and mental health services. These services may be integrated into nonstigmatizing frameworks or physical settings, such as primary care clinics, mother-child care units, community centers, and welfare offices. Families and women need to be better informed with regard to mental health problems, their consequences, and how these problems can be effectively treated. Professionals in these settings should be provided with knowledge about common mental health problems, so that they can play a role in increasing understanding and awareness of mental health issues, and they should also be equipped with contact information for mental health professionals and services that are readily available. Schools and community centers can play an important and unique role in detecting and addressing mental health problems of female adolescents. In the case of young mothers and older women, mother-child care units and primary care clinics are expected to play a major role in promoting mental health. Mental health services delivered in these settings may be more socially acceptable and less stigmatized.

The second recommendation is related to the development of and training for culturally competent and sociopolitically contextualized interventions to promote mental health among Palestinian women. One of the primary goals of cultural-competence and contextualized training is to introduce and reinforce the idea that cultural and sociopolitical contexts should be integral parts of interventions, as belief systems, value orientations, and sociopolitical contexts influence customs, norms, practices, and psychological processes (e.g., language, caretaking practices, etc.) (Fiske, Kitayama, Markus, & Nisbett, 1998). The broad concept of culture includes family acculturation and values and religious beliefs, as well as attitudes and beliefs about health and illness. It encompasses a way of living formed by the historical, economic, ecological, and political forces that exist within groups. Appropriate answers to the mental health needs of Palestinian women must consider the Arab culture as an integral part of every individual's development, mental health problems, and healing/care practices. For example, being familiar with the cultural dynamics that influence the professional/client relationship and behaving in a manner that enhances the mental health professional/patient relationship and employs a preferred pattern of communication may lead to more effective interventions and lower dropout rates. Furthermore, it is important to consider the sociopolitical context and its reflections (e.g., formal and informal racism, discrimination, and exclusion) and the implications of those factors on the quality of services and resource allocation for mental health. Research must acknowledge the sociopolitical context and the ethnic identity of both the mental health professionals and their clients. Any broad investigation should address different sociopolitical and cultural stressors among Palestinian women clients and not rely on stereotyping processes and/or culturally based, one-dimensional explanations (Kleinman & Benson, 2006).

Third, there is a need to raise awareness concerning mental health, especially among women, at the community level, mainly because Palestinian women tend to use informal sources of help. Family members with more mental health literacy can be effective sources of help and may encourage distressed women to get referrals to available mental health-care practitioners and services.

Finally, mental health interventions that address self-help strategies and techniques (e.g., the behavioral techniques associated with cognitive-behavioral therapy) may be useful and enrich the range of self-help activities that may be adopted by women in times of mental health distress.

SARAH ABU-KAF is Senior Lecturer in Cross-Cultural Psychology in the Conflict Management and Resolution Program at Ben-Gurion University of the Negev, Israel.

References

Abu-Baker, K. (1998). *A rocky road: Arab women as political leaders in Israel* [in Hebrew]. Ra'nana: Beit Berl, Institute for Israeli Arab Studies.

Abu-Kaf, S., & Braun-Lewensohn, O. (2015). Paths to depression among two different cultural contexts: Comparing Bedouin Arab and Jewish students. *Journal of Cross-Cultural Psychology, 46*(4), 612–630.

Abu-Kaf, S., & Priel, B. (2008). Dependent and self-critical vulnerabilities to depression in two different cultural contexts. *Personality and Individual Differences, 44*(3), 689–700.

Abu-Kaf, S., & Priel, B. (2012). Vulnerabilities to depression and sense of coherence among Bedouin Arab and Jewish students: A test of a mediation model. *International Journal of Psychology and Counselling, 4*(3), 31–40.

Abu-Kaf, S., & Shahar, G. (2017). Depression and somatic symptoms among two ethnic groups in Israel: Testing three theoretical models. *Israel Journal of Psychiatry and Related Sciences, 54*(2), 32–40.

Alfayumi-Zeadna, S., Kaufman-Shriqui, V., Zeadna, A., Lauden, A., & Shoham-Vardi, I. (2015). The association between sociodemographic characteristics and postpartum depression symptoms among Arab-Bedouin women in southern Israel. *Depression and Anxiety, 32*(2), 120–128.

Al-Haj, M. (1987). *Social change and family processes: Arab communities in Shefar-Am*. Boulder, CO: Westview.

Al-Haj, M. (1988). The changing Arab kinship structure: The effect of modernization in an urban community. *Economic Development and Cultural Change, 36*(2), 237–258.

Al-Haj, M. (2000). Identity and orientation among Israeli Arabs: A situation of double periphery [in Hebrew]. In R. Gavison & D. Hacker (Eds.), *The Jewish-Arab rift in Israel: A reader* (pp. 13–33). Jerusalem: Israel Democracy Institute.

Al-Haj, M. (2003). Higher education among the Arabs in Israel: Formal policy between empowerment and control. *Higher Education Policy, 16*(3), 351–368.

Al-Krenawi, A. (1998). Family therapy with a multiparental/multispousal family. *Family Process, 37*(1), 65–81.

Al-Krenawi, A. (1999). Women of polygamous marriages in primary health care centers. *Contemporary Family Therapy, 21*(3), 417–430.

Al-Krenawi, A. (2001). Women from polygamous and monogamous marriages in an out-patient psychiatric clinic. *Transcultural Psychiatry, 38*(2), 187–199.

Al-Krenawi, A. (2004). *Awareness and utilization of social, health/mental health services among Bedouin-Arab women, differentiated by type of residence and type of marriage.* Unpublished manuscript, The Spitzer Department of Social Work, Ben-Gurion University of the Negev, Beersheva, Israel.

Al-Krenawi, A., & Graham, J. R. (1999a). Gender and biomedical/traditional mental health utilization among the Bedouin-Arabs of the Negev. *Culture, Medicine and Psychiatry, 23*(2), 219–243.

Al-Krenawi, A., & Graham, J. R. (1999b). The story of Bedouin-Arab women in a polygamous marriage. *Women's Studies International Forum, 22*(5), 497–509.

Al-Krenawi, A., & Graham, J. R. (2006). A comparison of family functioning, life and marital satisfaction, and mental health of women in polygamous and monogamous marriages. *International Journal of Social Psychiatry, 52*(1), 5–17.

Al-Krenawi, A., & Graham, J. R. (2011). Mental health help-seeking among Arab university students in Israel, differentiated by religion. *Mental Health, Religion & Culture, 14*(2), 157–167.

Al-Krenawi, A., & Lev-Wiesel, R. (2002). Wife abuse among polygamous and monogamous Bedouin-Arab families. *Journal of Divorce & Remarriage, 36*(3–4), 151–165.

Al-Krenawi, A., & Slonim-Nevo, V. (2008). The psychosocial profile of Bedouin Arab women living in polygamous and monogamous marriages. *Families in Society: The Journal of Contemporary Social Services, 89*(1), 139–149.

Amara, A., & Yiftachel, O. (2014). *Confrontation in the Negev: Israel land policies and the indigenous Bedouin-Arabs.* Berlin: The Rosa Luxemburg Foundation.

Arar, K., & Abu-Asbah, K. (2010). Arab women's entrepreneurship in the triangle region of Israel: Characteristics, needs and difficulties [in Hebrew]. *Social Issues in Israel, 9*, 91–123.

Arar, K., & Mustafa, M. (2011). Access to higher education for Palestinians in Israel. *Education, Business and Society: Contemporary Middle Eastern Issues, 4*(3), 207–228.

Association for Civil Rights in Israel. (2014). *Annual state of human rights in Israel and the OPT, 2014.* Retrieved from http://www.acri.org.il/en/wp-content/uploads/2014/12/Situation -Report-2014.pdf.

Ayalon, L., Karkabi, K., Bleichman, I., Fleischmann, S., & Goldfracht, M. (2015). Between modern and traditional values: Informal mental health help-seeking attitudes according to Israeli Arab women, primary care patients and their providers. *International Journal of Social Psychiatry, 61*(4), 386–393.

Azaiza, F. (2006). Adolescent girls in distress: Views from Arab female adolescents living in Israel. *International Social Work, 49*(2), 188–197.

Azaiza, F. (2013). Processes of conservation and change in Arab society in Israel: Implications for the health and welfare of the Arab population. *International Journal of Social Welfare, 22*(1), 15–24.

Backer, B. (1983). Mother, sister, daughter, wife: The pillars of the traditional Albanian patriarchal society. In B. Utas (Ed.), *Women in Islamic societies: Social attitudes and historical perspectives* (pp. 48–65). London: Curzon.

Barakat, H. (1985). *Contemporary Arab society* [in Arabic]. Beirut: Center of Arab Union.

Barakat, H. (1993). *The Arab world: Society, culture, and state.* Los Angeles: University of California Press.

Ben-Ari, A. (2004). Sources of social support and attachment styles among Israeli Arab students. *International Social Work, 47*(2), 187–201.

Ben-Ari, A., & Azaiza, F. (1996). Minority group membership and perceptions of self-help: Evidence from Israel. *Journal of Community & Applied Social Psychology, 6*(2), 131–140.

Ben-Ari, A., & Gil, S. (2004). Well-being among minority students: The role of perceived social support. *Journal of Social work, 4*(2), 215–225.

Ben-Ari, A., & Pines, A. (2002). The changing role of family in utilization of social support: Views from Israeli Jewish and Arab students. *Families in Society: The Journal of Contemporary Social Services, 83*(1), 93–101.

Ben-Ari, R. (2004). Coping with the Jewish-Arab conflict: A comparison among three models. *Journal of Social Issues, 60*(2), 307–322.

Benbenishty, R., & Astor, R. A. (2005). *School violence in context: Culture, neighborhood, family, school, and gender.* New York: Oxford University Press.

Bener, A., & Ghuloum, S. (2011). Gender differences in the knowledge, attitude and practice towards mental health illness in a rapidly developing Arab society. *International Journal of Social Psychiatry, 57*(5), 480–486.

Branch, C. W. (2001). The many faces of self: Ego and ethnic identities. *Journal of Genetic Psychology, 162*(4), 412–429.

Braun-Lewensohn, O., Celestin-Westreich, S., Celestin, L.-P., Verleye, G., Verté, D., & Ponjaert-Kristoffersen, I. (2009). Coping styles as moderating the relationships between terrorist attacks and well-being outcomes. *Journal of Adolescence, 32*(3), 585–599.

Braun-Lewensohn, O., Sagy, S., & Roth, G. (2010). Coping strategies among adolescents: Israeli Jews and Arabs facing missile attacks. *Anxiety, Stress & Coping, 23*(1), 35–51.

Cogill, S., Caplan, H., Alexandra, H., Robson, K. M., & Kumar, R. (1986). Impact of maternal postnatal depression on cognitive development of young children. *British Medical Journal (Clinical Research Edition), 292*(6529), 1165–1167.

Cwikel, J., Lev-Wiesel, R., & Al-Krenawi, A. (2003). The physical and psychosocial health of Bedouin Arab women of the Negev area of Israel: The impact of high fertility and pervasive domestic violence. *Violence Against Women, 9*(2), 240–257.

Daeem, R., Mansbach-Kleinfeld, I., Farbstein, I., Khamaisi, R., Ifrah, A., Muhammad, A. S., . . . Apter, A. (2016). Help seeking in school by Israeli Arab minority adolescents with emotional and behavioral problems: Results from the Galilee study. *Israel Journal of Health Policy Research, 5*(1), 1–13. https://doi.org/10.1186/s13584-016-0109-0.

Daoud, N., Braun-Lewensohn, O., Eriksson, M., & Sagy, S. (2014). Sense of coherence and depressive symptoms among low-income Bedouin women in the Negev Israel. *Journal of Mental Health, 23*(6), 307–311.

Daoud, N., & Jabareen, Y. (2014). Depressive symptoms among Arab Bedouin women whose houses are under threat of demolition in southern Israel: A right to housing issue. *Health and Human Rights, 16*(1), 179–191.

Daoud, N., & Shoham-Vardi, I. (2016). *Different types of violence among Arab and Jewish women.* Manuscript in preparation.

Daoud, N., Shoham-Vardi, I., Urquia, M. L., & O'Campo, P. (2014). Polygamy and poor mental health among Arab Bedouin women: Do socioeconomic position and social support matter? *Ethnicity & Health, 19*(4), 385–405.

David, M. (2007). Equity and diversity: Towards a sociology of higher education for the twenty-first century? *British Journal of Sociology of Education, 28*(5), 675–690.

Desjarlais, R., Eisenberg, L., Good, B., & Kleinman, A. (1995). World mental health: Problems and priorities in developing countries. New York: Oxford University Press.

Douki, S., Zineb, S. B., Nacef, F., & Halbreich, U. (2007). Women's mental health in the Muslim world: Cultural, religious, and social issues. *Journal of Affective Disorders, 102*(1), 177–189.

Eilat-Tsanani, S., Merom, A., Romano, S., Reshef, A., Lavi, I., & Tabenkin, H. (2006). The effect of postpartum depression on women's consultations with physicians. *Israel Medical Association Journal, 8*(6), 406–409.

Eisikovits, Z., Winstok, Z., & Fishman, G. (2004). The first Israeli national survey on domestic violence. *Violence Against Women, 10*(7), 729–748.

Epel, O. B., Kaplan, G., & Moran, M. (2010). Perceived discrimination and health-related quality of life among Arabs and Jews in Israel: A population-based survey. *BMC Public Health, 10*(1), 282–291.

Fiske, A., Kitayama, S., Markus, H. R., & Nisbett, R. E. (1998). The cultural matrix of social psychology. In D. Gilbert, S. Fiske, & G. Lindzey (Eds.), *The handbook of social psychology* (4th ed., pp. 915–981). San Francisco: McGraw-Hill.

Folkman, S., & Lazarus, R. S. (1980). An analysis of coping in a middle-aged community sample. *Journal of Health and Social Behavior, 21*(3), 219–239.

Galilee Society: The Arab National Society for Health, Research and Services [Galilee Society]. (2013). *Annual report.* Retrieved from http://www.gal-soc.org/files/userfiles/GS_annual%20report_2013.pdf.

Garlow, S. J., Rosenberg, J., Moore, J. D., Haas, A. P., Koestner, B., Hendin, H., & Nemeroff, C. B. (2008). Depression, desperation, and suicidal ideation in college students: Results from the American foundation for suicide prevention college screening project at Emory University. *Depression and Anxiety, 25*(6), 482–488.

Gater, R., Tansella, M., Korten, A., Tiemens, B. G., Mavreas, V. G., & Olatawura, M. O. (1998). Sex differences in the prevalence and detection of depressive and anxiety disorders in general health care settings: Report from the World Health Organization collaborative study on psychological problems in general health care. *Archives of General Psychiatry, 55*(5), 405–413.

Geiger, B. (2013). Female Arab students' experience of acculturation and cultural diversity upon accessing higher education in the Northern Galilee-Israel. *International Journal of Higher Education, 2*(3), 91–106.

Ghanem, A. (2001). *The Palestinian-Arab minority in Israel, 1948–2000: A political study.* New York: State University of New York Press.

Gharrah, R. (2012). *Arab society in Israel* (5th ed.) [in Hebrew]. Jerusalem: Van Leer Jerusalem Institute.

Glasser, S. (2010). Postpartum depression: A chronicle of health policy development. *Israel Journal of Psychiatry and Related Sciences, 47*(4), 254–259.

Glasser, S., Stoski, E., Kneler, V., & Magnezi, R. (2011). Postpartum depression among Israeli Bedouin women. *Archives of Women's Mental Health, 14*(3), 203–208.

Glasser, S., Tanous, M., Shihab, S., Goldman, N., Ziv, A., & Kaplan, G. (2012). Perinatal depressive symptoms among Arab women in northern Israel. *Maternal and Child Health Journal, 16*(6), 1197–1205.

Goldberg, D. P., & Huxley, P. (1992). *Common mental disorders: A bio-social model.* London: Routledge.

Gottlieb, N., & Feder-Bubis, P. (2014). Dehomed: The impacts of house demolitions on the well-being of women from the unrecognized Bedouin-Arab villages in the Negev/Israel. *Health & Place, 29*, 146–153.

Grinstein-Weiss, M., Fishman, G., & Eisikovits, Z. (2005). Gender and ethnic differences in formal and informal help seeking among Israeli adolescents. *Journal of Adolescence, 28*(6), 765–779.

Guterman, N. B., Haj-Yahia, M. M., Vorhies, V., Ismayilova, L., & Leshem, B. (2010). Help-seeking and internal obstacles to receiving support in the wake of community violence exposure: The case of Arab and Jewish adolescents in Israel. *Journal of Child and Family Studies, 19*(6), 687–696.

Haj-Yahia, M. M. (1995). Toward culturally sensitive intervention with Arab families in Israel. *Contemporary Family Therapy, 17*(4), 429–447.

Haj-Yahia, M. M. (1997). Culturally sensitive supervision of Arab social work students in Western universities. *Social Work, 42*(2), 166–174.

Haj-Yahia, M. M. (2000). Wife abuse and battering in the sociocultural context of Arab society. *Family Process, 39*(2), 237–255.

Haj-Yahia, M. M. (2001). The incidence of witnessing interparental violence and some of its psychological consequences among Arab adolescents. *Child Abuse & Neglect, 25*(7), 885–907.

Haj-Yahia, M. M., & Peled, E. (2013). Guest editors' note [in Hebrew]. *Society and Welfare, 33,* 3–6.

Haj-Yahia-Abu Ahmad, N. (2006). *Couplehood and parenting in the Arab family in Israel: Processes of change and preservation in three generations* [in Hebrew] (Unpublished doctoral dissertation). University of Haifa, Israel.

Halperin, O., Sarid, O., & Cwikel, J. (2014). A comparison of Israeli Jewish and Arab women's birth perceptions. *Midwifery, 30*(7), 853–861.

Hamdi, E., Amin, Y., & Abou-Saleh, M. T. (1997). Problems in validating endogenous depression in the Arab culture by contemporary diagnostic criteria. *Journal of Affective Disorders, 44*(2), 131–143.

Hammen, C., Rudolph, K., Weisz, J., Rao, U., & Burge, D. (1999). The context of depression in clinic-referred youth: Neglected areas in treatment. *Journal of the American Academy of Child & Adolescent Psychiatry, 38*(1), 64–71.

Hassouneh-Phillips, D. (2001). Polygamy and wife abuse: A qualitative study of Muslim women in America. *Health Care for Women International, 22*(8), 735–748.

Hofstede, G., & Hofstede, G. J. (2005). *Cultures and organizations: Software of the mind* (2th ed). New York: McGraw-Hill.

Holahan, C. J., & Moos, R. H. (1987). Personal and contextual determinants of coping strategies. *Journal of Personality and Social Psychology, 52*(5), 946–955.

Hysenbegasi, A., Hass, S. L., & Rowland, C. R. (2005). The impact of depression on the academic productivity of university students. *Journal of Mental Health Policy and Economics, 8*(3), 145–151.

Israel Center for Disease Control [ICDC]. (2010). *Health status in Israel: Selected findings 2010* [in Hebrew] (Publication No. 333). Retrieved from http://www.health.gov.il /PublicationsFiles/Health_Status_in_Israel2010.pdf.

Israel Central Bureau of Statistics [Israel CBS]. (2015). *Statistical abstract of Israel 2015.* Retrieved from http://www.cbs.gov.il/reader/shnaton/shnatone_new.htm?CYear=2015&Vol=66 &CSubject=30.

Israel Central Bureau of Statistics [Israel CBS]. (2016). *Statistical abstract of Israel.* Retrieved from http://www.cbs.gov.il/reader/shnaton/shnatone_new.htm?CYear=2016&Vol=67 &CSubject=30.

Israel Ministry of Finance. (2015). *The second report on progress in implementing the recommendations of the Organization for Economic Cooperation and Development (OECD): The labor market and social policy—Israel* [in Hebrew]. Jerusalem: Brookdale Institute.

Jaber, L., & Halpern, G. J. (2006). Consanguinity among the Arab and Jewish populations in Israel. *Pediatric Endocrinology Reviews, 3*(3), 437–446.

Jackson, R. L. (1998). Tracing the evolution of "race," "ethnicity," and "culture" in communication studies. *Howard Journal of Communication, 9*(1), 41–55.

Janson, E. (2011). Stereotypes that define "us": The case of Muslim women. *ENDC [Estonian National Defense College] Proceedings, 14,* 181–196.

Joseph, S. (1994). *Gender and family in the Arab world.* Washington, DC: Middle East Research and Information Project.

Kaplan, G., Glasser, S., Murad, H., Atamna, A., Alpert, G., Goldbourt, U., & Kalter-Leibovici, O. (2010). Depression among Arabs and Jews in Israel: A population-based study. *Social Psychiatry and Psychiatric Epidemiology, 45*(10), 931–939.

Keinan, T., & Bar, D. (2007). *Mobility among Arab women in Israel* [in Hebrew]. Haifa: Kayan Feminist Organization.

Keshet, Y., & Popper-Giveon, A. (2016). Work experiences of ethnic minority nurses: A qualitative study. *Israel Journal of Health Policy Research, 5*(1), 18–28.

Khalaf, E., & Abu-Kaf, S. (2016). *Acculturation stress and adjustment among Arab students.* Manuscript in preparation.

King, N. J., & Bernstein, G. A. (2001). School refusal in children and adolescents: A review of the past 10 years. *Journal of the American Academy of Child & Adolescent Psychiatry, 40*(2), 197–205.

Kleinman, A. (2004). Culture and depression. *New England Journal of Medicine, 351*(10), 951–953.

Kleinman, A., & Benson, P. (2006). Anthropology in the clinic: The problem of cultural competency and how to fix it. *PLoS Med, 3*(10), 1673–1676. https://doi.org10.1371/journal .pmed.0030294.

Knesset Research and Information Center [Knesset RIC]. (2015). *Employment of Arab women: Data, barriers and recommendations* [in Hebrew]. Retrieved from https://www.knesset .gov.il/committees/heb/material/data/avoda2015-07-27-00-03.pdf.

Knesset Research and Information Center [Knesset RIC]. (2016). *Public transportation services in Arab communities: A snapshot* [in Hebrew]. Retrieved from http://knesset.gov.il /committees/heb/material/data/kalkala2016-02-22-00-02.pdf.

Lambert, V. A., Lambert, C. E., & Ito, M. (2004). Workplace stressors, ways of coping and demographic characteristics as predictors of physical and mental health of Japanese hospital nurses. *International Journal of Nursing Studies, 41*(1), 85–97.

Lazarus, R. S., & Folkman, S. (1984). *Stress, appraisal, and coping.* New York: Springer.

Levav, I., Ifrah, A., Geraisy, N., Grinshpoon, A., & Khwaled, R. (2007). Common mental disorders among Arab-Israelis: Findings from the Israel national health survey. *Israel Journal of Psychiatry and Related Sciences, 44*(2), 104–113.

Levinson, D. (1989). *Family violence in cross-cultural perspective.* Newbury Park, CA: Sage.

Lev-Wiesel, R., & Al-Krenawi, A. (1999). Attitude towards marriage and marital quality: A comparison among Israeli Arabs differentiated by religion. *Family Relations, 48*(1), 51–56.

Malley-Morrison, K., & Hines, D. (2004). *Family violence in a cultural perspective: Defining, understanding, and combating abuse.* Thousand Oaks, CA: Sage.

Mansbach-Kleinfeld, I., Farbstein, I., Levinson, D., Apter, A., Erhard, R., Palti, H., . . . Levav, I. (2010). Service use for mental disorders and unmet need: Results from the Israel survey on mental health among adolescents. *Psychiatric Services, 61*(3), 241–249.

Manzar, S. (1999). The English language and Arabic medical students. *Medical Education, 33*(5), 394–395.

Maziak, W., & Asfar, T. (2003). Physical abuse in low-income women in Aleppo, Syria. *Health Care for Women International, 24*(4), 313–326.

Mori, S. C. (2000). Addressing the mental health concerns of international students. *Journal of Counseling & Development, 78*(2), 137–144.

Nishimura, N. J. (1998). Assessing the issues of multiracial students on college campuses. *Journal of College Counseling, 1*(1), 45–53.

Okun, B. S., & Friedlander, D. (2005). Educational stratification among Arabs and Jews in Israel: Historical disadvantage, discrimination, and opportunity. *Population Studies, 59*(2), 163–180.

Patai, R., & DeAtkine, N. B. (1973). *The Arab mind.* New York: Scribner.

Patel, V., Kirkwood, B. R., Pednekar, S., Weiss, H., & Mabey, D. (2006). Risk factors for common mental disorders in women. *British Journal of Psychiatry, 189*(6), 547–555.

Physicians for Human Rights. (2008). *Annual report 2008.* Retrieved from http://d843006.bc470 .bestcms.com/uploaded/doch_2008_8_3_2009_final_www.pdf.

Piccinelli, M., & Wilkinson, G. (2000). Gender differences in depression. *British Journal of Psychiatry, 177*(6), 486–492.

Pines, A. M., Ben-Ari, A., Utasi, A., & Larson, D. (2002). A cross-cultural investigation of social support and burnout. *European Psychologist, 7*(4), 256–264.

Pines, A. M., & Zaidman, N. (2003). Gender, culture, and social support: A male-female, Israeli Jewish-Arab comparison. *Sex Roles: A Journal of Research, 49*(11–12), 571–586.

Pinson, H. (2007). At the boundaries of citizenship: Palestinian Israeli citizens and the civic education curriculum. *Oxford Review of Education, 33*(3), 331–348.

Renn, K. A. (2000). Patterns of situational identity among biracial and multiracial college students. *Review of Higher Education, 23*(4), 399–420.

RHA Center for Bedouin Studies and Development. (2010). *Statistical yearbook of the Bedouins in the Negev.* Beersheva, Israel: Ben-Gurion University of the Negev.

Righetti-Veltema, M., Conne-Perréard, E., Bousquet, A., & Manzano, J. (2002). Postpartum depression and mother-infant relationship at 3 months old. *Journal of Affective Disorders, 70*(3), 291–306.

Sandridge, A., Takeddin, J., Al-Kaabi, E., & Frances, Y. (2010). Consanguinity in Qatar: Knowledge, attitude and practice in a population born between 1946 and 1991. *Journal of Biosocial Science, 42*(01), 59–82.

Savaya, R. (1997). Political attitudes, economic distress, and the utilization of welfare services by Arab women in Israel. *Journal of Applied Social Sciences, 21*, 111–122.

Savaya, R. (1998). The under-use of psychological services by Israeli Arabs: An examination of the roles of negative attitudes and the use of alternative sources of help. *International Social Work, 41*(2), 195–209.

Sethi, B. (1986). Epidemiology of depression in India. *Psychopathology, 19*, 26–36.

Shechory-Bitton, M., & Kamel, D. (2014). Pathways to crime and risk factors among Arab female adolescents in Israel. *Children and Youth Services Review, 44*, 363–369.

Sheiner, E. K., Sheiner, E., Shoham-Vardi, I., Mazor, M., & Katz, M. (1999). Ethnic differences influence care giver's estimates of pain during labour. *Pain, 81*(3), 299–305.

Slonim-Nevo, V., & Al-Krenawi, A. (2006). Success and failure among polygamous families: The experience of wives, husbands, and children. *Family Process, 45*(3), 311–330.

Spitzer, R. L., Williams, J. B., Kroenke, K., Linzer, M., Verloin deGruy, F., Hahn, S. R., . . . Johnson, J. G. (1994). Utility of a new procedure for diagnosing mental disorders in primary care: The PRIME-MD 1000 study. *JAMA, 272*(22), 1749–1756.

State Comptroller of Israel. (2015). Report on the implementation of the education reform and reducing the gaps in early childhood education [in Hebrew] (Annual Report 65C). Retrieved from http://www.mevaker.gov.il/he/Reports/Report_290/ReportFiles/fullreport_2.pdf.

Tamres, L. K., Janicki, D., & Helgeson, V. S. (2002). Sex differences in coping behavior: A meta-analytic review and an examination of relative coping. *Personality and Social Psychology Review, 6*(1), 2–30.

Taylor, S. E., Klein, L. C., Lewis, B. P., Gruenewald, T. L., Gurung, R. A., & Updegraff, J. A. (2000). Biobehavioral responses to stress in females: Tend-and-befriend, not fight-or-flight. *Psychological Review, 107*(3), 411–429.

Taylor, S. E., Sherman, D. K., Kim, H. S., Jarcho, J., Takagi, K., & Dunagan, M. S. (2004). Culture and social support: Who seeks it and why? *Journal of Personality and Social Psychology, 87*(3), 354–362.

Triandis, H. C. (2001). Individualism-collectivism and personality. *Journal of Personality, 69*(6), 907–924.

Wickberg, B., & Hwang, C. P. (1996). Counselling of postnatal depression: A controlled study on a population based Swedish sample. *Journal of Affective Disorders, 39*(3), 209–216.

Williams, D. R. (1999). Race, socioeconomic status, and health. The added effects of racism and discrimination. *Annals of the New York Academy of Sciences, 896*(1), 173–188.

World Health Organization [WHO]. (1998). *The world health report 1998: Life in the 21st century—A vision for all.* Retrieved from http://www.who.int/whr/1998/en/.

World Health Organization [WHO]. (2000). *Women's mental health: An evidence-based review.* Retrieved from http://www.who.int/mental_health/publications/women_mh_evidence _review/en/.

World Health Organization [WHO]. (2001). *The world health report: Mental health—New understanding, new hope.* Retrieved from http://www.who.int/whr/2001/en/whr01_en.pdf?ua=1.

Yiftachel, O. (2009). Ghetto citizenship: Palestinian Arabs in Israel [In Hebrew]. In N. Rouhana & A. Sabagh (Eds.), *Israel and the Palestinians—Key terms* (pp. 56–60). Haifa: Mada Center for Applied Research.

Zeidner, M. (1992). Sources of academic stress: The case of first year Jewish and Arab college students in Israel. *Higher Education, 24*(1), 25–40.

Ziadna, G. (2013). *Report on demolition of houses of Arab-Bedouin in the Negev. International Human Rights Day 2013* [In Hebrew]. Beersheva: Negev Coexistence Forum for Civil Equality.

Zwingmann, C. A., Gunn, A. D., & WHO. (1983). *Uprooting and health: Psychosocial problems of students from abroad.* Geneva: World Health Organization.

8

MENTAL HEALTH IN OLDER ADULT
PALESTINIAN CITIZENS IN ISRAEL

Rabia Khalaila

MENTAL HEALTH DATA ON OLDER ADULT PALESTINIAN CITIZENS in Israel are generally sparse. Along with genetic determinants, other familial factors and health inequalities contribute to the development of mental and cognitive disorders (i.e., non-affective psychotic disorders, affective disorders, and dementia) (Bowirrat, Friedland, Farrer, Baldwin, & Korczyn, 2002; Werner, Friedland, & Inzelberg, 2015). In addition, several unique social, cultural, and political factors seem to affect the risk for cognitive and mental disorders in this population (Al-Krenawi, 2005; Levav, Ifrah, Geraisy, Grinshpoon, & Khwaled, 2007; Ponizovsky, Geraisy, Shoshan, & Kremer, 2007).

The Palestinian population in Israel tends to deny the existence of mental and cognitive disorders and therefore does not seek help from psychiatric professionals. Often, individuals in the Palestinian community only request treatment for symptoms expressed physically (Al-Krenawi, 2005). Thus, many of those with mental disorders in this population go undiagnosed and/or untreated. Several factors may underlie their reluctance to request help from mental health services, such as religious beliefs and degree of observance, perceived stigma, cultural sensitivity, and culturally inadequate mental services (Al-Krenawi, 2005; Al-Krenawi & Graham, 2000; Al-Krenawi, Graham, Dean, & Eltaiba, 2004; Al-Krenawi, Graham, Ophir, & Kandah, 2001; Nakash et al., 2012; Ponizovsky, Geraisy, Shoshan, & Kremer, 2007; Razali & Najib, 2000; Weatherhead & Daiches, 2010).

This chapter aims to shed light on the unique factors contributing to mental and cognitive disorders among older adult Palestinian citizens in Israel and their underutilization of the available mental health services. Recommendations are made to improve this situation.

The Older Adult Palestinian Population in Israel

The Palestinians are a minority in Israel, accounting for 20.7% of the population within the country's internationally recognized borders (Israel Central Bureau of Statisics [Israel CBS], 2011). Most of this minority group self-identify as Arab or Palestinian by nationality and Israeli by citizenship (Sa'di, 2002).

The Palestinian population of Israel is relatively young, with only 8% over the age of 65. This figure is expected to reach 12% by 2030 (Myers-JDC-Brookdale Institute, 2012). Almost 99% of these elderly reside with their families and relatives, and the rest live in long-term care institutions.

According to the Israel CBS (2011), life expectancy has risen over the past 10 years among Palestinian men and women in Israel, reaching 76.8 years and 81.0 years, respectively. These figures are lower than among Jewish men (80.4) and women (83.7).

Mental Health Problems among Elderly Palestinian Citizens in Israel

Only a few epidemiological studies of mental and cognitive disorders have been conducted among Palestinian citizens in Israel (Bowirrat, Friedland, Farrer, et al., 2002; Bowirrat, Friedland, & Korczyn, 2002; Bowirrat, Oscar-Berman, & Logroscino, 2006; Levav et al., 2007; Ponizovsky, Geraisy, Shoshan, & Kremer, 2007) and even fewer among the elderly (Bowirrat, Friedland, Farrer, et al., 2002; Bowirrat, Friedland, & Korczyn, 2002; Bowirrat et al., 2006; Shemesh et al., 2006). The situation is similar in most Arab countries and among ethnic Arabs around the world. Only a few community-based surveys on mental disorders have been published in English (Al-Krenawi & Graham, 2000; Bowirrat, Friedland, Farrer, et al., 2002; Bowirrat, Friedland, & Korczyn, 2002; Bowirrat et al., 2006; El-Islam, 2008; Hamdan, 2009).

For example, a high incidence of depressive symptoms, based on *DSM-IV* criteria, was found in a study of elderly Palestinians from Wadi Ara in Israel diagnosed with Alzheimer's disease (AD) and vascular dementia (VD) (Bowirrat, Friedland, Farrer, et al., 2002; Bowirrat, Friedland, & Korczyn, 2002; Bowirrat et al., 2006). The prevalence of depressive symptoms was higher among those with VD than in those with AD—86% and 57%, respectively (Bowirrat et al., 2006).

In addition, Bowirrat and colleagues (Bowirrat, Friedland, & Korczyn, 2002; Bowirrat, Friedland, Farrer, et al., 2002) reported an unusually high prevalence of AD (20.5%) in an epidemiological study of 821 Palestinian citizens in Israel, aged 60, from Wadi Ara. The incidence of VD in the same population was 6% (Bowirrat, Friedland, Farrer, et al., 2002), increasing sharply with age: from 8% up to the age of 70, to 33% among those aged 70–79, to 51% among those over 80 years old. Dementia was also more widespread among elderly Palestinian females than among males (25% and 15%, respectively) (Bowirrat, Friedland, & Korczyn, 2002). These findings were explained as a result of this group's unique characteristics, such as rural living conditions, environmental hardships, cigarette smoking, and their human genome data (Bowirrat et al., 2006).

In comparative studies in Israel, the incidence of mental/cognitive disorders was higher among Palestinian citizens in Israel than among Jewish Israelis (Al-Krenawi, 2000; Khalaila & Litwin, 2014; Ponizovsky, Geraisy, Shoshan, & Kremer, 2007; Ponizovsky, Geraisy, Shoshan, Kremer, & Smetannikov, 2007; Shemesh et al., 2006). For example, the prevalence of depression was significantly higher for Palestinian citizens in Israel than for Jewish citizens among those aged 21 or older (Kaplan et al., 2010; Levav et al., 2007; Levinson, Zilber, Lerner, Grinshpoon, & Levav, 2007) and in a community sample of those aged 50 or older (Khalaila & Litwin, 2014). Kaplan et al. (2010) found that depression rates increased with age in both ethnic groups. In addition, Shemesh et al. (2006) reported high scores of emotional distress among 824 Palestinians aged 60 and over: 43.4% among Muslims, followed by 37% for Christians and 17% for Druze, compared to 21.4% among Jewish respondents.

According to other studies based on the Israeli national community survey, in adults aged over 21, Palestinian citizens in Israel showed a higher rate of emotional distress compared to Jewish respondents (Gross, 2007; Levav et al., 2007; Levinson et al., 2007). In addition, Palestinian citizens in Israel gave lower self-appraisals of mental health compared to Jewish Israelis (Levav et al., 2007). However, in another study among 251 Israeli adult outpatients making their first visit to psychiatric clinics, Palestinian citizens in Israel reported emotional distress significantly less frequently than Jewish Israeli patients (68.4% and 89.7%, respectively) (Ponizovsky, Geraisy, Shoshan, Kremer, et al., 2007).

Risk Factors for Mental Health Problems

Sociopolitical Conditions

Several factors appear to have a unique impact on the mental health of elderly Palestinian citizens in Israel, including sociopolitical issues, such as the Arab-Israeli conflict (Al-Krenawi, 2005; Shemesh et al., 2006). The traumatic impact of social exclusion and various related socioeconomic factors (such as low educational levels, high unemployment, low income), and political problems within Palestinian society in Israel after the establishment of the state of Israel contributed significantly to their mental health problems, particularly among the elders of this group exposed to the negative effects of the Arab-Israeli conflict for the longest time (Rouhana & Ghanem, 1998; Sa'di, 2002).

Palestinian citizens in Israel experience stress stemming from their minority status (Al-Krenawi, 2005). They suffer from discrimination in various aspects of life, such as in the education, health, and economic domains (Somer, Maguen, Or-Chen, & Litz, 2009). These factors are strongly associated with mental ill-health, such as depression (Khalaila & Litwin, 2014; Williams, Yu, Jackson, & Anderson, 1997). For example, in general, depressive symptoms are more prevalent among older adults from ethnic minority groups (Duivis et al., 2011; Gelkopf, Solomon, Berger, & Bleich, 2008; Somer et al., 2009; Walsemann, Gee, & Geronimus, 2009). In Israel the rates are significantly higher among the elderly of the Palestinian minority than among the Jewish majority (Khalaila & Litwin, 2014; Shemesh et al., 2006).

Phone surveys were carried out among two distinct representative samples of the Israeli population aged 18 and over ($N = 512$ and $N = 501$) at two points in time: 19 months and 44 months after the eruption of the Al-Aqsa intifada, between September 2000 and 2004. Initially, Palestinian and Jewish Israelis reacted similarly to the situation, but subsequently, posttraumatic symptom disorders increased threefold among the Palestinian population, and their resilience fell significantly (Gelkopf et al., 2008).

Elder Neglect and Abuse

Mental and cognitive problems in later life were shown to be risk factors for elder abuse and neglect (Dong, Simon, Odwazny, & Gorbien, 2008), and vice versa (Roepke-Buehler, Simon, & Dong, 2015). The consequences of elder abuse include high levels of emotional distress and depression (Roepke-Buehler et al., 2015), as well as increased risks for developing fear and anxiety reactions, learned helplessness, and PTSD (Pillemer & Prescott, 1988). Indeed, according to the first national survey on elder abuse and neglect in Israel, carried out in 2004–2005, about 18.4% of the participants had been exposed to one or more kinds of abuse (physical, sexual, or psychological; limitation of freedom; or financial exploitation) during the preceding 12 months. Verbal abuse was the most frequent form, followed by financial exploitation (Lowenstein, Eisikovits, Band-Winterstein, & Enosh, 2009). The rates were quite similar among Jewish and Palestinian citizens in Israel. Women were more exposed to physical violence than men, and Palestinian women were the most vulnerable (Lowenstein et al., 2009). Abuse and neglect of seniors by family members within Palestinian society in Israel stands at 2.5% (Sharon & Zoabi, 1997). Litwin and Zoabi (2003) found increasing elder abuse among this population, with some cases going unreported. These results were attributed to the modernization process and the consequent family disruptions experienced by the Palestinian minority in Israel over the three decades prior to the study (Litwin & Zoabi, 2003).

Consanguineous Marriage

Consanguineous marriage, known to have adverse effects on morbidity and mortality, is a traditional practice in Arab Middle Eastern and North African countries, such as Tunisia and Egypt, with a frequency of more than 50% in some countries (Mansour et al., 2010; Othman & Saadat, 2009). Consanguinity may be associated with an increased risk of developing a wide range of genetically complex disorders, including cognitive and mental conditions such as depression and schizophrenia (Abu-Saad, Elbedour, Hallaq, Merrick, & Tenenbaum, 2014; Bener, Dafeeah, & Samson, 2012; Dobrusin et al., 2009). For example, Bener et al. (2012) found higher rates of parental consanguinity among persons with schizophrenia (41.3%) than among those free of the disorder (28.7%). Schizophrenia was also more common among the offspring of consanguineous than nonconsanguineous parents. A small but significant increase was noted in the rate of cousin marriages among the parents of persons with schizophrenia compared to the parents of infant controls among the Bedouin population in southern Israel (Dobrusin et al., 2009).

Consanguinity rates in the Palestinian population in Israel were the highest among the Druze (47%), followed by Muslims, including Bedouins (42%), and Christians (22%). Because the rate of first-cousin marriages was higher among Bedouins (37%) and Druze (37%) (Vardi-Saliternik, Friedlander, & Cohen, 2002), many of the Palestinian elderly in Israel are probably descendants of past consanguineous marriages and, therefore, carry a high risk of developing mental disorders. Many persons with schizophrenia in the Bedouin sector in southern Israel had consanguineous parents (Abu-Saad et al., 2014; Dobrusin et al., 2009; Na'amnih et al., 2015; Vardi-Saliternik et al., 2002), which is in keeping with the increased risk of developing schizophrenia in such marriages in Egypt (Mansour et al., 2010). Among Bedouin women, 45% were in consanguineous relationships, mainly between first cousins (Dobrusin et al., 2009). Data collected among Palestinian citizens in Israel between 2000 and 2009 indicate a steady decline in such marriages, from about 36% to 24% (Na'amnih et al., 2015).

Polygamy

Polygamy is another risk factor for mental disorders in Palestinian society in Israel, particularly among women. Islam permits men to marry up to four women, provided they deal justly with each (Qur'an Surah an-Nisa [The Women] 4:129). Polygamy may lead to co-wife jealousy, competition, and unequal distribution of household and emotional resources (Adams & Mburugu, 1994). Reviewing 22 relevant studies on polygamy spanning 15 countries, mainly in Africa and in the Muslim world, Shepard (2013) noted increased prevalence of somatization and psychiatric morbidity, including depression, anxiety, hostility, and psychoticism, among the older wives in polygamous marriages.

First wives, mostly senior wives, in polygamous families often experience major psychological crises (Al-Sherbiny, 2005). For example, among Syrian women, first wives reported more anxiety, paranoid ideation, and psychoticism than second and third wives (Al-Krenawi, 2013). In a cross-sectional study carried out in Turkey, there was a higher incidence of somatization disorder among polygamous senior wives than among junior or monogamous wives (Ozkan, Altindag, Oto, & Sentunali, 2006). In Kuwait psychiatric outpatients and inpatients included a disproportionate number of senior wives from polygamous marriages (Chaleby, 1985).

Similar studies have been carried out among Palestinian citizens in Israel. A qualitative study among a 69-member Bedouin family in Israel, consisting of one husband, 8 wives, and 60 offspring, showed extensive competition, hostility, and jealousy among the wives; lack of communication between the co-wives and the children of different wives; and a variety of behavioral and psychosocial problems among family members (Al-Krenawi, 1998). In a study among 10 polygamous families in a Bedouin town in Israel, this situation was perceived as emotionally painful, particularly for the wives (Slonim-Nevo & Al-Krenawi, 2006). In a cross-sectional statistical study of 352 Bedouin women in Israel, those in polygamous marriages exhibited significantly greater psychological distress, as well as higher levels of phobia, somatization, and other psychological problems (Al-Krenawi & Graham, 2006). Among women and their children, polygamy was associated with psychiatric morbidity, particularly depression and anxiety (Al-Krenawi, 2012; Al-Krenawi, Graham, & Al Gharaibeh, 2011).

Physical Health

Physical health also has an impact on mental health, and vice versa, particularly in later life. Frequently occurring chronic diseases and long-term illnesses in old age (such as cancer, hypertension, stroke, congestive heart failure, and diabetes mellitus) seem to be closely correlated with depressive symptoms in older adults (Duivis et al., 2011; Gale et al., 2011; Geerlings, Beekman, Deeg, & Van Tilburg, 2000; Khalaila & Litwin, 2014). Illness in old age may result in functional disabilities restricting mobility, possibly leading to the need for assistance with self-care, loss of dignity, and the onset of mental health disorders such as anxiety and depression (Gale et al., 2011; Geerlings et al., 2000).

Studies on health in Israel show large gaps in physical health status between the Palestinian and Jewish sectors, with higher rates of chronic morbidity symptoms associated with cancer and diabetes and greater physical disability among the former (Tarabeia et al., 2007; Tarabeia et al., 2008). Palestinian citizens in Israel generally engage in much less physical activity than Jewish Israelis, with high rates of obesity among the women (Khalaila & Litwin, 2014). Disability rates are significantly higher among adult and elderly Palestinian citizens in Israel than among the Jewish population (Myers-JDC-Brookdale Institute, 2012).

Attitudes toward Seeking Help from Mental Health Services

Seeking professional help is shunned in some sectors—for instance, Muslims tend to rely on religious practices to alleviate mental health problems. These practices are more prevalent among the elderly (Al-Krenawi & Graham, 1999b; Haque, 2004).

According to Al-Krenawi and Graham (1999b), Muslims in need of psychotherapeutic intervention often consult traditional healers. For example, among Bedouins in Israel, there are four types of traditional healers (Al-Krenawi, Graham, & Maoz, 1996): (1) *Khatibs* (sheikhs or imams) are male healers who make amulets to ward off evil spirits (*jinn*) and often prevent acknowledgment of medical or psychiatric problems (El-Islam, 2008). (2) Dervishes, both males and females, receive a *baraka* (a kind of emotional message perceived as a blessing from God). They are endorsed by socially recognized healers and treat mental disorders using a variety of religious and cultural rituals. (3) *Moalj Bel Koran* (Qur'anic healers) treat patients affected by evil spirits using religious principles derived from the Qur'an and prophetic traditions (Al-Krenawi, 1999; Al-Krenawi & Graham, 1999b). (4) *Al-Fataha* are fortune-tellers who use coffee grains to reveal the patients' secrets (Al-Krenawi, 1999; Al-Krenawi et al., 1996). All these healers tend to attribute illness to supernatural powers.

Because of the stigma surrounding mental illness, many Palestinians deny and keep mental illness secret for a long time, shunning professional treatment and intervention (Al-Krenawi, 2005). This leads to treatment lags and gaps, and poorer psychological adjustment, treatment adherence, clinical course, and outcomes (Nakash & Levav, 2012; Ponizovsky, Geraisy, Shoshan, Kremer, et al., 2007; Struch et al., 2008; Struch, Shereshevsky, Naon, Daniel, & Fischman, 2009). It also limits contacts with health-care options, treatment, social resources, and opportunities for recovery (Kadri & Sartorius, 2005; Nakash & Levav, 2012). Negative reactions from the community or shaming the family affect the individual's well-being and are perceived as barriers to seeking help for mental health problems (Al-Krenawi, 2005; Al-Krenawi & Graham, 1999a; Ponizovsky, Geraisy, Shoshan, Kremer, et al., 2007; Savaya, 1996; Struch et al., 2008).

Another reason for not seeking help for mental problems is the lack of adequate and affordable mental health services within Palestinian society in Israel. Access to services often necessitates traveling outside the community, reinforcing the system's estrangement from the patient's society (Al-Krenawi, 2005).

The scarcity of mental health professionals from minority backgrounds also contributes to the underutilization of these services (Weatherhead & Daiches, 2010). When mental health settings for Bedouins in Israel fail to use the same ethnic-national practitioners, or when Bedouins encounter professionals who cannot speak Arabic and do not use Arabic proverbs and have different values and beliefs, they are reluctant to seek mental help (Al-Krenawi, 1999, 2000). The cultural gap leads to mistrust between Palestinian clients and non-Palestinian mental health practitioners (Al-Krenawi, 2005). Thus, individuals with mental disorders in this society tend to seek treatment from traditional practitioners who share their identity and speak their language.

Lower levels of schooling and socioeconomic status, as well as being female and married, are related to delays in seeking psychiatric treatment because people in these categories are subject to stigmatizing attitudes with regard to mental disorders (Ponizovsky, Geraisy, Shoshan, Kremer, et al., 2007). Significant cultural differences with respect to gender may put women at a particularly high risk of not receiving timely diagnosis and treatment for mental health problems in Muslim communities (Al-Krenawi, 2005).

With respect to the rejection of mental health services, little distinction is made among the various mental health professionals: psychiatrists, psychologists, and marriage and family therapists (Al-Krenawi & Graham, 1999a). The roles of mental health practitioners and the nature of professional counseling are not well understood (Youssef & Deane, 2006). Mood symptoms, such as hopelessness, self-deprecatory thoughts, and worthlessness, are not commonly diagnosed, in particular among women. Service users frequently present conversion disorders that are defined by the DSM-IV as one or more symptoms or deficits that affect voluntary motor or sensory function suggestive of a neurological or other general medical condition (Dimsdale & Creed 2009), and do not show self-recognition of psychological distress or sadness but are ultimately diagnosed as suffering from depression (Al-Krenawi & Graham, 2000). While males tend to ascribe symptoms of mental illness to God's will, either directly or indirectly (through evil spirits), women often attribute them to sorcery, reflecting the integration of human behavior with supernatural powers (Al-Krenawi, 1999). Furthermore, as mentioned earlier, Palestinians often express such problems as physical or nonpsychiatric symptoms to avoid the stigma of mental symptoms (Al-Krenawi, 2005; Douki, Zineb, Nacef, & Halbreich, 2007; El-Islam, 2008; Ponizovsky, Geraisy, Shoshan, Kremer, et al., 2007).

Utilization of Mental Health Services

As noted throughout this book, Israel constitutes a multiethnic society with substantial interethnic and cultural differences among the various sectors. Many studies consider differences in attitudes toward utilization of mental health treatment services among diverse ethno-racial communities (Nakash & Levav, 2012; Nakash et al., 2012; Razali & Najib, 2000). For example, as Levav et al. (2007) found in the Israel National Health Survey, help-seeking rates from specialized health services were lower among Palestinians than among Jews in Israel. Despite their greater need, Palestinian users in Israel tend to underutilize mental health services (Al-Krenawi, 2005; Al-Krenawi & Graham, 1999a; Levav, 2009) and have higher therapy dropout rates compared to their Jewish counterparts (Al-Krenawi, 1999). Among those with mental illness, 2% of Palestinian citizens in Israel visited outpatient clinics compared to 70% of Jewish citizens, and only 7% of those treated were Palestinians compared to 67% of Jews (Struch et al., 2009).

Palestinian respondents generally expressed their desire to seek specialized health care only when their depression and anxiety disorders were accompanied by high distress scores (Levav et al., 2007; Ponizovsky, Geraisy, Shoshan, Kremer, et al., 2007).

Conclusions and Recommendations

The epidemiology of mental disorders among the older adult Palestinian population in Israel is still incomplete, and greater efforts should be focused on screening and treating such conditions in this population. As indicated in the literature, the prevalence of mental and cognitive disorders is higher among the Palestinian population in Israel than in the Jewish sector. In addition to genetic predisposition, various political, social, and cultural factors may underlie this phenomenon. Therefore, therapists should learn more about the religious affiliations, cultural practices, and national background of Palestinian service users before formulating treatment plans for them.

The Palestinian elderly and their families tend to avoid using mental health services and often hide mental or cognitive disorders from their society and from therapists, mainly because of negative views and stigma in their milieu. Therefore, interventions aimed at reducing fear and misconceptions relating to mental illness among the Palestinian population in Israel, including promotion of social interactions among potential service users, are recommended. In addition, decision makers should develop culturally competent psychogeriatric health services for the older population, which carry less stigma than psychiatric hospitalization and thus make them more acceptable to Palestinian society in Israel. Clinics should be established in these communities to provide individualized rehabilitation services, follow-ups, and referrals, as well as phone access to such services for the families of the mentally ill and specialized websites in Arabic.

It is also important to increase awareness among the clergy (e.g., sheikhs, imams, ministers) about the cognitive and mental disorders among older adults and the available pharmacological and psychological treatment for mental disorders. Interventions to change the perception of the psychiatrically ill as violent are important and might eventually lead to increased use of the biomedical services.

Specific interventions for dementia should include measures to educate the public about the need to show empathy and understanding toward older adults suffering from this condition. The public should also be informed about the biological basis of depression and the efficacy of the available treatments.

Future studies should examine the prevalence of mental and cognitive disorders among older adult Palestinian citizens in Israel and investigate the effects on mental health of sociocultural factors such as elder abuse, polygamy, and consanguinity. These studies should also take into account social, cultural, and political factors that possibly have an impact on the development of mental illness, as well as on the help-seeking patterns for mental health problems among this population.

RABIA KHALAILA is Associate Professor of Nursing and Gerontology and Vice President for Academic Affairs at Zefat Academic College, Israel.

References

Abu-Saad, H., Elbedour, S. M., Hallaq, E., Merrick, J., & Tenenbaum, A. (2014). Consanguineous marriage and intellectual and developmental disabilities among Arab Bedouins children of the Negev region in southern Israel: A pilot study. *Frontiers in Public Health, 2*(1–3). https://doi.org/10.3389/fpubh.2014.00003.

Adams, B. N., & Mburugu, E. (1994). Kikuyu bridewealth and polygyny today. *Journal of Comparative Family Studies, 25,* 159–166.

Al-Krenawi, A. (1998). Family therapy with a multiparental/multispousal family. *Family Process, 37*(1), 65–81.

Al-Krenawi, A. (1999). Explanations of mental health symptoms by the Bedouin-Arabs of the Negev. *International Journal of Social Psychiatry, 45*(1), 56–64.

Al-Krenawi, A. (2000). Bedouin-Arab clients' use of proverbs in the therapeutic setting. *International Journal for the Advancement of Counselling, 22*(2), 91–102.

Al-Krenawi, A. (2005). Socio-political aspects of mental health practice with Arabs in the Israeli context. *Israel Journal of Psychiatry and Related Sciences, 42*(2), 126–136.

Al-Krenawi, A. (2012). A study of psychological symptoms, family function, marital and life satisfactions of polygamous and monogamous women: The Palestinian case. *International Journal of Social Psychiatry, 58*(1), 79–86.

Al-Krenawi, A. (2013). Mental health and polygamy: The Syrian case. *World Journal of Psychiatry, 3*(1), 1.

Al-Krenawi, A., & Graham, J. R. (1999a). Gender and biomedical/traditional mental health utilization among the Bedouin-Arabs of the Negev. *Culture, Medicine, and Psychiatry, 23*(2), 219–243.

Al-Krenawi, A., & Graham, J. R. (1999b). Social work and Koranic mental health healers. *International Social Work, 42*(1), 53–65.

Al-Krenawi, A., & Graham, J. R. (2000). Culturally sensitive social work practice with Arab clients in mental health settings. *Health & Social Work, 25*(1), 9–22.

Al-Krenawi, A., & Graham, J. R. (2006). A comparison of family functioning, life and marital satisfaction, and mental health of women in polygamous and monogamous marriages. *International Journal of Social Psychiatry, 52*(1), 5–17.

Al-Krenawi, A., Graham, J. R., & Al Gharaibeh, F. (2011). A comparison study of psychological, family function, marital and life satisfactions of polygamous and monogamous women in Jordan. *Community Mental Health Journal, 47*(5), 594–602.

Al-Krenawi, A., Graham, J. R., Dean, Y. Z., & Eltaiba, N. (2004). Cross-national study of attitudes towards seeking professional help: Jordan, United Arab Emirates (UAE) and Arabs in Israel. *International Journal of Social Psychiatry, 50*(2), 102–114.

Al-Krenawi, A., Graham, J. R., & Maoz, B. (1996). The healing significance of the Negev's Bedouin Dervish. *Social Science & Medicine, 43*(1), 13–21.

Al-Krenawi, A., Graham, J. R., Ophir, M., & Kandah, J. (2001). Ethnic and gender differences in mental health utilization: The case of Muslim Jordanian and Moroccan Jewish Israeli out-patient psychiatric patients. *International Journal of Social Psychiatry, 47*(3), 42–54.

Al-Sherbiny, L. (2005). The case of first wife in polygamy: Description of an Arab culture-specific tradition. *Arabpsynet, 8,* 9–26. Retrieved from http://mail.arabpsynet.com/Archives/OP/apnJ8LotfiElsherbinie.pdf.

Bener, A., Dafeeah, E. E., & Samson, N. (2012). Does consanguinity increase the risk of schizophrenia? Study based on primary health care centre visits. *Mental Health in Family Medicine, 9*(4), 241–248.

Bowirrat, A., Friedland, R. P., Farrer, L., Baldwin, C., & Korczyn, A. (2002). Genetic and environmental risk factors for Alzheimer's disease in Israeli Arabs. *Journal of Molecular Neuroscience, 19*(1), 239–245.

Bowirrat, A., Friedland, R. P., & Korczyn, A. D. (2002). Vascular dementia among elderly Arabs in Wadi Ara. *Journal of the Neurological Sciences, 203*, 73–76.

Bowirrat, A., Oscar-Berman, M., & Logroscino, G. (2006). Association of depression with Alzheimer's disease and vascular dementia in an elderly Arab population of Wadi-Ara, Israel. *International Journal of Geriatric Psychiatry, 21*(3), 246–251.

Chaleby, K. (1985). Women of polygamous marriages in an inpatient psychiatric service in Kuwait. *The Journal of Nervous and Mental Disease, 173*(1), 56–58.

Dimsdale, J., & Creed, F. (2009). The proposed diagnosis of somatic symptom disorders in DSM-V to replace somatoform disorders in DSM-IV—a preliminary report. *Journal of Psychosomatic Research, 66*, 473–476.

Dobrusin, M., Weitzman, D., Levine, J., Kremer, I., Rietschel, M., Maier, W., & Belmaker, R. H. (2009). The rate of consanguineous marriages among parents of schizophrenic patients in the Arab Bedouin population in southern Israel. *The World Journal of Biological Psychiatry, 10*(4), 334–336.

Dong, X., Simon, M. A., Odwazny, R., & Gorbien, M. (2008). Depression and elder abuse and neglect among a community-dwelling Chinese elderly population. *Journal of Elder Abuse & Neglect, 20*(1), 25–41.

Douki, S., Zineb, S. B., Nacef, F., & Halbreich, U. (2007). Women's mental health in the Muslim world: Cultural, religious, and social issues. *Journal of Affective Disorders, 102*(1), 177–189.

Duivis, H. E., de Jonge, P., Penninx, B. W., Na, B. Y., Cohen, B. E., & Whooley, M. A. (2011). Depressive symptoms, health behaviors, and subsequent inflammation in patients with coronary heart disease: Prospective findings from the heart and soul study. *American Journal of Psychiatry, 168*(9), 913–920.

El-Islam, F. M. (2008). Arab culture and mental health care. *Transcultural Psychiatry, 45*(4), 671–682.

Gale, C., Sayer, A. A., Cooper, C., Dennison, E., Starr, J., Whalley, L., . . . Hardy, R. (2011). Factors associated with symptoms of anxiety and depression in five cohorts of community-based older people: The HALCyon (healthy ageing across the life course) programme. *Psychological Medicine, 41*(10), 2057–2073.

Geerlings, S. W., Beekman, A. T., Deeg, D. J., & Van Tilburg, W. (2000). Physical health and the onset and persistence of depression in older adults: An eight-wave prospective community-based study. *Psychological Medicine, 30*(2), 369–380.

Gelkopf, M., Solomon, Z., Berger, R., & Bleich, A. (2008). The mental health impact of terrorism in Israel: A repeat cross-sectional study of Arabs and Jews. *Acta Psychiatrica Scandinavica, 117*(5), 369–380.

Gross, R. (2007). Psychiatric epidemiology in Israel, 2007: Reflections on the Israel national health survey. *Israel Journal of Psychiatry and Related Sciences, 44*(2), 152–157.

Hamdan, A. (2009). Mental health needs of Arab women. *Health Care for Women International, 30*(7), 593–611.

Haque, A. (2004). Religion and mental health: The case of American Muslims. *Journal of Religion and Health, 43*(1), 45–58.

Israel Central Bureau of Statistics [Israel CBS]. (2011). *Israel in numbers* [in Hebrew]. Retrieved from http://www.cbs.gov.il/publications/isr_in_n11h.pdf.

Myers-JDC-Brookdale Institute. (2012). *The Arab population of Israel: Facts and figures 2012*. Retrieved from http://www.iataskforce.org/sites/default/files/resource/resource-1114.pdf.

Kadri, N., & Sartorius, N. (2005). The global fight against the stigma of schizophrenia. *PLoS Med, 2*(7), e136, 597–599. http://doi.org/10.1371/journal.pmed.0020136.

Kaplan, G., Glasser, S., Murad, H., Atamna, A., Alpert, G., Goldbourt, U., & Kalter-Leibovici, O. (2010). Depression among Arabs and Jews in Israel: A population-based study. *Social Psychiatry and Psychiatric Epidemiology, 45*(10), 931–939.

Khalaila, R., & Litwin, H. (2014). Changes in health behaviors and their associations with depressive symptoms among Israelis aged 50+. *Journal of Aging and Health, 26*(3), 401–421.

Levav, I. (2009). *Psychiatric and behavioral disorders in Israel: From epidemiology to mental health action.* Jerusalem: Gefen.

Levav, I., Ifrah, A., Geraisy, N., Grinshpoon, A., & Khwaled, R. (2007). Common mental disorders among Arab-Israelis: Findings from the Israel national health survey. *Israel Journal of Psychiatry and Related Sciences, 44*(2), 104–113.

Levinson, D., Zilber, N., Lerner, Y., Grinshpoon, A., & Levav, I. (2007). Prevalence of mood and anxiety disorders in the community: Results from the Israel national health survey. *Israel Journal of Psychiatry and Related Sciences, 44*(2), 94–103.

Litwin, H., & Zoabi, S. (2003). Modernization and elder abuse in an Arab-Israeli context. *Research on Aging, 25*(3), 224–246.

Lowenstein, A., Eisikovits, Z., Band-Winterstein, T., & Enosh, G. (2009). Is elder abuse and neglect a social phenomenon? Data from the first national prevalence survey in Israel. *Journal of Elder Abuse & Neglect, 21*(3), 253–277.

Mansour, H., Fathi, W., Klei, L., Wood, J., Chowdari, K., Watson, A., . . . Salah, H. (2010). Consanguinity and increased risk for schizophrenia in Egypt. *Schizophrenia Research, 120*(1), 108–112.

Na'amnih, W., Romano-Zelekha, O., Kabaha, A., Rubin, L. P., Bilenko, N., Jaber, L., . . . Shohat, T. (2015). Continuous decrease of consanguineous marriages among Arabs in Israel. *American Journal of Human Biology, 27*(1), 94–98.

Nakash, O., & Levav, I. (2012). Mental health stigma in a multicultural society: The case of Israel. *Psychology, Society & Education, 4*(2), 195–209.

Nakash, O., Nagar, M., Mandel, R., Alon, S., Gottfried, M., & Levav, I. (2012). Ethnic differentials in mental health needs and service utilization among persons with cancer. *Supportive Care in Cancer, 20*(9), 2217–2221.

Othman, H., & Saadat, M. (2009). Prevalence of consanguineous marriages in Syria. *Journal of Biosocial Science, 41*(5), 685–692.

Ozkan, M., Altindag, A., Oto, R., & Sentunali, E. (2006). Mental health aspects of Turkish women from polygamous versus monogamous families. *International Journal of Social Psychiatry, 52*(3), 214–220.

Pillemer, K., & Prescott, D. (1988). Psychological effects of elder abuse: A research note. *Journal of Elder Abuse & Neglect, 1*(1), 65–73.

Ponizovsky, A. M., Geraisy, N., Shoshan, E., & Kremer, I. (2007). Emotional distress among first-time patients attending outpatient mental health clinics in Israel: An Arab-Jewish comparative study. *Israel Journal of Psychiatry and Related Sciences, 44*(1), 62–70.

Ponizovsky, A. M., Geraisy, N., Shoshan, E., Kremer, I., & Smetannikov, E. (2007). Treatment lag on the way to the mental health clinic among Arab-and Jewish-Israeli patients. *Israel Journal of Psychiatry and Related Sciences, 44*(3), 234–243.

Razali, S., & Najib, M. (2000). Help-seeking pathways among Malay psychiatric patients. *International Journal of Social Psychiatry, 46*(4), 281–289.

Roepke-Buehler, S. K., Simon, M., & Dong, X. (2015). Association between depressive symptoms, multiple dimensions of depression, and elder abuse: A cross-sectional, population-based analysis of older adults in urban Chicago. *Journal of Aging and Health, 27*(6), 1003–1025.

Rouhana, N., & Ghanem, A. (1998). The crisis of minorities in ethnic states: The case of Palestinian citizens in Israel. *International Journal of Middle East Studies, 30*(3), 321–346.

Sa'di, A. H. (2002). Catastrophe, memory and identity: Al-Nakbah as a component of Palestinian identity. *Israel Studies, 7*(2), 175–198.

Savaya, R. (1996). Attitudes towards family and marital counseling among Israeli Arab women. *Journal of Social Service Research, 21*(1), 35–51.

Sharon, N., & Zoabi, S. (1997). Elder abuse in a land of tradition: The case of Israel's Arabs. *Journal of Elder Abuse & Neglect, 8*(4), 43–58.

Shemesh, A. A., Kohn, R., Blumstein, T., Geraisy, N., Novikov, I., & Levav, I. (2006). A community study on emotional distress among Arab and Jewish Israelis over the age of 60. *International Journal of Geriatric Psychiatry, 21*(1), 64–76.

Shepard, L. D. (2013). The impact of polygamy on women's mental health: A systematic review. *Epidemiology and Psychiatric Sciences, 22*, 47–62.

Slonim-Nevo, V., & Al-Krenawi, A. (2006). Success and failure among polygamous families: The experience of wives, husbands, and children. *Family Process, 45*(3), 311–330.

Somer, E., Maguen, S., Or-Chen, K., & Litz, B. T. (2009). Managing terror: Differences between Jews and Arabs in Israel. *International Journal of Psychology, 44*(2), 138–146.

Struch, N., Levav, I., Shereshevsky, Y., Baidani-Auerbach, A., Lachman, M., Daniel, N., & Zehavi, T. (2008). Stigma experienced by persons under psychiatric care. *Israel Journal of Psychiatry and Related Sciences, 45*(3), 210–218.

Struch, N., Shereshevsky, Y., Naon, D., Daniel, N., & Fischman, N. (2009). People with severe mental disorders in Israel: An integrated view of the service systems [in English]. Jerusalem: Myers-JDC-Brookdale Institute. Retrieved from https://brookdale.jdc.org.il /wp-content/uploads/2018/01/549-09-SevereMentalDisorders-ES-ENG.pdf.

Tarabeia, J., Baron-Epel, O., Barchana, M., Liphshitz, I., Ifrah, A., Fishler, Y., & Green, M. S. (2007). A comparison of trends in incidence and mortality rates of breast cancer, incidence to mortality ratio and stage at diagnosis between Arab and Jewish women in Israel, 1979–2002. *European Journal of Cancer Prevention, 16*(1), 36–42.

Tarabeia, J., Green, M. S., Barchana, M., Baron-Epel, O., Ifrah, A., Fishler, Y., & Nitzan-Kaluski, D. (2008). Increasing lung cancer incidence among Israeli Arab men reflects a change in the earlier paradox of low incidence and high smoking prevalence. *European Journal of Cancer Prevention, 17*(4), 291–296.

Vardi-Saliternik, R., Friedlander, Y., & Cohen, T. (2002). Consanguinity in a population sample of Israeli Muslim Arabs, Christian Arabs and Druze. *Annals of Human Biology, 29*(4), 422–431.

Walsemann, K. M., Gee, G. C., & Geronimus, A. T. (2009). Ethnic differences in trajectories of depressive symptoms: Disadvantage in family background, high school experiences, and adult characteristics. *Journal of Health and Social Behavior, 50*(1), 82–98.

Weatherhead, S., & Daiches, A. (2010). Muslim views on mental health and psychotherapy. *Psychology and Psychotherapy: Theory, Research, and Practice, 83*(1), 75–89.

Werner, P., Friedland, R. P., & Inzelberg, R. (2015). Alzheimer's disease and the elderly in Israel: Are we paying enough attention to the topic in the Arab population? *American Journal of Alzheimer's Disease and Other Dementias, 30*(5), 448–453.

Williams, D. R., Yu, Y., Jackson, J. S., & Anderson, N. B. (1997). Racial differences in physical and mental health: Socio-economic status, stress and discrimination. *Journal of Health Psychology, 2*(3), 335–351.

Youssef, J., & Deane, F. P. (2006). Factors influencing mental-health help-seeking in Arabic-speaking communities in Sydney, Australia. *Mental Health, Religion & Culture, 9*(1), 43–66.

PART III
PSYCHIATRIC AND BEHAVIORAL HEALTH DISORDERS AMONG PALESTINIAN CITIZENS IN ISRAEL

9

ATTITUDES, BELIEFS, AND STIGMA TOWARD MENTAL HEALTH ISSUES AMONG PALESTINIAN CITIZENS IN ISRAEL

Alean Al-Krenawi

ACCORDING TO THE WORLD HEALTH ORGANIZATION (WHO) (2015), mental disorders are one of the leading causes of the current global disease burden (GDB). The GDB provides data on the main causes of death and disability worldwide. As a measure, it uses the Disability-Adjusted Life-Years (DALY), which shows the potential years of life lost due to premature death and the years of life lost because of disability or ill health (Barratt, Kirwan, 2009; Shantikumar, 2018). The impact of mental disorders is expected to increase in coming decades, making it critical to deal with stigma in the efforts to reduce this burden.

Stigma is a socially powerful phenomenon that fuels a strong negative perception about individuals with mental disorders. It has been recognized as the most significant barrier to seeking care, adhering to treatment, and recovering from mental illness (Schulze & Angermeyer, 2003). The impact of stigma can be far-reaching and profound. Its consequences include unemployment, homelessness, diminished self-esteem, and weak social support. These issues pose major obstacles to recovery, affect long-term prognosis, and induce disability. Additionally, stigma can disrupt relationships and reduce normal social interactions because of the desire for secrecy with which it is associated.

Stigma as a Universal Phenomenon

Stigma presents people with specific features in a negative light and leads to their exclusion as a result of race, religion, nationality, physical disabilities, and/or mental illness. With reference to the latter, stigma perpetuates the perception of the population with severe mental disorders as an unusual and dangerous group in society.

The sources of stigma are diverse, and so are its effects. Individuals with mental illness as well as their families may experience both direct discrimination from others within the community, in the form of unfair social policies, and internalized stigma, resulting from negative attitudes toward mental illness that resonate with the individual diagnosed.

Public conceptions about people with mental illness may lead to prejudice, discrimination, and stereotyping (Corrigan, 2004). The stigmatizing behavior that often accompanies mental illness can create complex barriers to recovery, making it difficult for those struggling with this disease to deal with everyday demands in romantic and family relationships, communication, employment, and achieving life goals. Another aspect of stigma that influences the daily routine of people with mental illness is the damage it may do to their confidence and sense of self.

It is not uncommon for those suffering from mental illness to try to avoid being subjected to stigma by hiding their problems and not seeking professional care (Corrigan, 2004; Gary, 2005). Such individuals may adopt two different behavioral repertoires: one for being among those who are aware of their illness and another for those who are not. This trend leaves sick people, who would under different circumstances seek treatment and live a more fulfilling and healthier life, untreated and at risk of perpetuating their illness. Stigma-related perceptions about mental illness can be tackled from many angles. For example, educational programs dedicated to addressing and refuting the social stigma linked with mental illness could be constructed, thus diminishing negative associations. A further direction would be to encourage those with mental illness to publicly share their struggles and advocate against prejudice. Such a course would reflect the positive capabilities and strength of people with mental illness and even elevate their confidence as they take a stand against the prejudice that stigmas produce (Corrigan, Watson, & Barr, 2006; Karnieli-Miller et al., 2013).

Double Stigma and Courtesy Stigma

Studies on relatives of individuals with mental illness report that family members may experience a "double stigma" (Angermeyer, Schulze, & Dietrich, 2003, p. 600). Focus group interviews have revealed that in addition to experiencing stigma directly because of their familial relationship, relatives of individuals diagnosed with schizophrenia also shared some of the disapproval of the stigmatized person by identifying themselves with him or her. Family members encountered stigma toward themselves as well as their mentally ill relatives in four areas: interpersonal interaction, structural discrimination, public images of mental illness, and access to social roles (Angermeyer et al., 2003; Schulze & Angermeyer, 2003). Additionally, it has been found that families may further contribute to stigma by overprotecting their mentally ill relative (Angermeyer et al., 2003; González-Torres, Oraa, Arístegui, Fernández-Rivas, & Guimon, 2007).

Goffman (1963, p. 30) introduced the notion of "courtesy stigma" to describe the devaluation of family members of individuals with a mental disorder. While the symptoms of mental illness do not always present in a clear way, courtesy stigma can contribute to the delay of treatment for psychiatric symptoms until they reach crisis proportions (Gerson et al., 2009). Parents dealing with the mental illness of a child have the added burden of dealing with the predominant view that mental disorders stem from faulty parental discipline or socialization (Hinshaw, 2005). Parental blame is a legacy of twentieth-century conceptions of mental illness and still remains one of its major tenets, which contributes to parents' continued reluctance to seek evaluation and treatment for emotional and behavioral abnormalities of their offspring (Hinshaw, 2008).

Public Stigma and Self-Stigma

Stigma here and elsewhere is defined as a mark or flaw resulting from a personal or physical characteristic that is viewed as socially unacceptable (Blaine, 1999). Corrigan (2004) described two types: public stigma and self-stigma. Public stigma is the perception held by a group or society that an individual is socially unacceptable and often leads to negative associations toward him or her, whereas self-stigma is the decline of an individual's self-esteem or self-worth caused by the individual self-labeling him- or herself as an unacceptable person (Vogel, Wade, & Haake, 2006).

Cultural, Religious, and Societal Perceptions of Mental Illness among Palestinian Citizens in Israel

Although stigma appears to be a universal phenomenon, its meanings, practices, and outcomes differ across cultures. Western culture tends to be less stigmatizing and more accepting of people with mental illness and their families, while non-Western cultures show little tolerance toward mentally ill people and their relatives (Al-Krenawi & Graham, 2000). In Eastern cultures, there is a common conception that mentally ill people are dangerous and aggressive, which leads to them being discriminated against (Lauber & Rössler, 2007).

Mental illness is perceived as a taboo among the Palestinian population in Israel. For this population, public stigma results from the view held by the family and ethnic community that the individual is socially unacceptable. In addition, self-stigma can occur when individuals internalize public stigma and begin to view themselves as socially unacceptable.

Thus, the association between public stigma and attitudes toward therapy may be mediated by self-stigma or by the internalization of the negative messages of the community or family with regard to mental illness. Self-stigma can reduce or increase the role of public stigma in predicting attitudes toward psychiatric treatment.

Across traditional cultures worldwide, mental illness has long been understood as spiritually based. Many Muslim Arabs, for example, believe that there are two spirits; one is good, and the other, called *Iblis* (the devil), is bad (Ibn-Tymiah, 1957). In this perspective, the bad spirit seduces humankind to commit sins against God, and therefore the sinners are punished physically and psychologically (El-Shamy, 1977; Ibn-Tymiah, 1957). This belief is revealed in everyday language—a common Arabic term used to describe mental illness is *majnun*, which is derived from the term *jinn*, meaning "a supernatural spirit" (Al-Krenawi & Graham, 2000).

According to some religious leaders, illness is one method of connection with God and should not be considered as alien but "rather . . . an event, a mechanism of the body, that is serving to cleanse, purify, and balance us on the physical, emotional, mental, and spiritual planes" (Rassool, 2000, p. 1479). This core belief has been reported in numerous studies on the perspectives of Muslim community members toward physical and mental illnesses. Mental illness is considered to be divine punishment or the will of God (Al-Krenawi, 1995; Eickelman, 1966). Muslim culture places great weight on *qader*, or destiny, and illness may be seen as an opportunity to restore faith or a connection to Allah through regular prayer and a sense of self-responsibility.

Palestinian citizens in Israel are in a state of acculturation, "a process of adaptation and change whereby a person or an ethnic, social, religious, language or national group integrates with or adapts to the cultural values and patterns of the majority group" (Al-Krenawi & Graham, 2005, pp. 310–311). Although the collectivity of Palestinian citizens in Israel is quite strong and the population still feels attached to its community, religion, and history, they are gradually adapting to different features of Israeli Jewish culture. Arab citizens who are in a state of transition from Eastern to Western culture tend to consider the use of mental health care and to show less stigmatizing behavior toward persons with mental illness (Al-Krenawi, 2002) than traditional and religious Arabs, who tend to ignore the illness, stigmatize the ill person, and consider only the most traditional treatments. Despite the significant societal changes that occurred in Israel, the attitude of its Palestinian citizens toward mental health has resisted modification, which leads to treatment challenges.

Gender Roles as They Relate to Stigma

One of the most salient features in the life of Palestinian citizens of Israel concerns gender roles. While women are responsible for bearing and nurturing children, men are expected to support the family financially and make the important familial decisions. Many women still do not have careers outside of the home (Al-Krenawi, 2013). In addition, the mother is often tasked with the children's religious education and observance (Abu-Ras, 2007; Al-Krenawi, Graham, Dean, & Eltaiba, 2004). It is worth mentioning that, despite the Western perception that Arab women are oppressed (Erickson & Al-Timimi, 2001), they may have equal or even more influential roles in the family that are practiced in a more discreet way (Mahmood, 2005).

Mental health services can be particularly stigmatizing for Palestinian women because they are considered more vulnerable than men. Douki, Zineb, Nacef, and Halbreich (2007) found that women are at a greater risk of developing mental disorders than men. According to Islam, women are more readily influenced by "the evil spirit"—mental illness—than men, a belief that might be an outcome of gender differences (El-Shamy, 1977; Ibn-Tymiah, 1957).

Palestinian citizens of Israel who seek mental health services, like those in other non-Western societies, can find psychiatric and psychological intervention (Fabrega, 1991) and family and marital therapies (Savaya, 1998) stigmatizing. This is particularly true for women in the Muslim world, as the stigma of mental health services have the potential to damage their marital prospects, increase the likelihood of separation or divorce, or be used by a husband or his family as leverage for obtaining a second wife (Al-Krenawi, 1998; Bazzoui & Al-Issa, 1966; Okasha & Lotaif, 1979).

Help-Seeking Behavior among Palestinian Citizens in Israel

"Help seeking" is the process of looking for assistance from others during a time of personal crisis or chronic psychological discomfort, including distress caused by mental illness (Lifeline Australia, 2017). Perceptions of help-seeking behavior vary widely; thus, some view help seeking as a sign of weakness or failure, and therefore reach out for psychological or psychiatric help only as a last resort. Others turn to therapy as an answer to more everyday problems. Such radically different attitudes toward help seeking can be associated with factors such as gender, social norms, and cultural beliefs, as well as personal characteristics, such as one's personal beliefs about psychological therapy, the extent of support one gets from his or her family or friends, the self- and public stigma regarding psychological care, the ability to expose oneself to others, the individual's economic situation, and the urgency of the problem (Mojaverian, Hashimoto, & Kim, 2013). With respect to the influence of stigma on help seeking, a growing body of literature demonstrates that people fear the stigma that is associated with seeking psychological or psychiatric treatment (Baptista & Zanon, 2017; Corrigan, Watson, & Barr, 2006). Effective help-seeking strategies may be collective and collaborative (Committee on the Science of Changing Behavioral Health Social Norms; Board on Behavioral, Cognitive, and Sensory Sciences; Division of Behavioral and Social Sciences and Education, 2016).

Importantly, while the individual may him- or herself perceive a mental health problem, it may be the family of the sufferer that initiates its articulation and resolution. The collective (*hamula*-based) nature of Palestinian society is a vital feature of the help-seeking process, as the family exerts a strong influence on the individual's perception and the way in which he or she decides to deal with his or her problems (Al-Krenawi, 1995; Al-Krenawi & Graham, 1999a, 1999b, 1999c).

Cultural influences on presentation of symptoms and mental health problems also warrant consideration. Because of the lesser stigma of physical symptoms as well as cultural idioms of distress revolving around the physical body, mental health problems are often expressed as physical symptoms. At the same time, explicit mood symptoms such as hopelessness, self-deprecatory thoughts, and worthlessness are uncommon. In particular, women ultimately diagnosed with depression often first present with conversion disorders (neurological symptoms that cause distress and impairment but cannot be linked to a neurological disease) and no self-recognition of psychological distress or sadness (Al-Krenawi & Graham, 2000; Al-Krenawi & Jackson, 2014).

Mental Health Services and Barriers

A range of factors may contribute to the stigmatization of mental health services among Palestinian citizens in Israel. First, cultural expectations may complicate the healing procedure. For example, men may resist receiving help from a female social worker or psychologist because of the gender differences in status in Palestinian society. A related difficulty could arise if the mental health practitioner is male and the patient is female. There are clear perceptions in the Arab world about gender: males are expected to play the dominant role and exercise power across life areas. Second, as a result of the abiding collectivist orientation in Palestinian society in Israel, family members expect a high level of involvement in the healing process; this approach may run counter to that of the practitioner. The family unit is sacred in the Arab world, and family members expect to be consistently consulted in times of crisis. The patient's family might even terminate treatment if they do not trust the therapist or if they look to the therapist to provide a solution and such a solution is not forthcoming.

A further feature that applies particularly to the Palestinian community in Israel and that has a major impact on help seeking and treatment is the political component. Therapists' national affiliation has the potential to impact strongly on their relationship with their patients. The ongoing geopolitical conflict between Jewish Israelis and Palestinians leaves Palestinian citizens in Israel ambivalent toward modern Israeli mental health services, despite the fact that mental health intervention might improve their lives (Al-Krenawi & Graham, 1996). Some Palestinians residing in Israel perceive Israeli mental health services as culturally insensitive to them. In addition, political motivations can be erroneously ascribed to these services and, as a consequence, spur the Palestinian population in Israel to avoid mental health services (Lee, 2001).

Religion plays a major role in the lives of many Palestinian citizens in Israel. Accordingly, Palestinians tend to choose traditional religious treatments and consult traditional healers over professional therapists. Muslim healers—sheikhs—base their work on the Qu'ran (Al-Krenawi & Graham, 1999c). Palestinians tend to rely on these healers because both the patient and the healer live in the same community and share the same traditions, values, and religious practices. Moreover, the healers offer treatments without labelling diagnoses (Al-Krenawi, 2005).

Reducing Stigma and Other Treatment Barriers

One way that stigma can be reduced or avoided is by integrating mental health services into stigma-free settings, such as general medical clinics (as facilitated by the 2015 Israeli psychiatry reform) and general hospitals (Al-Krenawi, 1996).

In addition, the therapist should strive to prevent politics from influencing the course of the treatment by self-educating about the religious, cultural, and national background of the patient. Before formulating a treatment plan, the therapist must take a thorough history of the patient and family, the family dynamics, and the patient and family's degree of religious affiliation. Alongside this, the therapist must gain an understanding of the views of the patient and his or her family on health and medicine, and Western society. As noted above, religion is a cornerstone in the lives of many Palestinian Arabs, and in Israel, religion is one of the most salient markers of cultural differences among citizens (Al-Abdul-Jabbar & Al-Issa, 2000, p. 278).

Across cultures and treatment modalities, the therapeutic alliance has been identified as a major predictor of treatment efficacy (Knobloch-Fedders, 2008). Crucially, among Palestinian citizens of Israel, this alliance must be extended to the patient's family. This goal of a more expansive trust relationship follows from the enduring communal orientation of the Arab population.

Guidelines for Treatment of Diverse Populations: The Arab Case

Beyond gaining a clear history of the patient and his or her family and showing sensitivity toward the values of the Arab world, specific methods should be developed for treating Palestinian citizens of Israel who are suffering from mental illness.

The treatment of Arab patients with Western methods often exposes two distinct worldviews. The practitioner has acquired globalized knowledge that allows him or her to take care of people and approach treatment from this viewpoint, while the patient has localized knowledge and constructs reality from his or her own perception. The practitioner is actually coding a specific perception to the patient; however, the patient is decoding the perception from a different point of view (Van der Wel et al., 2018). Perceptual misunderstandings between the practitioner and patient have the potential to derail treatment. When the globalized knowledge of the therapist and the localized knowledge of the patient meet head on, the collision can create confusion that damages therapeutic communication. Some Palestinian citizens in Israel are experiencing acculturation and adapting to the common culture of the majority. Acculturation has a direct impact on both the treatment and the relationship of the practitioner and patient. An acculturated service user is better equipped to understand the terms and perspective of the globalized knowledge of the practitioner, which reduces misunderstandings and allows the construction of a trusting and helping therapeutic relationship.

Before treatment begins, the practitioner must formulate a culturally attuned and efficient plan for the patient. Al-Krenawi and Graham (2005) have proposed several guidelines and recommendations for treating patients from Palestinian society. Their suggestions highlight the importance of developing less stigmatizing services while working collaboratively with the patient, his or her immediate and extended family, traditional healers, and key stakeholders in the community. All interventions with Palestinian patients should be made in the broader context of family, community, and tribal background. As such, they necessitate knowledge of customs and cultural norms. Treatment planning must take into account the patient's identity as it is situated within the family's collective identity. Additionally, religion should be considered a foundational context in which problems are constructed and resolved. Palestinian patients' communication may be restrained and formal, and their idioms of distress might rely on a complex system of metaphors and proverbs. As such, cultural sensitivity is needed to communicate effectively. Treatments tend to be most successful when they are short term and directive, offering specific strategies and solutions (Al-Krenawi & Graham, 2005).

In sum, for the success of the mental health intervention, the therapist must consider the patient's history, gender, and family, as well as other features of Palestinian citizens in Israel. Practitioners must be culturally sensitive to and build trust with both the service user and the family. The treatment plan should be short term and directive. At the same time, the practitioner must remember that treating a person from a changing society is a complex process that calls for creative flexibility.

Conclusion

People with mental illness and their families deal with a strong negative perception derived from a socially dominant construct known as stigma. The stigma associated with mental disorders is the most significant barrier to seeking care, adhering to treatment, and recovering from mental illnesses. The collective nature of Arab society, in which the family has a marked influence on the individual's perception and the way he or she chooses to confront problems, is another factor affecting stigma and the help-seeking process. Research on health and social service utilization among minority Arab individuals in advanced industrialized countries points to lower rates of utilization of mental health services compared to their nonminority fellow citizens. Moreover, many obstacles for services delivery exist, including gender dynamics, language barriers, culturally inappropriate services, and communication style (Al-Krenawi & Graham, 2000). The practitioner must formulate a treatment plan that is both culturally attuned and highly efficient. This chapter presents several guidelines and recommendations for treating patients from Arab societies.

ALEAN AL-KRENAWI is Professor of Social Work; Director of the Center for Bedouin Studies and Development at Ben-Gurion University, Israel; and

Dean of the School of Social Work at Memorial University, Newfoundland, Canada. He is editor (with John Graham) of *Multicultural Social Work in Canada: Working with Diverse Ethno-racial Communities* and author of *Building Peace through Knowledge: The Israeli-Palestinian Case.*

References

Abu-Ras, W. (2007). Cultural beliefs and service utilization by battered Arab immigrant women. *Violence Against Women, 13*(10), 1002–1028.

Al-Abdul-Jabbar, J., & Al-Issa, I. (2000). Psychotherapy in Islamic society. In I. Al-Issa (Ed.), *Al-Junun: Mental illness in the Islamic world* (pp. 277–293). Madison, CT: International Universities Press.

Al-Krenawi, A. (1995). *A study of dual use of modern and traditional mental health systems by the Bedouin of the Negev.* Canada: University of Toronto.

Al-Krenawi, A. (1996). Group work with Bedouin widows of the Negev in a medical clinic. *Affilia, 11*(3), 303–318.

Al-Krenawi, A. (1998). Family therapy with a multiparental/multispousal family. *Family Process, 37*(1), 65–81.

Al-Krenawi, A. (2002). Mental health service utilization among the Arabs in Israel. *Social Work in Health Care, 35*(1–2), 577–589.

Al-Krenawi, A. (2005). Socio-political aspects of mental health practice with Arabs in the Israeli context. *Israel Journal of Psychiatry and Related Sciences, 42*(2), 126–136.

Al-Krenawi, A. (2013). Mental health and polygamy: The Syrian case. *World Journal of Psychiatry, 3*(1), 1–7.

Al-Krenawi, A., & Graham, J. R. (1996). Tackling mental illness: Roles for old and new disciplines. *World Health Forum, 17*(3), 246–248.

Al-Krenawi, A., & Graham, J. R. (1999a). Conflict resolution through a traditional ritual among the Bedouin Arabs of the Negev. *Ethnology, 38*(2), 163–174.

Al-Krenawi, A., & Graham, J. R. (1999b). Gender and biomedical/traditional mental health utilization among the Bedouin-Arabs of the Negev. *Culture, Medicine and Psychiatry, 23*(2), 219–243.

Al-Krenawi, A., & Graham, J. R. (1999c). Social work and Koranic mental health healers. *International Social Work, 42*(1), 53–65.

Al-Krenawi, A., & Graham, J. R. (2000). Culturally sensitive social work practice with Arab clients in mental health settings. *Health & Social Work, 25*(1), 9–22.

Al-Krenawi, A., & Graham, J. R. (2003). Social work with Canadians of Arab background: Insight into direct practice. In A. Al-Krenawi & J. R. Graham (Eds.), *Multicultural social work in Canada: Working with diverse ethno-racial communities* (pp. 174–201). Toronto: Oxford University Press.

Al-Krenawi, A., & Graham, J. R. (2005). Marital therapy for Arab Muslim Palestinian couples in the context of reacculturation. *The Family Journal, 13*(3), 300–310.

Al-Krenawi, A., Graham, J. R., Dean, Y. Z., & Eltaiba, N. (2004). Cross-national study of attitudes towards seeking professional help: Jordan, United Arab Emirates (UAE) and Arabs in Israel. *International Journal of Social Psychiatry, 50*(2), 102–114.

Al-Krenawi, A., & Jackson, S. O. (2014). Arab American marriage: Culture, tradition, religion, and the social worker. *Journal of Human Behavior in the Social Environment, 24*(2), 115–137.

Angermeyer, M. C., Schulze, B., & Dietrich, S. (2003). Courtesy stigma. *Social Psychiatry and Psychiatric Epidemiology, 38*(10), 593–602.

Baptista, M. N., & Zanon, C. (2017). Why not seek therapy? The role of stigma and psychological symptoms in college students. *Paidéia (Ribeirão Preto) 27*(67), 76–77. Retrieved from http://www.scielo.br/pdf/paideia/v27n67/1982-4327-paideia-27-67-00076.pdf.

Barrett, H., & Kirwan, M. (2009). Measures of disease burden (event-based and time-based) and population attributable risks including identification of comparison groups appropriate to public health. *Health Knowledge,* 1. Retrieved from https://www.healthknowledge.org.uk/public-health-textbook/research-methods/1c-health-care-evaluation.

Bazzoui, W., & Al-Issa, I. (1966). Psychiatry in Iraq. *British Journal of Psychiatry, 112*(489), 827–832.

Blaine, B. (1999). *The psychology of diversity: Perceiving and experiencing social difference.* Mountain View, CA: Mayfield.

Committee on the Science of Changing Behavioral Health Social Norms; Board on Behavioral, Cognitive, and Sensory Sciences; Division of Behavioral and Social Sciences and Education; National Academies of Sciences, Engineering, and Medicine. (2016). *Ending discrimination against people with mental and substance use disorders: The evidence for stigma change.* Washington, DC: National Academies Press. Retrieved from https://www.ncbi.nlm.nih.gov/books/NBK384914/.

Corrigan, P. (2004). How stigma interferes with mental health care. *American Psychologist, 59*(7), 614–625.

Corrigan, P., Watson, A. C., & Barr, L. (2006). The self-stigma of mental illness: Implications for self-esteem and self-efficacy. *Journal of Social and Clinical Psychology, 25*(8), 875–884.

Douki, S., Zineb, S. B., Nacef, F., & Halbreich, U. (2007). Women's mental health in the Muslim world: Cultural, religious, and social issues. *Journal of Affective Disorders, 102*(1), 177–189.

Eickelman, D. (1966, March). *The Islamic attitude towards possession states.* Paper presented at the Proceedings of the Second Annual Conference, Trance and Possession States, R. M. Bucke Memorial Society, Montreal, Canada.

El-Shamy, H. (1977). *The supernatural belief-practice system in the contemporary folk cultures of Egypt.* Bloomington, IN: Folklore Publications Group.

Erickson, C. D., & Al-Timimi, N. R. (2001). Providing mental health services to Arab Americans: Recommendations and considerations. *Cultural Diversity and Ethnic Minority Psychology, 7*(4), 308–327.

Fabrega, H. (1991). Psychiatric stigma in non-Western societies. *Comprehensive Psychiatry, 32*(6), 534–551.

Gary, F.A. (2005). Stigma: Barrier to mental health care among ethnic minorities. *Issues in Mental Health Nursing, 26*(10), 979–999.

Gerson, R., Davidson, L., Booty, A., McGlashan, T., Malespina, D., Pincus, H. A., & Corcoran, C. (2009). Families' experience with seeking treatment for recent-onset psychosis. *Psychiatric Services, 60*(6), 812–816.

Goffman, E. (1963). *Stigma: Notes on the management of spoiled identity.* Englewood Cliffs, NJ: Prentice Hall.

González-Torres, M. A., Oraa, R., Arístegui, M., Fernández-Rivas, A., & Guimon, J. (2007). Stigma and discrimination towards people with schizophrenia and their family members. *Social Psychiatry and Psychiatric Epidemiology, 42*(1), 14–23.

Hinshaw, S. P. (2005). The stigmatization of mental illness in children and parents: Developmental issues, family concerns, and research needs. *Journal of Child Psychology and Psychiatry, 46*(7), 714–734.

Hinshaw, S. P. (2008). *Breaking the silence: Mental health professionals disclose their personal and family experiences of mental illness.* New York: Oxford University Press.

Ibn-Tymiah, A. (1957). *The task of the Jinn* [in Arabic]. Cairo: Maatbaat Al-Sunna Al-Muhammadeh.

Karnieli-Miller, O., Perlick, D. A., Nelson, A., Mattias, K., Corrigan, P., & Roe, D. (2013). Family members' of persons living with a serious mental illness: Experiences and efforts to cope with stigma. *Journal of Mental Health, 22*(3), 254–262.

Knobloch-Fedders, L. (2008). The importance of the relationship with the therapist. *Clinical Science Insights: Knowledge Families Count On, 1,* 1–3. Retrieved from https://www.family-institute.org/sites/default/files/pdfs/csi_fedders_relationship_with_therapist.pdf.

Lauber, C., & Rössler, W. (2007). Stigma towards people with mental illness in developing countries in Asia. *International Review of Psychiatry, 19*(2), 157–178.

Lee, S. (2001). Who is politicising psychiatry in China? *British Journal of Psychiatry, 179*(2), 178–179.

Lifeline Australia. What is help-seeking? Retrieved from https://www.lifeline.org.au/static/uploads/files/what-is-help-seeking-wfwydudaixnf.pdf.

Mahmood, S. (2005). *Politics of piety: The Islamic revival and the feminist subject.* Princeton, NJ: Princeton University Press.

Mojaverian, T., Hashimoto, T., and Kim, H. S. (2013). Cultural differences in professional help seeking: A comparison of Japan and the U.S. *Front Psychol, 3,* 615. Retrieved from https://doi.org/10.3389/fpsyg.2012.00615.

Okasha, A., & Lotaif, F. (1979). Attempted suicide: An Egyptian investigation. *Acta Psychiatrica Scandinavica, 60*(1), 69–75.

Rassool, G. H. (2000). The crescent and Islam: Healing, nursing and the spiritual dimension. Some considerations towards an understanding of the Islamic perspectives on caring. *Journal of Advanced Nursing, 32*(6), 1476–1484.

Savaya, R. (1998). The under-use of psychological services by Israeli Arabs: An examination of the roles of negative attitudes and the use of alternative sources of help. *International Social Work, 41*(2), 195–209.

Schulze, B., & Angermeyer, M. C. (2003). Subjective experiences of stigma. A focus group study of schizophrenic patients, their relatives and mental health professionals. *Social Science & Medicine, 56*(2), 299–312.

Shantikumar, S. (2018). Measures of disease burden (event-based and time-based) and population attributable risks including identification of comparison groups appropriate to public health. *Health Knowledge, 1.* Retrieved from https://www.healthknowledge.org.uk/public-health-textbook/research-methods/1a-epidemiology/measures-disease-burden.

Van der Wel, Robrecht P.R.D., et al. Action perception from a common coding perspective. Donders Institute for Brain, Cognition, and Behavior, Radboud University Nijmegen, Netherlands, 35–36. Retrieved from https://somby.ceu.edu/sites/somby.ceu.edu/files/attachment/basicpage/6/inpressrobchapter.pdf.

Vogel, D. L., Wade, N. G., & Haake, S. (2006). Measuring the self-stigma associated with seeking psychological help. *Journal of Counseling Psychology, 53*(3), 325.

World Health Organization (WHO). (2015). Disease burden and mortality estimates. Retrieved from http://www. who.int/healthinfo/global_burden_disease/estimates.

10

MENTAL HEALTH STATUS, SERVICE USE, AND HELP-SEEKING PRACTICES OF CHILDREN AND ADOLESCENTS AMONG PALESTINIAN CITIZENS IN ISRAEL

Ivonne Mansbach-Kleinfeld and Raida Daeem

IN THEIR COMPREHENSIVE REVIEW OF ISRAELI STUDIES, STERNE and Porter (2013) claimed that the Israel Survey of Mental Health among Adolescents (ISMEHA), carried out in 2004–2005, had filled a prolonged void in epidemiological information on children and adolescents. This nationwide study assessed the prevalence rates of mental disorders and treatment gaps in a representative sample of 14- to 17-year-old Israeli adolescents (Mansbach-Kleinfeld, Levinson, et al., 2010). The study yielded information on a wide range of issues, such as prevalence rates of common mental disorders (Farbstein et al., 2010), use of mental health services in the community by mothers of adolescents with a mental disorder (Mansbach-Kleinfeld, Farbstein, et al., 2010), and visits to the primary care practitioner (PCP) (Mansbach-Kleinfeld, Palti, Ifrah, Levinson, & Farbstein, 2011).

By comparing Palestinian minority youth in Israel with Jewish Israeli majority adolescents, the ISMEHA provided an empirical estimate of the seldom measured large disparity in mental health service utilization that exists to the detriment of Palestinian youth (Mansbach-Kleinfeld, Farbstein, et al., 2010). This considerable treatment gap among Palestinian youth led the researchers, as well as the Israel National Institute for Health Policy Research (NIHP), to undertake further examination of the mental health status and mental health service needs and utilization of these adolescents, with particular emphasis on structural and cultural obstacles to help seeking. The Galilee Study, carried out between September 2012 and May 2014, was designed to address these questions. However, unlike the ISMEHA, which combined all Palestinian youth into one pooled group, the Galilee Study, which included Palestinian ninth-grade students living in the Galilee and surrounding regions, distinguished among the different subpopulations comprising the Palestinian minority.

The precondition presented by the NIHP for funding the Galilee Study was that Mental Health Services of the Israel Ministry of Health complete a mapping of the services available for the minority population by 2011 (Mansbach-Kleinfeld et al., 2013). This would allow a baseline on the availability of public mental health clinics for children and adolescents to be established. Data were analyzed according to geographic districts and population groups. Most of the Palestinian population is concentrated in the Northern District (53.1%), followed by the Haifa District (17.8%), the Southern District (15.8%), the Central District (11.9%), and Jaffa (1.4%). Palestinians living in East Jerusalem (nearly 300,000 inhabitants in 2011), were not included in this mapping given that most have a resident status and not citizenship, and their rights and the services they receive are not comparable to those of the rest of the Israeli population.

The mapping showed the geographic, structural, and ethnic-national disparities in the provision of professional mental health care by the state. It revealed that, on the whole, 49.9% of all Israeli children and adolescents in need of mental health care received treatment in a public mental health clinic in 2011, in contrast to 19.8% among Palestinian children. "Need for care" was calculated based on the estimate of the Israel Ministry of Health that 2% of the general child and adolescent population will need care for a mental health problem each year, once the 2015 Mental Health Reform is enacted (Tabibian-Mizrahi, 2007). The treatment gap—that is, the percentage of adolescents who need treatment but do not receive it—for Palestinian adolescents was particularly high in the Northern District (83.2%), the Haifa District (62.2%), and the Southern District (95.7%), compared to 34.5%, 34%, and 42.2% for Jewish Israelis, respectively (Mansbach-Kleinfeld et al., 2013).

By 2011, only two public mental health clinics for children and adolescents in which the clinical professionals spoke Arabic existed in Palestinian localities: one in the Galilee (Northern District) and one in the Triangle region (Haifa District). Clinics serving the majority population, where the spoken language is Hebrew, are less accessible to Palestinian youth. The language barrier is a strong obstacle when caring for children and adolescents who have little or no knowledge of Hebrew and their communication with professionals who do not speak Arabic or are not acquainted with their cultural codes is deficient.

Several factors influence the great disparity in public mental health clinics and number of clinicians by region and population group. One factor accounting for the shortage of available services staffed by Arabic-speaking mental health professionals is that Palestinian professionals are underrepresented in Israel. An unpublished report from the Department of Information of the Israel Ministry of Health listed the number of new licenses approved for the different clinical mental health professions between 2000 and 2013: of the 487 licenses approved for psychiatrists, 2.2% were granted to Palestinians; of the 117 licenses approved for child and adolescent psychiatrists, 2.6% were granted to Palestinians; and of the 5,664 licenses approved for clinical psychologists, 6.2% were granted to Palestinians. In 2011 Palestinian children and adolescents under 18 years of age represented nearly 26% of all Israeli children and adolescents. Clearly, the number of clinical professionals licensed by the Israel Ministry of Health is inadequate.

The fact that so few Palestinian professionals complete the requirements to obtain a clinician's license calls for a revision of the Israeli public educational system regarding the Palestinian sector. But this may not be an easy task. In Israel, the educational system is segregated, and Jewish and Palestinian students attend separate schools, have different curricula, learn in different languages, and have a different budget allocation, biased against the Palestinian sector (Hesketh, Bishara, Rosenberg, & Zaher, 2011). According to a report of the Israel Central Bureau of Statistics (2004), in the school year 2000/2001, the Israeli government invested NIS 534 for each Palestinian student in the educational system compared to NIS 1,779 for each Jewish student. In 2012 about 28% of the Palestinian students completed their high school diploma compared with 51% among the Jewish students, and only 22% of the Palestinian students reached the minimum requirement to be accepted by a university compared with 44% among Jewish students. In addition, in 2011 only 11% of the BA students, 7% of the MA students, and 3% of the PhD students were Palestinians (Nesher, 2012).

It seems, then, that a couple of factors may be responsible for the low number of Arabic-speaking mental health professionals and the low number of child and adolescent mental health clinics available for this minority population: (1) Insufficient public mental health clinics have been established in areas populated mainly by Palestinian citizens, based on the claim that, although great efforts are made to find suitable staff, there are not enough Arabic-speaking mental health professionals to work in these clinics (G. Lubin, former director of Mental Health Services, Ministry of Health, Israel, personal communication). (2) The educational system in the Palestinian sector has low standards, and therefore the academic level of students does not allow them to compete with their Jewish counterparts when applying for higher education slots. This vicious circle may be severed only by modifying education policies to increase excellence and competitiveness of Palestinian students or by other policy decisions such as affirmative action.

Another popular argument supported by studies (Struch et al., 2007) and presented by those who believe there is no need for the establishment of more services for the Arabic-speaking population maintains that it is not the lack of public services but rather stigma or other cultural constraints that prevent Palestinians in need of care from seeking help. Yet changes have been occurring in recent years, and the opposite has been increasingly found to be the case, according to the heads of the mental health clinics for children and adolescents located in Palestinian localities that have Arabic-speaking professionals. An interlocutor reported that the demands far exceed the capacity of the staff to provide care (G. Karmon, director of the Mental Health Clinic for Children and Adolescents, Umm—Al Fahm, personal communication).

This chapter presents the findings of the two major epidemiological studies that provide data on Palestinian adolescents' mental health status and help-seeking patterns—that is, the ISMEHA and the Galilee Study. It also presents findings of other selected studies carried out among distinct Palestinian minority groups. We present the findings of each study separately in order to first provide a short description of the methodology used and thus highlight both the strengths and limitations of the findings.

The ISMEHA

Objectives and Methods

The specific objectives of the ISMEHA were to estimate the prevalence rates of behavioral, emotional, and psychiatric disorders among adolescents according to the *International Classification of Diseases, Tenth Edition* (*ICD-10*) (World Health Organization, 1993), and the *DSM-IV* (American Psychiatric Association, 1994), and patterns of comorbidity. Additionally, it aimed to identify help-seeking patterns in the adolescents and their mothers, assess the extent of unmet needs, and identify protective and risk factors for mental disorders (Mansbach-Kleinfeld et al., 2010).

This cross-sectional survey included a representative sample of all adolescents who were residents of Israel and born between July 1, 1987, and June 30, 1990. Localities with a minimum of 30 adolescents in this age group were included in the sampling and were distributed into strata according to population group (Jewish/mixed or mainly Palestinian-populated localities) and by geographic region, then ordered within each stratum according to their size. Adolescents within each of the sampled localities were ordered according to age, gender, and residential distribution within them, so that they would represent all socioeconomic groups; adolescents in each locality were sampled using a systematic random method. The sampling probability within each locality was calculated so that the final sampling fraction would be the same for the total sample. Ten localities with exclusively Palestinian populations were included in the study, nine from the Northern, Haifa, and Central Districts and one from the Southern District.

The sociodemographic characteristics of the study population were as follows: 77% were Jewish Israelis and 23% were Druze, Christian, or Muslim Palestinians. Palestinian youth were more likely than Jewish Israeli youth to come from two-parent families with three or more siblings, their mothers were more likely to have less than 12 years of education, their fathers were more likely to be unemployed, and their families were more likely to be under the care of a welfare agency.

Adolescents and their mothers were interviewed at length in their homes between January 2004 and March 2005, when the adolescents were between 14 and 17 years of age. The diagnostic instruments used were the Strengths and Difficulties

Questionnaire (SDQ) (Goodman, 1999); the Development and Well-Being Assessment (DAWBA) inventory (Goodman, Ford, Richards, Gatward, & Meltzer, 2000); and ad hoc questions regarding service utilization, health status, and sociodemographic traits. The overall response rate for the total population was 68.2%, but among those living in exclusively Palestinian localities it was 89.6%.

Findings

PREVALENCE RATES OF INTERNALIZING AND
EXTERNALIZING MENTAL DISORDERS

The rate of any mental disorder among the total Israeli population was 11.7%, and for internalizing and externalizing mental disorder, 8.1% and 4.8%, respectively (Farbstein et al., 2010). Internalizing disorders refers broadly to emotional and social problem areas, and externalizing disorders to hyperactivity and behavioral problems. The rate of internalizing disorders among Palestinian adolescents was 9.1%, a non-statistically significant difference from the 7.9% rate among Jewish adolescents. Externalizing disorders were significantly lower for Palestinian adolescents than for Jewish adolescents (1.9% vs. 5.7%, respectively). Risk factors for an externalizing disorder were being male, living with a divorced or single parent, and having only one or no siblings. These risk factors may explain some of the variance between Jewish and Palestinian adolescents as most of the latter live in two-parent families and have many siblings. Sagy, Orr, Bar-On, and Awwad (2001) offered an explanation for the lower prevalence rate of externalizing disorders among Palestinian adolescents. They claimed that the strong family values and a community orientation, favor control and surveillance over children's behavior, so that they conform to group norms.

Table 10.1 shows the prevalence rates of specific mental disorders by population group (Farbstein et al., 2010). Palestinian adolescents had higher rates of any anxiety disorder, separation anxiety, specific phobias, panic attacks, and obsessive-compulsive disorder (OCD) than Jewish Israeli adolescents. The latter had higher rates of depression, attention-deficit/hyperactivity disorder (ADHD), oppositional defiant disorder (ODD), and conduct disorder (CD). The number of subjects presenting with the specific mental disorders were small; no statistical tests for significance were carried out. Regarding comorbidity, 25% of Palestinian but only 10% of Jewish adolescents were diagnosed with comorbidity of internalizing disorders with a learning disability and a hearing or visual impairment.

Although the ISMEHA researchers found that rates of any mental disorder were similar for Palestinian and Jewish adolescents, they expressed their reservations and concluded that it might be possible that with the inclusion of a larger number of minority adolescents in the study, which would have given more statistical power to the analysis, significant differences might have been found (Farbstein et al., 2010).

Table 10.1. Prevalence Rates of Specific Mental Disorders of Adolescents by Population Group (Percentage and Standard Error)

Specific Disorder	Population group					
	Jewish citizens		Palestinian citizens		Total	
	(*n* = 654)		(*n* = 300)		(*N* = 954)	
	%	SE	%	SE	%	SE
Any anxiety disorder	5.3	0.9	9.3	2.9	6.1	0.9
Separation anxiety	0.3	0.2	3.1	1.4	0.8	0.9
Specific phobia	2.1	0.5	4.3	1.6	2.5	0.5
Social phobia	1.0	0.6	0.6	0.4	0.9	0.5
Panic disorder	—	—	1.8	0.8	0.4	0.2
PTSD	0.6	0.3	1.6	1.0	0.8	0.3
OCD	0.9	0.4	2.6	1.8	1.2	0.5
GAD	1.6	0.5	1.1	0.7	1.5	0.4
Depression	3.8	0.8	1.3	0.7	3.3	0.6
ADHD	3.4	0.8	1.2	0.9	3.0	0.6
ODD	2.1	0.7	0.5	0.5	1.8	0.6
Conduct disorder	0.8	0.3	1.4	0.7	0.9	0.3
Any internalizing disorder	7.9	1.3	9.1	2.8	8.1	1.1
Any externalizing disorder	5.7	1.0	1.9	0.9	4.8	0.8

Note. SE, standard error; PTSD, posttraumatic stress disorder; OCD, obsessive compulsive disorder; GAD, general anxiety disorder; ADHD, attention-deficit/hyperactivity disorder; ODD, oppositional defiant disorder.
Source: I. Farbstein, I. Mansbach-Kleinfeld, D. Levinson, R. Goodman, I. Levav, I. Vograft, . . . A. Apter. (2010). Prevalence and correlates of mental disorders in Israeli adolescents: Results from a national mental health survey. *Journal of Child Psychology and Psychiatry, 51*(5), 630–639.

PREVALENCE OF ADHD

In general, 3% of the Israeli adolescents met the *DSM-IV* criteria for ADHD; 3.4% among Jewish adolescents and 1.2% among Palestinian adolescents (Farbstein, Mansbach-Kleinfeld, Auerbach, Ponizovsky, & Apter, 2014). ADHD was significantly associated with gender, with higher prevalence rates in boys than girls (3.9% vs. 2.0%), and with being an only child or having only one sibling compared to two or more siblings (5.9% vs. 2.2%, respectively). This may partly explain the lower rates of ADHD reported among minority adolescents, as almost all the Palestinian adolescents (96.6%) had two or more siblings compared to 71.5% of the Jewish adolescents.

Concerns have been raised about the risk of possible overdiagnosis and overmedication in the general population in developed countries but also about underdiagnosis and undermedication among minority populations (Coghill et al., 2014; McCabe & West, 2013). The ISMEHA found that the low prevalence rate of ADHD and lack of use of medication (i.e., methylphenidate) among Palestinian minority adolescents was very striking when compared with that of the Jewish Israeli majority. This may represent "a true discrepancy due to genetic or environmental factors. Alternatively, it may be at least partly attributable to possible cultural sensitivity of the instrument used, which could have led to missing some cases" (Farbstein et al., 2014, p. 572). Another possible cause may be underdiagnosis as a result of low availability of mental health services in the Palestinian sector. A previous Israeli study (Fogelman, Vinker, Guy, & Kahan, 2003) that examined a one-year prevalence of methylphenidate prescriptions dispensed between 1999 and 2001 to children living in central or northern Israel by the four health management organizations (HMOs) also found a significant difference between the Palestinian minority and the Jewish majority with a prescription rate of 0.2% in Palestinian cities compared with 6.0% in Jewish *kibbutzim*. A community psychiatric survey carried out in the United Arab Emirates, where the Arab adolescents are a majority, and using a similar methodology, reported findings similar to those of the ISMEHA: a 0.9% prevalence of ADHD in a mixed sample of children and adolescents (Eapen, Jakka, & Abou-Saleh, 2003).

Farbstein et al. (2014) found that very few Palestinian adolescents were referred by an authoritative figure from school or the community to seek medical attention. They explained this as possibly resulting from "less tolerance for excessive activity in the classroom at the Palestinian/Druze schools than at the Jewish schools, and thus teachers . . . might not refer their students for ADHD diagnosis as they mistakenly interpret symptoms as bad behavior" (p. 572). The authors concluded that more studies are needed to establish to what extent underdiagnosis and undermedication are because of structural factors related to service provision and to what extent they are related to cultural perceptions of this minority population.

USE OF SERVICES AND HELP-SEEKING PATTERN

The ISMEHA found that 22% of all Israeli adolescents and 11% of their mothers sought help regarding emotional or behavioral problems of the adolescents in the 12 months preceding the survey (Mansbach-Kleinfeld, Farbstein, et al., 2010). These results are within the range of studies in North America, Europe, and Australia, which span from 7% to 30% (Meltzer, Gatward, Goodman, & Ford, 2003; Sawyer et al., 2001; Simpson, Cohen, Pastor, & Reuben, 2008).

The ISMEHA obtained independent reports on help-seeking practices from the adolescents and their mothers, given that exclusive reliance on parents' information may not cover the adolescents' help-seeking practices in school. Adolescents were specifically asked about help seeking in school and not from other community sources as access to mental health care is usually mediated by parents who make appointments, transport the adolescent to the clinic, and pay for services, whereas school-based services are available all the time and free of cost (Costello, Egger, & Angold, 2005).

The study compared Palestinian adolescents living in almost exclusively Palestinian localities with Jewish adolescents living in almost exclusively Jewish localities. As previously mentioned, locality of residence in Israel is strongly associated with ethnic-national affiliation, thus more than 91% of Palestinians reside in exclusively Palestinian localities while a small percentage live in mixed Jewish-Palestinian cities such as Haifa, Lod, Akko, and Ramle (Mansbach-Kleinfeld, Levinson, et al., 2010).

Regarding mothers' help-seeking practices, we found strong differences between Palestinian and Jewish mothers: 9% of Palestinian mothers of adolescents with a mental disorder, compared to 46% of Jewish mothers, consulted a mental health professional or paraprofessional in the community (Mansbach-Kleinfeld, Farbstein, et al., 2010). This discrepancy may be related to structural elements as mentioned earlier, such as referral bias or lack of access to or availability of mental health specialists or public family counseling services in the Palestinian localities. Other elements common in traditional societies such as failure to acknowledge the problem and pessimistic attitudes about treatment or stigma must also be considered (Eapen & Ghubash, 2004; Youssef & Deane, 2006).

Severity of psychopathology is the strongest predictor of service use (Ford, Hamilton, Meltzer, & Goodman, 2008). At the same time, a great proportion of those who need care do not seek help. However, the opposite is also true: adolescents with no diagnosed disorder do seek help. In all, 25% of Palestinian adolescents, compared to 21% among Jewish adolescents, consulted someone in school (Mansbach-Kleinfeld, Farbstein, et al., 2010). The fact that one-quarter of all Israeli adolescents included in the ISMEHA—regardless of psychopathological status—consulted a school source may suggest, according to the authors, that a considerable proportion of adolescents with subthreshold problems seek help before a full-fledged problem arises.

Half of adolescents with a mental disorder among the Palestinians in Israel consulted a school-based source compared to 30% among the Jewish adolescents. Among those consulting, there were more adolescents with an internalizing than with an externalizing disorder. According to the authors, it seems that the Palestinian adolescents have "higher awareness of their need for help than their more conservative parents and thus sought it from accessible, Arabic-speaking school sources" (Mansbach-Kleinfeld, Farbstein, et al., 2010, p. 248).

MENTAL HEALTH CARE AND THE PCP

The ISMEHA found that nearly 69% of Israeli adolescents visited a PCP in the 12 months preceding the interview, although there were significant differences by ethnic-national group. Among the Palestinian adolescents, 44.7% visited a PCP in the preceding 12 months, while among the Jewish majority adolescents, 75.8% did

(Mansbach-Kleinfeld et al., 2011). This study also found that among adolescents with a mental disorder whose mothers did not consult any mental health service provider, the proportion who visited the PCP in the preceding 12 months was even higher: 82.2% among Jewish adolescents and 60% among Palestinian adolescents. These data clearly show that the PCP has the opportunity to identify, treat, or, when unable to treat, refer adolescents to specialized services.

The lower rate of PCP visits by minority adolescents in Israel cannot be explained by structural problems, as the universal National Health Insurance (NHI) Law enacted in 1995 ensures universal access to primary health care and facilitates service utilization. Studies have shown that there is a strong association between underutilization of services, minority status, and poverty (Funk, Drew, Freeman, & Faydi, 2010). In 2004, at the time ISMEHA data were gathered, about 50% of Palestinian households were below the poverty line compared with 20% among Jewish households (Manna, 2008). Nevertheless, "it is encouraging that 60% of these minority adolescents diagnosed with a mental disorder who did not seek help from any professional mental health provider contacted a PCP who then had the opportunity to assess their mental health needs" (Mansbach-Kleinfeld et al., 2011, p. 154). Given the accessibility of the PCP in the Israeli universal health care system and in view of the high treatment gap, particularly for Palestinian minority adolescents, it seems important "to examine the feasibility of involving PCPs, with specialty backup, in the identification, referral and monitoring of children and adolescents with mental problems, a policy supported by other countries" (Mansbach-Kleinfeld et al., 2011, p. 151).

The treatment gap for mental disorders is universally large, though it varies across regions (Kohn, Saxena, Levav, & Saraceno, 2004). In Israel, as elsewhere, more parents seek help for externalizing disorders that cause a significant burden on family and teachers than for internalizing disorders that can remain undetected (Mansbach-Kleinfeld, Farbstein, et al., 2010), and therefore it is particularly important to look for the more elusive internalizing disorders among adolescents visiting the PCP.

The case for action is even stronger among the Palestinian population, where so few mothers of adolescents with a mental disorder seek help from professional or paraprofessional sources and the treatment gap is high. It is recommended that parents' and PCPs' awareness of adolescents' problems be improved. Tabenkin and Gross (2000) claimed that in Israel "health care policymakers have an ambivalent attitude to strengthening the role of primary care" (p. 73) because of a lack of faith in PCPs' capacities, training, and availability. Goldfracht, Shalit, Peled, and Levin (2007), in their study of attitudes of Israeli PCPs regarding mental health care, reported that lack of knowledge regarding diagnosis and treatment, lack of specialists' support, or of interest or personal difficulties in relating to mental health problems were some of the barriers to PCPs' identification and treatment of mental disorders. This is relevant for PCP care among the Jewish majority as well as the Palestinian minority.

The Galilee Study

Objectives and Methods

The Galilee Study was designed to examine mental health status and mental health service needs and utilization by Palestinian adolescents, with particular emphasis on structural (e.g., accessibility) and cultural (e.g., stigma) obstacles to help seeking by the adolescents and their parents (Daeem et al., 2016). The findings of this epidemiological study were to allow for rational planning of services and prevention programs for this underserved population. This cross-sectional study included 1,639 adolescent ninth graders living in four Palestinian localities in the Galilee in northern Israel and one in the Triangle region, representative of the Muslim and Druze populations.

The study was carried out in two stages. During the first stage—the screening stage, which took place between September 2012 and June 2013—all ninth-grade students in the five localities completed the SDQ (Goodman, 1999) in the classroom. During the second stage, between October 2013 and May 2014, students were categorized according to their SDQ scores from the first stage, and all students in the higher twenty-fifth percentile (at high risk for emotional and behavioral problems) and a simple systematic sample without replacement of the remaining 75% (low risk) were included: $N = 704$ students and their mothers. This preference (oversampling) for high-risk adolescents, to ensure enough statistical power for the analyses, yielded a sample composed of 51.7% in the high-risk group and 48.3% in the low-risk group. Because this is not representative of the normal distribution of risk in a general population, all results were analyzed according to risk category.

The adolescents and their mothers were interviewed at home by two interviewers, simultaneously but independently in separate rooms. Total response rate during the screening stage was 69.3% and during the follow-up stage, 84.4%. Differences in response rates were found by gender, with more girls than boys participating in the study in each locality, but not by religion.

Background for Help Seeking in School

The ISMEHA showed that nearly half of the Palestinian minority adolescents with mental disorders sought help in school (Mansbach-Kleinfeld, Farbstein, et al., 2010), while other studies reported that about half of adolescents expressed their intention to seek help from teachers and educational counselors (Gilat, Ezer, & Sagee, 2010). Grinstein-Weiss, Fishman, and Eisikovits (2005) explained this result as a function of the accessibility of school-based services, which are always available, cost little, do not require transportation, and have an essential language and cultural fit between students and school staff. In addition, it seems that Israeli adolescents perceive school staff as more acquainted with their lives and better able to understand their difficulties than mental health professional sources (Gilat et al., 2010). However, although expert mental health professionals are needed, there are few school psychologists in the Palestinian educational system, mostly because of a shortage of Palestinian educational psychologists (Ashkenazi, Angel, & Topolsky, 2014). Most mental health problems are dealt with by school counselors who are not supervised by the school psychology services of the Israel Ministry of Education (Erhard & Erhard-Weiss, 2007). To date no government agency has been in charge of coordinating the ministries involved in mental health service provision to children and adolescents—that is, the Israel Ministries of Health, Education, or Social Affairs. In fact, no decision has been reached as to whether school mental health services should be integrated with the rest of the services provided to children and adolescents or whether mental health services should remain separate from the other service providers (Aviram & Azary-Viesel, 2015).

Several known factors encourage help seeking, among them high emotional distress (Schiff et al., 2010) and social or family support. The question of who is more likely to seek professional help, whether those who enjoy social support or those who do not, is relevant for the Palestinian adolescents who live mainly in a traditional family setting. Some studies claim that adolescents who enjoy higher levels of social and family support will more willingly seek help from teachers and not only from peers and family members (Sheffield, Fiorenza, & Sofronoff, 2004). Grinstein-Weiss et al. (2005) identified positive satisfaction with school, family, and friends as predictors of willingness to ask for help from school sources. Sears (2004), however, offered the opposite view and claimed that "youths who sought professional help were less likely to talk to others when they have problems than those who had not sought professional help" (p. 401)—that is, when family support is weak or when the family is perceived to be the problem and not part of the solution, the adolescents will be more likely to seek help in school or in the community.

Findings

RISK FOR EMOTIONAL AND BEHAVIORAL PROBLEMS

The classification of the study population into high- and low-risk categories proved reliable as these two categories were significantly distinct in many ways: mean scores in each one of the SDQ scales were higher for the high-risk than the low-risk group, significantly more adolescents at high risk than at low risk were cared for by the welfare services, and paternal education was significantly lower for the high-risk group than for the low-risk group. All subsequent analyses were carried out while comparing adolescents in the high-risk group with those in the low-risk group (Daeem et al., 2016). The Galilee Study used the question, "How comfortable do you feel at home?" as a proxy measure for family support. As a whole, most adolescents reported feeling very comfortable at home, although 23% among those in the high-risk group, compared with 8% in the low-risk group, did not feel very comfortable at home (Daeem et al., 2016).

HELP SEEKING IN SCHOOL

Daeem et al. (2016) found that 27% of adolescents in the high-risk group consulted a school source in the 12 months preceding the interview compared with 15% in the low-risk group. When attempting to characterize those adolescents who consulted in school, they found more students belonging to the high-risk group and more Muslim students living in the larger localities than Druze, who live in smaller localities: "The size of the city may be a factor encouraging help-seeking in school, as in the larger cities there is relatively less familiarity between the student and the staff providing care, as compared with the intimacy between students and school staff in the smaller communities" (Daeem et al., 2016, p. 8). The possible association between increased familiarity with the school staff and a decrease in help seeking in school may indicate that stigma or shame plays a role in the help-seeking practices.

A strong association was also found between feeling uncomfortable at home and seeking help in school: nearly 35% of those who felt uncomfortable at home consulted someone in school, regardless of risk category. The findings of the Galilee Study seem to conform more to the view of Sears (2004), who claimed that those who seek professional help are less likely to talk to peers or family members when they have problems. Feeling uncomfortable at home seems to be a very strong indicator of distress, associated with the risk category as well as with help seeking. This study found that less than 10% of adolescents living in smaller Druze localities felt uncomfortable at home compared with between 20% and 30% in the larger cities with a mainly Muslim population. This may partly explain the lower help-seeking practices in the Druze localities as adolescents in those localities might be able to rely on family sources at times of distress. Alternatively, it is likely that in smaller, closed communities, students may fear that information in the school system might leak from the source of consultation to teachers and administrative staff, and this might discourage them from opening up.

Severity of the distress, as shown by the higher SDQ mean total difficulties scores among the Muslim students in the Galilee Study, may also be a function of socioeconomic scarcity (Daeem et al., 2016). In 2009 the larger, mainly Muslim localities were classified as having a lower socioeconomic status than the smaller Druze localities (Gharrah, 2013). Mean wages in the Muslim cities are much lower than those in the smaller Druze localities, as a large segment of Druze citizens are employed by the Israeli military and security establishment in which wages are relatively high.

PREFERRED SCHOOL CONSULTATION SOURCES

The Galilee Study found that 43% of adolescents in the high-risk group consulted the school counselor and 38%, their grade teacher. However, "only 3.2% reported having consulted a school psychologist, the specialized mental health professional source available at the school, probably due to the fact that there are very few psychologists in the Palestinian educational system" (Daeem et al., 2016, p. 7).

Previous findings also showed that the school counselor is the most common source of advice for Palestinian students as well as for their mothers (Mansbach-Kleinfeld, Farbstein, et al., 2010). In Israel the role of the school counselor was determined two decades ago, and it included a large range of responsibilities such as individual counseling, group counseling within the classroom setting, crisis intervention, improvement of learning skills, preventive education, and life skills programs (Karayanni, 1996). Over the years, the paradigm in counseling has changed; the focus turned to prevention rather than curing and, more recently, to a wellness paradigm (Erhard & Klingman, 2004). The comprehensive role of the counselor noted earlier is not nearly fulfilled for Palestinian students. One consequence of segregation in the educational system is a disparity in resource allocation: in 1999 only 20% of the Palestinian schools had a counselor compared to 80% of the Jewish schools. Although between 2000 and 2007 the number of school counselors in the Palestinian sector increased as a result of investment in professional training (Erhard & Erhard-Weiss, 2007), a large gap still remains and the challenges faced by the counselors in Palestinian schools have not diminished, mainly because of the need to work with very disadvantaged youth.

According to the National Insurance Institute of Israel (2015), in 2013, at the time of the Galilee Study data collection, 63.5% of Palestinian children and adolescents were living below the poverty line compared with 21.6% of Jewish children and adolescents. Habib, King, Shoham, Wolde-Tsadick, and Lasky (2010) and Khamaisi (2013) stressed that Palestinian minors have lower living standards, their parents have less educational and employment opportunities, and they have fewer recreational options than their Jewish counterparts. Therefore, school counselors must sometimes deal with very basic survival needs of their students (i.e., food and clothing), rather than with their formal tasks (M, classroom teacher at a school in a Palestinian locality in northern Israel, personal communication).

Emotional and Behavioral Problems among Bedouin Children Living in Unrecognized Villages in Southern Israel

Background

The socioeconomic status of Bedouin Palestinian citizens living in southern Israel is lower than that of all other Israeli citizens (Hesketh et al., 2011; Svirsky & Hason, 2006). About 76,000 Bedouins live in 45 unrecognized Bedouin villages, and a high proportion of them, 37%, are children between the ages of 4 and 10 (Sheikh Muhammad & Khatib, 2010). The Israeli government has branded these Bedouin villages as illegal entities. The population is distinctly rural and makes its livelihood mainly from grooming and selling sheep. These citizens are not supplied with basic municipal services such as electricity, sewage, running water, educational institutions, or public transportation. Like all other citizens, they do have access to primary care clinics, hospital care, and mental health facilities that are available in other localities. In this particular population, 78.1% of children, between 4 and 10 years of age, were below the poverty line in 2010, and their parents suffered from high unemployment and illiteracy rates (Sheikh Muhammad & Khatib, 2010).

The scarcity of all government services is accompanied by a dearth of information regarding the educational and health needs of these children. One of the few studies, carried out by Auerbach, Goldstein, and Elbedour (2000), compared a sample of Bedouin elementary schoolchildren living in officially recognized villages with an American sample and found that the former had higher levels of internalizing problems, particularly anxiety and depression, than the latter, while Bedouin boys had lower scores on externalizing problems than their American peers. Other studies have focused on the effects of polygamy on the mental health of Bedouin children and adolescents (Hamdan, Auerbach, & Apter, 2009). Al-Krenawi and Slonim-Nevo (2008) claimed that women who live in polygamous families suffer from higher rates of fear, anxiety/depression, and somatic symptoms and report less life satisfaction than women in monogamous families. According to Elbedour, Onwuegbuzie, Caridine, and Abu-Saad (2002), children from polygamous families report more mental distress, social difficulties, externalizing problems, and low achievement and greater conflict with parents.

Given the distinct socioeconomic profile and very low status of these adolescents, national estimates of emotional and behavioral problems among Israeli children cannot be generalized to the Bedouin Palestinian children living in the unique conditions of the unrecognized Bedouin villages. The findings of a preliminary study on emotional and behavioral problems among Bedouin children in unrecognized villages (Sheikh Muhammad, Mansbach-Kleinfeld, & Khatib, 2017), therefore, present specific information that could be of assistance to policy makers in charge of the well-being of underserved children and serve as a baseline for future research.

Methods

The study by Sheikh Muhammad et al. (2017) assessed emotional and behavioral problems among children in four unrecognized Bedouin villages between April and May 2012. All children between the ages of 4 and 10 in these villages were included in the study. Mothers provided basic sociodemographic information and also reported on the child's exposure to traumatic events (because of the precarious physical surroundings, these Bedouin children are prone to be exposed to home and road accidents). They were also asked to rate each one of their children with the SDQ (Goodman, 1999). In all, 205 mothers participated in the study. The response rate was 95%.

Complex sample analysis was used to take into consideration the potential correlation between mothers within one village and between children within one family, as each mother rated one or more of her children. The three-stage cluster sampling included four villages and 205 mothers, who scored 548 children. Maternal scoring was found to be independent of the number of children for which the mother scored and of the village where she lived.

Findings

Mothers attributed more conduct problems, peer problems, hyperactivity, and higher total difficulties scores to boys than to girls. Polygamy was associated only with limited prosocial behavior (i.e., positive acts such as caring, sharing, and helping others).

Indeed, children living in monogamous households have higher prosocial behavior scores than those living in polygamous families. This might be explained by studies that have found that, after controlling for the effect of socioeconomic factors, there were no differences between offspring of polygamous marriages and those of monogamous marriages regarding behavioral, emotional, or academic adjustment scales: "When polygamy is the accepted practice in a particular social milieu, it does not have a deleterious psychological effect on adolescents" (Hamdan et al., 2009, p. 755).

Maternal education is known to be one of the most influential factors in the development of a child (Sonego, Llácer, Galán, & Simón, 2013). In this study, more highly educated mothers attributed less emotional and conduct problems to their children. It is possible that educated mothers have different expectations regarding the behavior of their children or different norms regarding discipline or inquisitiveness and therefore are more accepting of behaviors that are somewhat different. Another explanation may be that they are more able and available for child-rearing.

The relation between emotional and behavioral problems and the child's exposure to a traumatic life event was assessed. An association was found between the total difficulties scores and having been exposed or not to a home accident (15.2 vs. 12.8; $F = 10.8$; $p = .001$), to a road accident (15.3 vs. 13.1; $F = 5.8$; $p = .001$), to an attack by a family member or a stranger (17.0 vs. 13.1; $F = 13.1$; $p = .000$), to acts of violence in the family (15.3 vs. 12.8; $F = 13.2$; $p = .000$), and to a death in the family (14.9 vs. 12.8; $F = 9.0$; $p = .003$). These traumatic life events were found to be associated with higher total difficulties scores.

The higher SDQ total difficulties scores among the Bedouin children living in unrecognized villages could be explained by their dismal living conditions, lack of basic services, and exposure to home and road accidents. However, one must also consider the possibility that minority groups and residents of rural communities tend to express extreme answers (Baron-Epel, Kaplan, Weinstein, & Green, 2010), so that their response style may be responsible for the high scores: "It is possible that lack of familiarity with rating scales or cultural factors that make them understand the question differently, or understand what is required from them differently than mainstream populations, are responsible for the high scores attributed to these children" (Sheikh Muhammad et al., 2017).

But even when considering response styles of mothers, one must remember that underdevelopment and poverty are strongly related to distress and maternal feelings of despondence that will surely affect the children's mental state (Ford, Goodman, & Meltzer, 2004). Therefore, it is very difficult to separate the response style of mothers from the context of poverty and distress in which they live that would actually lead to higher SDQ scores in the problem scales. Dire socioeconomic conditions, low household income, and high rates of poverty among children have been associated with increased psychiatric and academic problems (Scharte & Bolte, 2013). Thus, it is to be expected that Bedouin children living in unrecognized villages and under great hardship experience significantly more stressors than children living in less disadvantaged communities.

There are no published SDQ normative data for 4- to 10-year-olds in an Israeli population or in Arabic-speaking countries, including the Gaza Strip. Children in Gaza were assessed with the SDQ, but the published results did not include normative data (Thabet, Stretch, & Vostanis, 2000). The comparison among population groups residing in different parts of the world and enjoying different lifestyles and socioeconomic conditions is complicated because of the plethora of different variables that affect each population group. Nevertheless, the analyses of Sheikh Muhammad et al. (2017) showed that the Bedouin children had higher mean scores in the emotional and behavioral problem scales and higher total difficulties scores when rated with the SDQ than children in other comparative studies carried out in Europe (Meltzer et al., 2003), the United States (Bourdon, Goodman, Rae, Simpson, & Koretz, 2005), China (Du, Kou, & Coghill, 2008), and Australia (Hawes & Dadds, 2004). Norms for Israeli children in general in this age group, as well as for specific subpopulations, are needed.

General Discussion

The studies reviewed here reveal a complex picture regarding mental health problems among the different subpopulations comprising the Palestinian minority. The ISMEHA, for instance, has contributed in two ways. First, it has provided baseline data of diagnosed mental disorders for Palestinian adolescents with a standardized instrument and has compared their prevalence of mental disorders with those among Jewish majority adolescents. Second, the ISMEHA identified the limited help-seeking practices of Palestinian mothers of adolescents with a mental disorder in the health system, with a treatment gap of 91% compared with the higher consultation rates of their children in school.

The mapping of the public mental health clinics for children and adolescents carried out in 2011, which shows the strong geographic and ethnic disparities in service provision, provides part of the answer for the low consultation rates of

Palestinian families. But questions remain regarding the discrepancy between mothers' and adolescents' consultation rates. Is the difference owing to a generation gap that makes younger students, who have gone through a process of acculturation and are exposed to international media, more open to consult and share their problems with professionals outside of the family? Or is it that the school services, with their availability, accessibility, and language fit, offer much-needed care for adolescents who do not receive it elsewhere? The ISMEHA also noted the potential role of the PCP to identify, treat, or refer adolescents with a mental disorder who have not received care by any professional source but do visit the PCP.

The Galilee Study has also offered several important contributions. For one, it is the first epidemiological study on mental health and service use to deal exclusively with a large and representative sample of Palestinian adolescents living in the north of Israel. In its comparison of Muslim and Druze adolescents, two distinct population groups in terms of locality, religion, and national identity, but both identified as part of the Palestinian minority, the Galilee Study found that Muslim adolescents, living in poorer and larger cities than the Druze, under more stressful conditions and with less feeling of support at home, had higher rates of emotional and behavioral problems. They also had higher rates of help seeking in school. The Galilee Study shows the need for quality school mental health services for these minority adolescents.

The studies carried out among the Bedouin children and adolescents, the most underprivileged citizens of Israel, show enhanced rates of emotional and behavioral problems and a lack of access to needed services. The mapping carried out in 2011 emphasized the fact that in the Southern District, only 4.3% of the population of Palestinian children and adolescents in need received cared through the public mental health clinics.

Policy Recommendations

The comprehensive Israeli Mental Health Reform has been in effect since July 2015. One of its main objectives is to "improve the link between mental and physical care by enhancing [PCPs'] capacity to diagnose and treat mental illness, and by strengthening the consultation and referral relationships between the PCPs and mental health specialists" (Rosen, Nirel, Gross, Bramali, & Ecker, 2008, p. 203). The ISMEHA showed that nearly 60% of Palestinian adolescents with a mental disorder who did not receive care from any mental health professional visited the PCP in the year preceding the interview. Therefore, it is encouraging that the Mental Health Reform articulates the need for involvement of PCPs in the treatment of mild problems or referral of moderate or severe problems to a secondary tier.

However, the Mental Health Reform does not articulate the linkage between community mental health services and school mental health services. Given the important role that the school plays as a first and sometimes sole consultation option for minority adolescents with a high risk for mental disorders—as seen in both the ISMEHA and the Galilee Study—one of the possible strategies to enhance mental health provision for these students, particularly in the larger and poorer Muslim communities, implies integrating the educational system with the child and adolescent mental health services in Israel. This would require the systematic involvement of educators, counselors, and school psychologists in school-based mental health programs. Sterne and Porter (2013) suggest following the model of the child and adolescent mental health (CAMH) services in the United Kingdom, which propose an integrated system of mental health services in which teachers receive additional training to recognize and deal with simple emotional and behavioral issues and also have adequate knowledge and awareness to make referrals for further care. To date, the quality of the care students receive in school in the Palestinian sector has not been examined, and the issue of referral is dependent on the availability of specialized services to which children and adolescents can be referred. It is necessary to invest in special training for educators and to increase the number of school counselors and school psychologists in the Palestinian sector, particularly in middle and high schools.

Rosen et al. (2008) claimed that not enough attention has been paid to mild and moderate psychiatric problems, and most of the resources are directed toward a small proportion of the severely mentally ill. These mild and moderate psychiatric problems are those that appear frequently among adolescents attending the educational system and are likely to become severe problems if they remain untreated.

Lastly, there is a definite need to increase the number of public mental health clinics for Palestinian children and adolescents in Israel as well as the number of Palestinian mental health clinicians. A concerted effort is needed by the Israel Ministry of Health and Israel Ministry of Education, as well as Israeli universities and colleges. The Israel Ministry of Health needs to request that HMOs open more clinics in Palestinian localities. The Israel Ministry of Education needs to improve the educational level of Palestinian children and adolescents. The heads of Israeli universities and colleges need to promote affirmative action and open the clinical professions to the Palestinian minority in order to increase the number of Palestinian professionals in the field. At the school level, coordination and cooperation between school counselors and educational staff at the school, in the welfare system, and among professional staff at mental health clinics is essential.

IVONNE MANSBACH-KLEINFELD is Senior Research Fellow of the Feinberg Child Study Center at the Schneider Children's Medical Center, Petah Tikva, Israel.

RAIDA DAEEM is Director of Maghar Child and Adolescent Mental Health Clinic and senior clinical psychologist at Ziv Medical Center, Safed, Israel.

References

Al-Krenawi, A., & Slonim-Nevo, V. (2008). The psychosocial profile of Bedouin Arab women living in polygamous and monogamous marriages. *Families in Society: The Journal of Contemporary Social Services, 89*(1), 139–149.

American Psychiatric Association. (1994). *Diagnostic and statistical manual of mental disorders* (4th ed.). Washington, DC: American Psychiatric Association.

Ashkenazi, Y., Angel, M., & Topolsky, T. (2014). *Psychological services in elementary schools in normal times and in emergencies.* Jerusalem: Engelberg Center for Children and Youth, Smokler Center for Health Policy Research, Myers-JDC-Brookdale. Retrieved from http://brookdale.jdc.org.il/_Uploads/PublicationsFiles/Summary_eng(10).pdf.

Auerbach, J. G., Goldstein, E., & Elbedour, S. (2000). Behavior problems in Bedouin elementary schoolchildren. *Transcultural Psychiatry, 37*(2), 229–241.

Aviram, U., & Azary-Viesel, S. (2015). *Mental health reform in Israel: Challenge and opportunity. Policy paper No. 2015.02.* Jerusalem: Taub Center for Social Policy Studies in Israel.

Baron-Epel, O., Kaplan, G., Weinstein, R., & Green, M. S. (2010). Extreme and acquiescence bias in a bi-ethnic population. *European Journal of Public Health, 20*(5), 543–548. Retrieved from https://doi.org/10.1093/eurpub/ckq052.

Bourdon, K. H., Goodman, R., Rae, D. S., Simpson, G., & Koretz, D. S. (2005). The strengths and difficulties questionnaire: US normative data and psychometric properties. *Journal of the American Academy of Child & Adolescent Psychiatry, 44*(6), 557–564.

Coghill, D. R., Seth, S., Pedroso, S., Usala, T., Currie, J., & Gagliano, A. (2014). Effects of methylphenidate on cognitive functions in children and adolescents with attention-deficit/hyperactivity disorder: Evidence from a systematic review and a meta-analysis. *Biological Psychiatry, 76*(8), 603–615.

Costello, E. J., Egger, H., & Angold, A. (2005). 10-year research update review: The epidemiology of child and adolescent psychiatric disorders: I. Methods and public health burden. *Journal of the American Academy of Child & Adolescent Psychiatry, 44*(10), 972–986.

Daeem, R., Mansbach-Kleinfeld, I., Farbstein, I., Khamaisi, R., Ifrah, A., Muhammad, A. S., . . . Apter, A. (2016). Help seeking in school by Israeli Arab minority adolescents with emotional and behavioral problems: Results from the Galilee study. *Israel Journal of Health Policy Research, 5*(1), 49. Retrieved from https://doi.org/10.1186/s13584-016-0109-0.

Du, Y., Kou, J., & Coghill, D. (2008). The validity, reliability and normative scores of the parent, teacher and self report versions of the strengths and difficulties questionnaire in China. *Child and Adolescent Psychiatry and Mental Health, 2*(1), 8. Retrieved from https://doi.org/10.1186/1753-2000-2-8.

Eapen, V., & Ghubash, R. (2004). Help-seeking for mental health problems of children: Preferences and attitudes in the United Arab Emirates. *Psychological Reports, 94*(2), 663–667.

Eapen, V., Jakka, M. E., & Abou-Saleh, M. T. (2003). Children with psychiatric disorders: The Al Ain community psychiatric survey. *Canadian Journal of Psychiatry, 48*(6), 402–407.

Elbedour, S., Onwuegbuzie, A. J., Caridine, C., & Abu-Saad, H. (2002). The effect of polygamous marital structure on behavioral, emotional, and academic adjustment in children: A comprehensive review of the literature. *Clinical Child and Family Psychology Review, 5*(4), 255–271.

Erhard, R., & Erhard-Weiss, D. (2007). The emergence of counseling in traditional cultures: Ultra-orthodox Jewish and Arab communities in Israel. *International Journal for the Advancement of Counselling, 29*(3), 149–158.

Erhard, R., & Klingman, A. (2004). Introduction: School counseling–professional ecology. In R. Erhard & A. Klingman (Eds.), *School counseling in a changing society* (pp. 9–26). Ramot: Tel-Aviv University.

Farbstein, I., Mansbach-Kleinfeld, I., Auerbach, J. G., Ponizovsky, A. M., & Apter, A. (2014). The Israel survey of mental health among adolescents: Prevalence of attention-deficit/hyperactivity disorder, comorbidity, methylphenidate use, and help-seeking patterns. *Israel Medical Association Journal, 16*(9), 568–573.

Farbstein, I., Mansbach-Kleinfeld, I., Levinson, D., Goodman, R., Levav, I., Vograft, I., . . . Apter, A. (2010). Prevalence and correlates of mental disorders in Israeli adolescents: Results from a national mental health survey. *Journal of Child Psychology and Psychiatry, 51*(5), 630–639.

Fogelman, Y., Vinker, S., Guy, N., & Kahan, E. (2003). Prevalence of and change in the prescription of methylphenidate in Israel over a 2-year period. *CNS Drugs, 17*(12), 915–919.

Ford, T., Goodman, R., & Meltzer, H. (2004). The relative importance of child, family, school and neighbourhood correlates of childhood psychiatric disorder. *Social Psychiatry and Psychiatric Epidemiology, 39*(6), 487–496.

Ford, T., Hamilton, H., Meltzer, H., & Goodman, R. (2008). Predictors of service use for mental health problems among British schoolchildren. *Child and Adolescent Mental Health, 13*(1), 32–40.

Funk, M., Drew, N., Freeman, M., & Faydi, E. (2010). *Mental health and development: Targeting people with mental health conditions as a vulnerable group*. Geneva: World Health Organization.

Gharrah, R. (2013). The quality of life. In R. Gharrah (Ed.), *Arab society in Israel*. Vol. 6: *Population, society, economy* [in Hebrew]. Jerusalem: Van Leer Jerusalem Institute, Hakibbutz Hameuchad.

Gilat, I., Ezer, H., & Sagee, R. (2010). Help-seeking attitudes among Arab and Jewish adolescents in Israel. *British Journal of Guidance & Counselling, 38*(2), 205–218.

Goldfracht, M., Shalit, C., Peled, O., & Levin, D. (2007). Attitudes of Israeli primary care physicians towards mental health care/commentary-attitudes. *Israel Journal of Psychiatry and Related Sciences, 44*(3), 225–230.

Goodman, R. (1999). The extended version of the strengths and difficulties questionnaire as a guide to child psychiatric caseness and consequent burden. *Journal of Child Psychology and Psychiatry, 40*(5), 791–799.

Goodman, R., Ford, T., Richards, H., Gatward, R., & Meltzer, H. (2000). The development and well-being assessment: Description and initial validation of an integrated assessment of child and adolescent psychopathology. *Journal of Child Psychology and Psychiatry, 41*(5), 645–655.

Grinstein-Weiss, M., Fishman, G., & Eisikovits, Z. (2005). Gender and ethnic differences in formal and informal help seeking among Israeli adolescents. *Journal of Adolescence, 28*(6), 765–779.

Habib, J., King, J., Shoham, A. B., Wolde-Tsadick, A., & Lasky, K. (2010). *Labour market and socio-economic outcomes of the Arab-Israeli population*. OECD Social, Employment and Migration Working Papers, No. 102. Paris: Organization for Economic Co-operation and Development.

Hamdan, S., Auerbach, J., & Apter, A. (2009). Polygamy and mental health of adolescents. *European Child & Adolescent Psychiatry, 18*(12), 755–760.

Hawes, D. J., & Dadds, M. R. (2004). Australian data and psychometric properties of the strengths and difficulties questionnaire. *Australian and New Zealand Journal of Psychiatry, 38*(8), 644–651.

Hesketh, K., Bishara, S., Rosenberg, R., & Zaher, S. (2011). *The inequality report*. Haifa: Adalah: The Legal Center for Arab Minority Rights in Israel.

Israel Central Bureau of Statistics. (2004). *New survey: Inputs in education* [in Hebrew]. Retrieved from http://www.cbs.gov.il/hodaot2004/06_04_205.pdf.

Karayanni, M. (1996). The emergence of school counseling and guidance in Israel. *Journal of Counseling and Development, 74*(6), 582–587.

Khamaisi, R. (2013). Housing transformation within urbanized communities: The Arab Palestinians in Israel. *Geography Research Forum, 33*, 184–209.

Kohn, R., Saxena, S., Levav, I., & Saraceno, B. (2004). The treatment gap in mental health care. *Bulletin of the World Health Organization, 82*(11), 858–866.

Manna, A. (2008). Introduction: Change and continuity in the experience of the Arab citizens in Israel. In A. Manna (Ed.), *Arab society in Israel* [in Hebrew] (2th ed.). Jerusalem: Van Leer Jerusalem Institute and Hakibbutz Hameuchad.

Mansbach-Kleinfeld, I., Farbstein, I., Levinson, D., Apter, A., Erhard, R., Palti, H., . . . Levav, I. (2010). Service use for mental disorders and unmet need: Results from the Israel survey on mental health among adolescents. *Psychiatric Services, 61*(3), 241–249.

Mansbach-Kleinfeld, I., Farbstein, I., Saragusti, I., Karmon, G., Apter, A., Ifrah, A., & Lubin, G. (2013, June). *Mapping of mental health clinics for children and adolescents in Israel: Geographic and structural disparities*. Paper presented at the 5th International Jerusalem Conference of Health Policy.

Mansbach-Kleinfeld, I., Levinson, D., Farbstein, I., Apter, A., Levav, I., Kanaaneh, R., . . . Ponizovsky, A. M. (2010). The Israel survey of mental health among adolescents: Aims and methods. *Israel Journal of Psychiatry and Related Sciences, 47*(4), 244–253.

Mansbach-Kleinfeld, I., Palti, H., Ifrah, A., Levinson, D., & Farbstein, I. (2011). Missed chances: Primary care practitioners' opportunity to identify, treat and refer adolescents with mental disorders. *Israel Journal of Psychiatry and Related Sciences, 48*(3), 150–156.

McCabe, S. E., & West, B. T. (2013). Medical and nonmedical use of prescription stimulants: Results from a national multicohort study. *Journal of the American Academy of Child & Adolescent Psychiatry, 52*(12), 1272–1280.

Meltzer, H., Gatward, R., Goodman, R., & Ford, T. (2003). Mental health of children and adolescents in Great Britain. *International Review of Psychiatry, 15*(1–2), 185–187.

National Insurance Institute of Israel. (2015). *Poverty and social gaps annual report 2014*. Retrieved from https://www.btl.gov.il/English%20Homepage/Publications/AnnualSurvey/2014/Pages/default.aspx.

Nesher, T. (2012, October 21). Only about 11% of undergraduate students are Arabs [in Hebrew]. *Haaretz*. Retrieved from http://www.haaretz.co.il/news/education/1.1846561.

Rosen, B., Nirel, N., Gross, R., Bramali, S., & Ecker, N. (2008). The Israeli mental health insurance reform. *Journal of Mental Health Policy and Economics, 11*(4), 201–208.

Sagy, S., Orr, E., Bar-On, D., & Awwad, E. (2001). Individualism and collectivism in two conflicted societies comparing Israeli-Jewish and Palestinian-Arab high school students. *Youth & Society, 33*(1), 3–30.

Sawyer, M. G., Arney, F. M., Baghurst, P. A., Clark, J. J., Graetz, B. W., Kosky, R. J., . . . Raphael, B. (2001). The mental health of young people in Australia: Key findings from the child and adolescent component of the national survey of mental health and well-being. *Australian and New Zealand Journal of Psychiatry, 35*(6), 806–814.

Scharte, M., & Bolte, G. (2013). Increased health risks of children with single mothers: The impact of socio-economic and environmental factors. *European Journal of Public Health, 23*(3), 469–475.

Schiff, M., Pat-Horenczyk, R., Benbenishty, R., Brom, D., Baum, N., & Astor, R. A. (2010). Do adolescents know when they need help in the aftermath of war? *Journal of Traumatic Stress, 23*(5), 657–660.

Sears, H. A. (2004). Adolescents in rural communities seeking help: Who reports problems and who sees professionals? *Journal of Child Psychology and Psychiatry, 45*(2), 396–404.

Sheffield, J. K., Fiorenza, E., & Sofronoff, K. (2004). Adolescents' willingness to seek psychological help: Promoting and preventing factors. *Journal of Youth and Adolescence, 33*(6), 495–507.

Sheikh Muhammad, A., & Khatib, M. (2010). *The Palestinians in Israel. 3rd Socio-economic survey* [in Arabic]. Shefa Amr, Israel: The Galilee Society. Retrieved from http://www.rikaz.org/en/publication/SE3/Third%20Socio%20Economic%20Survey.pdf.

Sheikh Muhammad, A., Mansbach-Kleinfeld, I., & Khatib, M. (2017). A preliminary study of emotional and behavioral problems among Bedouin children in "unrecognized villages" in Southern Israel. *Mental Health and Prevention, 6*, 12–18.

Simpson, G. A., Cohen, R. A., Pastor, P. N., & Reuben, C. A. (2008). Use of mental health services in the past 12 months by children aged 4–17 years: United States, 2005–2006. NCHS Data Brief No. 8. Atlanta, GA: Centers for Disease Control and Prevention. Retrieved from https://www.cdc.gov/nchs/products/databriefs/db08.htm.

Sonego, M., Llácer, A., Galán, I., & Simón, F. (2013). The influence of parental education on child mental health in Spain. *Quality of Life Research, 22*(1), 203–211.

Sterne, A., & Porter, B. (2013). *Overview of child and adolescent mental health services in Israel.* Jerusalem: Myers-JDC-Brookdale Institute.

Struch, N., Shereshevsky, Y., Baidani-Auerbach, A., Lachman, M., Zehavi, T., Sagiv, N. (2007). *Stigma, discrimination, and mental health in Israel: Stigma against people with psychiatric illnesses and against mental health care.* RR-478-07. Jerusalem: Myers-JDC-Brookdale Institute, Center for Research on Disability and Special Populations.

Svirsky, S., & Hason, Y. (2006). *Invisible citizens: Government's policy regarding the Bedouin in the Negev.* Tel Aviv: Adva Center.

Tabenkin, H., & Gross, R. (2000). The role of the primary care physician in the Israeli health care system as a "gatekeeper": The viewpoint of health care policy makers. *Health Policy, 52*(2), 73–85.

Tabibian-Mizrahi, M. (2007). *The mental health reform* [in Hebrew]. Jerusalem: Knesset Research and Information Center.

Thabet, A. A., Stretch, D., & Vostanis, P. (2000). Child mental health problems in Arab children: Application of the strengths and difficulties questionnaire. *International Journal of Social Psychiatry, 46*(4), 266–280.

World Health Organization. (1993). *The ICD-10 classification of mental and behavioural disorders: Diagnostic criteria for research.* Genevah: World Health Organization.

Youssef, J., & Deane, F. P. (2006). Factors influencing mental-health help-seeking in Arabic-speaking communities in Sydney, Australia. *Mental Health, Religion & Culture, 9*(1), 43–66.

11

THE PSYCHIATRIC EPIDEMIOLOGICAL PORTRAIT OF PALESTINIAN CITIZENS IN ISRAEL

A Review of Community Studies

Giora Kaplan, Itzhak Levav, and Ora Nakash

THIS CHAPTER RELIES ON PREVIOUSLY PUBLISHED COMMUNITY-BASED STUDIES on the adult Palestinian population in Israel.[1] Importantly, they were conducted by different teams of epidemiologists using different diagnostic instruments and methods and targeting different population samples. Yet all arrived at analogous findings and conclusions. The convergence of the findings strengthens the robustness of these studies.

The chapter that follows describes a study on psychiatric hospitalizations specifically designed for this book. That study, together with the community studies discussed here, constitute an important set of inputs for rational mental health programs and service planning intended to answer the psychiatric needs of Palestinian citizens in Israel.

The Current Status of Epidemiologic Studies on Palestinian Citizens in Israel

As noted earlier in this book, Palestinians constitute a sizable minority of the Israeli population. However, except for a few studies (Al-Krenawi, Graham, Dean, & Eltaiba, 2004; Department of Information and Evaluation, 2004; Shemesh et al., 2006), psychiatric epidemiological research data based on the Palestinian population remains wanting.

Parenthetically, an analogous situation is found in most Middle Eastern countries (Ghubash, 2001; Ghubash, Hamdi, & Bebbington, 1992; Weissman et al., 1996). One exception is Lebanon, a country in which epidemiologic research has thrived even in the midst of armed internal and external conflicts. For example, in the early 1990s, 500 community respondents were interviewed with the Diagnostic Interview Schedule, version III (DIS-III). The lifetime rates for major depression were the highest of a group of 10 countries outside the Middle East that coparticipated in an international study. The overall estimated rate was 19.0%; women, 23.1%; men, 14.7%. These relatively high rates were attributed to the effects of the civil war raging in that country at the time of the fieldwork (Weissman et al., 1996). Additional psychiatric epidemiological surveys in the Middle East have focused on selected, relatively small populations—for example, primary medical care visitors (El-Rufaie & Daradkeh, 1996).

In recent years, the World Mental Health (WMH) Survey, launched and co-ordinated by the WHO and Harvard University in 28 countries (Demyttenaere et al., 2004), has investigated the prevalence of several psychiatric disorders as well as the use of mental health services. This global effort that includes Iraq, Israel, and Lebanon broadens a still narrow psychiatric epidemiological window into Arab populations (Ghubash, 2001). The Lebanese WMH study yielded the following 12-month prevalence rates: anxiety, 11.2% (95% CI, 8.9–13.5); and mood disorders, 6.6% (95% CI, 4.9–8.2) (Demyttenaere et al., 2004). The Israeli WMH study provided the rates of any affective or anxiety disorder. As shown in greater detail in the discussion that follows, these rates were higher among Palestinians (11.1%, 95% CI, 8.7–14.2) than among Jewish Israelis (9.3%, 95% CI, 8.3–10.3), and higher among women (Palestinian women: 12.0%, 95% CI, 8.6–16.7; Jewish women: 10.1%, 95% CI, 8.6–11.7) than among men (Palestinian men: 10.2%, 95% CI, 7.0–14.7; Jewish men: 8.4%, 95% CI, 7.2–9.8) (Levav, Ifrah, Geraisy, Grinshpoon, & Khwaled, 2007).

Help-Seeking Practices

Other authors in this book discuss the assumptive world (Al-Issa & Al-Junun, 2002) that orients some Arab population groups with regard to both the etiology of mental disorders and the sources of care. In many Arab countries, the assumptive world has had limited interaction with Western psychiatry, while in Israel, as a result of the development of the field and the relatively higher supply of services, the interaction has been greater. However, the expression of such a set of concepts with reference to the use of mental health services in Israel remains generally unknown, except for national data on psychiatric hospitalizations for all Palestinian citizens in Israel and cultural psychiatric data on the Bedouin population (Department of Information and Evaluation, 2004). With regard to the latter population group, a study reported on in other chapters found that men were more familiar with the biomedical model, while women relied on traditional practitioners. In addition, female service users were more aware of the stigma associated with seeking psychiatric services, inasmuch as women are the repository of the honor of their families. Importantly, psychiatric contacts for unmarried women risk jeopardizing both their honor and their marital prospects (Al-Krenawi & Graham, 1999). Conceivably, such avoidance may give room to symptom substitution (presenting with physical complaints instead of mental health concerns) (Racy, 1980) because physical complaints are perceived as a more legitimate pathway to care as individuals are assumed to have no control over them (Al-Krenawi, 1998).

The extent of the treatment gap, defined as the difference between the true and treated prevalence rates of mental disorder (Kohn, Saxena, Levav, & Saraceno, 2004), is probably one measurable reflection of the assumptive world. The WMH Survey, in addition to data on morbidity, also provides useful information on treatment gap, as reported by the Israeli studies discussed next (Demyttenaere et al., 2004).

The Targeted Population

As noted in other chapters, the Palestinian population in Israel includes three major groups often classified by their religious affiliation: Muslims (including Bedouins), Christians, and Druze. Although different in many regards other than religion—for example, age (median age: 18.5, 27.9, and 22.7, respectively) and health status (for 2003, infant mortality rates were 8.6, 3.2, and 7.1 per 1,000 live births, respectively) (Israel Center for Disease Control [ICDC], 2005)—empirical studies aggregate them because of power analysis constraints.

Relevant for mental health, including the use of services, it is important to note that the Palestinian minority in Israel, which enjoys legally sanctioned citizenship rights and has made remarkable progress in health and life expectancy over the years (ICDC, 2005), still suffers from a disadvantaged position within the larger society (Smooha, 1999). As for Palestinian women, their social disadvantage is further compounded by their subordinate position in a patriarchal community (Elnekave & Gross, 2004). They share this plight with women in most Arab countries (Kadri & Moussaoui, 2001; Saif Al Dawla, 2001). To these sociopolitical and psychological factors, one may add other variables of the same domains, such as the rapid process of social change taking place in the Palestinian population, analogous to that described by Ghubash, Hamdi, and Bebbington (1994) in Dubai and in other chapters in this book, in which tradition and modernity clash daily. Another crucial psychosocial determinant, particularly for the Muslim and Christian groups, is the experience of the Nakba, which followed the establishment of the state of Israel and the defeat of Arab armies from surrounding countries in the 1948–1949 war. Conceivably, these factors have had an effect on the prevalence rates of anxiety and depression disorders, as measured by the Composite International Diagnostic Instrument (CIDI), and/or on emotional distress, as determined by the General Health Questionnaire (GHQ). For women, social stress may be further amplified. Seif El Dawla (2001) noted that Palestinian women's position in society is a major factor contributing to their higher prevalence of depression and anxiety."

Community Study I

The most recent of the community-based studies reported on in this chapter (Baron-Epel, Kaplan, & Moran, 2010) was designed to assess the levels of perceived discrimination on the basis of origin and ethnic-national affiliation and their association with physical and mental health.

A cross-sectional random telephone survey was performed including 1,004 Israelis aged 35–65. Of these, 400 were Palestinians, 404 were nonimmigrant Jews, and 200 were immigrants from the former Soviet Union. The perceived discrimination questionnaire was adapted from the instrument developed and validated by Krieger, Smith, Naishadham, Hartman, and Barbeau (2005). The 12-item Short Form (SF-12) questionnaire (Ware, Kosinski, & Keller, 1996), previously validated in Hebrew (Amir, Lewin-Epstein, Becker, & Buskila, 2002), was used to measure quality of life with regard to physical and mental health.

The Hebrew questionnaire was translated into Arabic and back-translated into Hebrew to ensure accuracy. Bilingual professionals familiar with Palestinian culture validated the translation and confirmed that the questions had equal meaning as in Hebrew. Emphasis was made on the exact wording to decrease differential understanding of the questions. A pretest confirmed the cultural adaptation of the questionnaire, which was subsequently administered by telephone by trained interviewers from the relevant population group.

The SF-12 scores were transformed into a scale of 0 to 100, with 0 indicating poor health and 100, optimal health; a mean score was calculated for each individual. Since physical and mental health variables were not normally distributed, they were dichotomized around the median. Both mental and physical health statuses were categorized as suboptimal (0) with scores from 0.0 to 79.9 and optimal with scores of 80.0 and above. About half of the respondents were classified as having optimal health. Table 11.1 shows that the Palestinian respondents had lower mean scores than Jewish respondents, but their scores were similar to Jewish immigrants from the former Soviet Union.

Perceived discrimination, particularly in education and employment, was higher among Jewish Israeli immigrants and Palestinians than in the majority group (nonimmigrant Jewish Israelis). However, after adjusting for socioeconomic variables, discrimination was not significantly associated with poor physical or mental health among Palestinians. Importantly, for immigrants and Palestinians, the health-care services seem to be a national system with comparatively little perceived discrimination.

With regard to the finding that among Palestinians perceived discrimination was not associated with health status, Baron-Epel et al. (2010) have proposed some possible explanations. First, the Palestinians' residential segregation decreases the level of contact with the majority group and thus reduces ongoing perceived discrimination, including exposure to everyday hassles and elevated stress. As a result, the Palestinians' health measures could be less affected. Second, Palestinians do

Table 11.1. Results of Short Form Health Survey (SF-12) by Population Group

Dimension	Measure	Nonimmigrant Israeli Jews	Immigrant Israeli Jews	Palestinian citizens in Israel
Physical health-related quality of life*	Mean (*SD*) (range 1–100)	82.3 (20.9)	72.3 (24.4)	71.5 (29.0)
Mental health-related quality of life*	Mean (*SD*) (range 1–100)	77.8 (20.5)	66.8 (24.6)	68.2 (25.6)

Note. SD, standard deviation.
* (*p* < 0.0001).
Source: O. Baron-Epel, G. Kaplan, & M. Moran. (2010). Perceived discrimination and health-related quality of life among Arabs and Jews in Israel: A population-based survey. *BMC Public Health, 10*(1), 282.

not expect to be part of Israeli Jewish society, and their ethnic identity serves as a key resource in their coping mechanisms, thus reducing exposure to the prolonged stress of discrimination. This may obviate ill effects on health. Interestingly, an analogous condition was found among African Americans, in whom racial identity was a protective factor in buffering the negative impact of discrimination (Sellers, Caldwell, Schmeelk-Cone, & Zimmerman, 2003).

Community Study II

A population-based cross-sectional study (Kaplan et al., 2010) estimated the prevalence of depression among Israeli Jews and Muslim Palestinians in a random sample of the general urban population of the Hadera district in northern Israel. The district population (about 300,000 residents), mostly urbanite, comprises about 60% Jews and 40% Palestinians, living in separate towns. The study sample (*N* = 880) was stratified into groups of equal size according to ethnic-national affiliation (Palestinian or Jewish), gender, and four age groups (overall age range: 25–67 years).

The overall response rate to the interviews in the original sample was 79.0%; 90.0% among Palestinians and 68.0% among Jews (*p* = 0.001). Nonresponders (who could not be traced or refused to participate) were on average three years younger than the participants (*p* = 0.07). The proportion of men among the nonresponders was 44.0% compared to 51.0% among participants (*p* = 0.08). Nonresponders were substituted by others drawn from a random sample, matched by gender, age, national-ethnic affiliation, and town of residence.

Depression was measured using the Harvard Department of Psychiatry National Depression Screening Day Scale (HANDS) (Baer, Jacobs, et al., 1999) following permission received for its translation and use. The HANDS is a 10-question screening instrument for assessing depression symptoms over the previous two weeks, developed and tested in a community population of adults with and without depression. Symptom scores range from 0 (occurring none or a little of the time) to 3 (occurring all of the time), for total scores ranging from 0 to 30. Internal consistency reliability was satisfactory; Cronbach's alpha coefficient was 0.87. Validation in the general population suggested that a cutoff score greater than or equal to 9 had a sensitivity of 0.95 and a specificity of 0.94 for meeting *DSM-IV-TR* criteria for a major depressive episode (American Psychiatric Association, 2000). Further distinction regarding severity was as follows: 0–8 indicated that the presence of a major depressive episode was unlikely; 9–16, that the presence of a major depressive episode was likely; and 17–30, that the presence of a major depressive episode was very likely (Baer et al., 1999). The authors recommend that persons with a score of 9 or higher undergo a complete mental health evaluation to determine whether a diagnosis of clinical depression is indicated. Since there were very few scores at the extremes of the scoring range, for the current analysis, the HANDS score was dichotomized into "not likely" to be suffering from depression (0–8) and "likely/very likely" to be suffering from depression (9–30).

The rate of scores in the likely/very likely range was 2.4 times higher among Palestinians than among Jewish Israelis (24.9% vs. 10.6%; $p = 0.001$). Palestinian respondents were more likely to report depression than were Jewish respondents in almost every strata of the variables associated with depression (e.g., age, gender, number of chronic diseases). No difference in the depression rate was found among those employed in the highest professional prestige percentile. Among those with at least 13 years of education, the rate was lower among Palestinians than among Jews; 1.4 versus 7.7%, respectively.

The differences in the depression prevalence rates between both groups were maintained after controlling for each potential confounding variable separately, except for years of education ($p = 0.77$). After adjusting for all variables in the multivariate analysis, no significant association remained between ethnic-national affiliation and depression (odds ratio [OR] = 0.80; 95% CI, 0.45–1.40). There were no significant interactions between age, gender, or ethnic-national affiliation and any of the other variables.

The increase in depression by age differed by gender, rising more steeply for women than for men. The age/gender differential was not identical for the two ethnic-national groups. In all age groups, Palestinian men had higher rates than Jewish men. While among Jewish women the rate rose from 7.7% in the youngest group and peaked at 19.0% among the 46- to 55-year-olds, the rate among Palestinian women rose steadily with age, from 14.0% to 51.7%. The finding that over half of the older Palestinian women (aged ≥ 56) were likely to suffer depressive symptoms indicates that attention should be given to the mental health needs of this at-risk group—for example, by screening and early intervention in primary care. The fact that rates of depression rise among older Palestinians while dropping among older Jews should prompt further research into the health, social, and cultural factors that could explain this rise specifically (fig. 11.1).

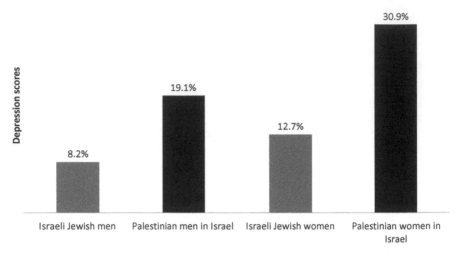

Figure 11.1. Depression scores by ethno-national group and gender. *Source:* Based on data from G. Kaplan, S. Glasser, H., Murad, A. Atamna, G. Alpert, U. Goldbourt, & O. Kalter-Leibovici. (2010). Depression among Arabs and Jews in Israel: A population-based study. *Social Psychiatry and Psychiatric Epidemiology, 45*(10), 931–939.

These findings concur with the Israeli National Health Interview Survey (INHIS) 2003–2004, which included a single question, "[I have been/ Have you been] feeling depressed most or all of the time during the past 4 weeks?" The IN-HIS found that for Palestinian men the age-adjusted rate of positive responses was 1.5 times greater than that of Jewish men, while Palestinian women's rates were 1.7 times higher than that of Jewish women (ICDC, 2006). The INHIS 2003–2004 (Levav et al., 2007) found more expressions of emotional distress among Palestinians compared to Jews, according to the GHQ, with rates of depressive symptoms during the preceding 12 months also higher, albeit of borderline significance. Although the prevalence of depressive symptoms is similar to the latter study (Levav et al., 2007), the multivariate analysis indicates that the Palestinian ethnic-national variable in itself did not enter as an independent significant factor. Rather, the differences between the ethnic-national groups were better explained by disparities in their educational level and health status.

Two methodological issues should be raised. First, when analyzing health data based on surveys, it is necessary to consider the potential effect of respondents' biases in answering questionnaires, particularly when looking at cross-cultural differences between population groups. A study conducted in Israel in 2006 (Baron-Epel, Kaplan, Weinstein, & Green, 2010) empirically measured the extent of choosing the extreme values of the scale and acquiescence biases. In a random telephone survey including 809 Palestinians and 2,322 Jewish Israelis, three attitude questions were presented twice with opposite wording to measure extreme and acquiescence biases. Extreme bias ranged from 2.0% to 14.0% among Jewish Israelis and from 6.0% to 29.0% among Palestinians, depending on the question. The respective acquiescence bias ranged from 2.0% to 10.0% and 5.0% to 19.0%. After adjusting for age and education, the odds ratio of giving more extreme biased answers was higher among Palestinians compared to Jewish Israelis for all three questions (OR = 2.49, 95% CI, 1.87–3.31; OR = 2.33, 95% CI, 1.75–3.10; and OR = 2.94, 95% CI, 1.83–4.71, respectively for each question).

Many researchers regard extreme and acquiescence bias simply as a nonsystematic error. It has been suggested that this type of bias is an expression of cultural orientation and differing styles of communication (Cheung & Rensvold, 2000). However, caution is needed in drawing conclusions about differences between Palestinians and Jews based on survey data.

The second methodological issue is the validation process of translating mental health research instruments into the Arabic language and culture. A limited number of papers focusing on their validation is available. A recent example of such an effort is the validation in Hebrew and Arabic of the Outcome Questionnaire-45 (OQ-45) to measure the progress of mental health treatment, which aids in assessing and monitoring psychotherapeutic outcomes (Gross et al., 2014). More research is needed to get a clear epidemiological portrait of the mental health of the Palestinian population in Israel, and high-quality research on the subject must be encouraged.

Community Study III

This study, taken in part from the article "Common Mental Disorders among Arab-Israelis: Findings from the Israel National Health Survey" (Levav et al., 2007), was conducted under the umbrella of the WHO-Harvard WMH Survey. The objective was to investigate the rates of common mental disorders and the use of services and their respective correlates. This household survey followed the procedures established by the WMH Survey Initiative (Demyttenaere et al., 2004; Kessler & Üstün, 2004).

Sampling Procedure

The sample population was extracted from the Israeli National Population Register (NPR) and comprised noninstitutionalized de jure residents aged 21 and over. The sample was designed to reflect a fixed distribution of respondents combining the following characteristics: population groups, Palestinian and Jewish (Israel-born and pre- and post-1990 immigrants); age groups in the range 21–75 years and over; and gender.

In large localities ($n = 73$), where approximately 80% of the total population live, a one-stage stratified sample was drawn. Each stratum was defined as a combination of population group, age, and gender. The records in each stratum were sorted by geographic characteristics and a systematic sample was drawn. In small localities ($n = 1,113$), a two-stage sample was drawn. First, the localities were assigned to 33 strata according to localization, size, and type (e.g., village, city). A systematic sample of localities was drawn from each stratum with probability proportional to their size; 89 localities were selected, at least two localities in each stratum. In the second stage, the sampling rate was set so that the final probability of individuals was fixed across localities. A systematic sample of individuals in the sampled localities was drawn from the NPR after sorting the records by population group, age, and gender. On average, 15 respondents were selected in each locality.

Weighting Procedures

The interviewed sample was weighted back to the total population to compensate for unequal selection probabilities resulting from disproportionate stratification, clustering effects, and nonresponse. The weights were adjusted to make weighted sample totals conform to known population totals taken from reliable Israel Central Bureau of Statistics sources.

The Questionnaire

The five-part survey instrument was a detailed, computerized schedule that included a number of questionnaires and appraisals.

1. Respondents were asked to provide sociodemographic information.
2. The 12-item GHQ (GHQ-12), which had previously been used both locally (Shemesh et al., 2006) and in Arab countries (El-Rufaie & Daradkeh, 1996) is a scale that screens for psychiatric disorders and measures emotional distress. Scores range between 12 and 48, where higher scores indicate increased distress.
3. The WMH-CIDI, a fully structured diagnostic instrument, assesses lifetime and recent prevalence of disorders according to both the *ICD-10* and the US-originated *DSM-IV* psychiatric classification systems. The following disorders were assessed: anxiety disorders (panic disorder, generalized anxiety disorder, agoraphobia without panic disorder, and PTSD); mood disorders (major depressive disorder, dysthymia, bipolar I and II disorders); and substance use disorders (alcohol and drug abuse and dependence). Prevalence estimates of mental disorder were determined by whether the respondent's past or current symptoms met the 12-month and/or lifetime diagnostic criteria for *DSM-IV* disorder. For each disorder, a screening section was administered to all respondents. All participants that answered positively to a specific screening question were referred to the respective diagnostic section of the questionnaire. Whenever appropriate, organic exclusion criteria were taken into account in the evaluation of the *DSM-IV* diagnoses.

4. Several items explored the use of general and mental health services. Respondents were asked whether they had consulted with any one of a list of professionals for problems related to their mental health. The professionals included those in specialized mental health services (psychologists, psychiatrists, social workers), general medical professionals (such as family physicians), religious counselors (rabbis, sheikhs), and other healers (e.g., naturopaths). Respondents who never used professional or traditional services were asked whether they ever thought they needed such services or whether they intended to consult.
5. In a self-appraisal of mental health, all respondents were asked to appraise their mental health using a 1–5 scale, from excellent to poor.
6. In a self-appraisal of social status, respondents were asked to rate their social status on a 1–10 scale in relation to that of the general society, from the lowest, 1, to the highest, 10.

The original English schedules were translated into Arabic and Hebrew following a translation and back-translation procedure. Special attention was given to the cultural adequacy of terms and their acceptability to respondents with different educational backgrounds. A panel of experienced clinicians, whose mother tongue was Arabic or Hebrew, discussed the equivalence of terms.

Field Operation

The interviews were conducted from 2003 to 2004. The survey was administered using laptop computer-assisted personal interview (CAPI) methods. The interviews were conducted in the respondent's preferred language. The overall response rate was 73.0%; 88.0% among Palestinians and 71.0% among Jewish Israelis, totaling 4,864 completed interviews. There were no replacements.

Statistical Analysis

The analysis was based on the two main subgroups of the entire sample: Palestinians (men, 324; women, 335) and Jewish Israelis, local-born or immigrants who arrived before 1990 (men, 1,662; women, 1,670). For the analysis, age was classified into two groups, 21–49 years and 50 and over. Marital status was classified as married; separated, divorced, or widowed; and never married. Educational level was dichotomized as lower (0–9 years) and higher (10 years and above). Income was dichotomized as below and above the median national income. Number of persons in the household and number of children were grouped as follows: 1–3, 4–6, and 7 and over. Employment was classified into three groups: employed, unemployed in the last 12 months, and not in the workforce. Twelve-month prevalence rates and standard errors were calculated. GHQ scores were analyzed by population group (Palestinians and Jewish Israelis), gender, and education using analysis of variance (MANOVA). The association between help-seeking practices and sociodemographic variables was analyzed by means of univariate and multivariate tests.

Findings

SAMPLE CHARACTERISTICS

Table 11.2 describes the sample by selected sociodemographic features. In comparison with Jewish Israeli respondents, Palestinians were younger, more likely to be

Table 11.2. Sociodemographic Characteristics of the Palestinian and Jewish Israeli Study Samples (Raw Figures and Weighted Proportions)

Variables	Palestinian Israelis				Jewish Israelis			
	Males		Females		Males		Females	
	N	(%)	N	(%)	N	(%)	N	(%)
Age groups								
21–49	1,003	(63)	961	(61)	251	(78)	247	(76)
50+	659	(37)	709	(39)	73	(22)	88	(24)
Family status								
Married	1,139	(70)	1,066	(66)	255	(77)	241	(73)
Separated/Divorced/ Widowed	135	(7)	335	(18)	6	(2)	35	(9)
Never married	388	(23)	269	(16)	63	(21)	59	(18)
Educational level								
Lower, 0–9 years	161	(9)	226	(13)	110	(34)	152	(45)
Higher, 10+ years	1,495	(91)	1,438	(87)	211	(66)	183	(55)
Income								
Below the median	618	(41)	661	(45)	244	(78)	271	(84)
Above the median	1,044	(59)	1,009	(55)	80	(22)	64	(16)
No. of persons in household								
1–3	869	(48)	967	(53)	74	(19)	99	(23)
4–6	721	(46)	636	(42)	181	(56)	170	(52)
7+	72	(6)	67	(6)	69	(25)	66	(25)
No. of children								
1–3	868	(70)	951	(70)	96	(42)	100	(39)
4–6	277	(24)	298	(25)	104	(42)	103	(41)
7+	53	(5)	59	(5)	37	(16)	53	(20)
Employment status								
Employed	1,123	(64)	936	(54)	212	(62)	90	(22)
Unemployed	90	(6)	98	(7)	36	(7)	23	(4)
Out of the workforce	449	(30)	636	(39)	76	(31)	222	(74)

Source: I. Levav, A. Ifrah, N. Geraisy, A. Grinshpoon, & R. Khwaled. (2007). Common mental disorders among Arab-Israelis: Findings from the Israel National Health Survey. *Israel Journal of Psychiatry and Related Sciences, 44*(2), 104–113.

married, with lower incomes, with lower levels of education, and with larger families. In addition, they were less likely to be employed full-time and, for women, less likely to be in the workforce.

EMOTIONAL DISTRESS

The GHQ-12 scale showed high internal consistency reliability; Cronbach's alpha coefficient was 0.76 for Palestinians and Jewish Israelis of both genders.

Univariate analysis. Palestinian respondents, both men and women, had higher mean scores—overall score, 10.8 (standard error [SE] 0.35); men, 10.2 (SE 0.5); women, 11.5 (SE 0.41)—than their Jewish counterparts: overall score, 7.3 (SE 0.11); men, 6.4 (SE 0.14); women, 8.1 (SE 0.15). Both differences were statistically significant ($p < 0.0001$). Mean GHQ scores were significantly higher among older adults (aged 50 and over), respondents with lower levels of education, those with incomes below the median, and individuals outside of the workforce or who had been unemployed during the past year (table 11.3).

Multivariate analysis. In the analysis (MANOVA), population group (Palestinians/Jews), gender, age, and education were included in the model (table 11.4). In all categories, GHQ scores were higher among Palestinians than among Jewish Israelis, among women than among men, and among those of lower rather than higher educational status. Older age (50 and over) was found to be a significant risk factor only among those of lower educational status. The highest GHQ mean score was found among older Palestinian women of lower educational status (15.1; 95% CI, 12.5–17.7). Younger Jewish Israeli men of higher educational status had the lowest score (5.5; 95% CI, 5.1–5.9).

PREVALENCE RATES OF COMMON MENTAL DISORDERS

Anxiety Disorders. Overall, there were no statistically significant differences between Palestinians and Jewish Israelis in the 12-month prevalence rates of any anxiety disorder (table 11.5). Among men, Palestinians had higher rates than Jewish Israelis, 3.7% (95% CI, 2.1–6.5) and 2.8% (95% CI, 2.1–3.8), respectively. The findings went in the opposite direction for women: Palestinians, 3.0% (95% CI, 1.5–5.8); and Jewish Israelis, 3.6% (95% CI, 2.8–4.6).

Depressive Disorders. The overall 12-month prevalence rates for any affective disorder were, for Palestinians, 8.2% (95% CI, 6.2–11.0) and, for Jewish Israelis, 5.9% (95% CI,5.1–6.8). The respective rates for men were 6.2% (95% CI, 3.8–9.4) and 4.7% (95% CI, 3.8–5.8), and for women, 10.5% (95% CI, 7.3–14.8) and 7.1% (95% CI, 5.9–8.5). Differences between Palestinians and Jewish Israelis were of borderline statistical significance ($p = 0.06$).

The combined rates of any depressive or anxiety disorder (common mental disorders) were higher among Palestinians than among Jewish Israelis and higher among women than among men. These differences, however, did not reach statistical significance (table 11.5).

Table 11.3. Univariate Analysis of Emotional Distress: Mean GHQ Scores by Demographic Variables

Variables	Sample *N*	Mean score	*SE*
Total	3,889	7.9	0.11
Population groups*			
Palestinian Israelis	632	10.8	0.35
Jewish Israelis	3,257	7.3	0.11
Gender*			
Male	1,943	7.0	0.15
Female	1,946	8.6	0.15
Age groups*			
21–49	2,435	7.4	0.13
50+	1,454	8.6	0.19
Family status*			
Married	2,637	7.5	0.13
Separated/divorced/widowed	479	10.4	0.38
Never married	773	7.4	0.2
Median income*			
Below	1,741	8.6	0.17
Above	2,148	7.0	0.12
Educational level*			
Lower, 0–9 years	2,162	9.0	0.16
Higher, 10+ years	1,713	6.3	0.12
Employment status*			
Employed	2,338	6.4	0.1
Unemployed in past 12 months	239	9.3	0.47
Out of the workforce	1,312	9.7	0.22

Note. SE, standard error. * $p < 0.0001$
Source: I. Levav, A. Ifrah, N. Geraisy, A. Grinshpoon, & R. Khwaled, R. (2007). Common mental disorders among Arab-Israelis: Findings from the Israel National Health Survey. *Israel Journal of Psychiatry and Related Sciences, 44*(2), 104–113.

GHQ AND ANY ANXIETY OR DEPRESSIVE DISORDER

Mean GHQ scores for respondents who were diagnosed with any disorder, affective or anxiety, were considerably higher for Palestinian men (18.9; *SE* 1.5) than for Jewish men (13.6; *SE* 0.7). Findings were similar for women: Palestinians, 18.6 (*SE* 1.3); and Jews, 15.4 (*SE* 0.6).

HELP-SEEKING BEHAVIOR

A considerably higher proportion of Jewish Israeli than Palestinian respondents, both men and women, sought help from the medical or psychiatric health systems

Table 11.4. Multivariate Analysis of Emotional Distress: Mean GHQ Scores by Population Group, Gender, Age Group, and Educational Level (95% Confidence Intervals)

Mean GHQ (95% CI) Population groups*	Palestinian Citizens in Israel				Jewish Israelis			
Gender*	Males		Females		Males		Females	
Age groups*	21–49	50+	21–49	50+	21–49	50+	21–49	50+
Educational level*								
Lower, 0–9	9.9	14.7	11.3	15.1	6.7	7.8	8.6	10.2
	(8.3–11.5)	(12.3–17.0)	(10.3–12.3)	(12.5–17.7)	(6.2–7.2)	(7.0–8.6)	(8.0–9.3)	(9.4–10.8)
Higher, 10+ years	7.1	5.6	8.9	8.3	5.5	5.7	6.6	7.0
	(5.5–8.8)	(2.9–8.2)	(7.6–10.3)	(0.5–16.0)	(5.1–5.9)	(5.0–6.4)	(6.2–7.0)	(6.3–7.7)

Note. GQH, General Health Questionnaire; CI, confidence interval.
* $p < 0.0001$.
Source: I. Levav, A. Ifrah, N. Geraisy, A. Grinshpoon, & R. Khwaled. (2007). Common mental disorders among Arab-Israelis: Findings from the Israel National Health Survey. *Israel Journal of Psychiatry and Related Sciences, 44*(2), 104–113.

Table 11.5. Twelve-Month Prevalence Rates of *DSM-IV* Any Affective Disorder and Anxiety Disorder by Population Group and Gender (Percent)

Population groups	N	Any affective disorder* % (95% CI)	Any anxiety disorder** % (95% CI)	Any affective or anxiety disorder** % (95% CI)
Palestinian citizens in Israel		8.2 (6.2–11.0)	3.3 (2.2–5.0)	11.1 (8.7–14.2)
Males	324	6.2 (3.8–9.4)	3.7 (2.1–6.5)	10.2 (7.0–14.7)
Females	335	10.5 (7.3–14.8)	3.0 (1.5–5.8)	12.0 (8.6–16.7)
Jewish Israelis		5.9 (5.1–6.8)	3.2 (2.6.2–3.9)	9.3 (8.3–10.3)
Males	1,662	4.7 (3.8–5.8)	2.8 (2.1–3.8)	8.4 (7.2–9.8)
Females	1,670	7.1 (5.9–8.5)	3.6 (2.8–4.6)	10.1 (8.6–11.7)

Note. CI, confidence interval; NS, not significant.
* Overall gender difference, $p = 0.0008$; overall Palestinian Israeli/Jewish Israeli difference, $p = 0.06$. ** Overall gender difference, NS; overall Palestinian Israeli/Jewish Israeli difference, NS.
Source: I. Levav, A. Ifrah, N. Geraisy, A. Grinshpoon, & R. Khwaled. (2007). Common mental disorders among Arab-Israelis: Findings from the Israel National Health Survey. *Israel Journal of Psychiatry and Related Sciences, 44*(2), 104–113.

Table 11.6. Presence of Anxiety or Mood Disorder and Expressed Need for Care: Mean GHQ Scores by Population Group

Population group Expressed need for care	Palestinian citizens in Israel				Jewish Israeli citizens			
	Affective or anxiety disorder		No affective or anxiety disorder		Affective or anxiety disorder		No affective or anxiety disorder	
	n	Mean GHQ (*SE*)	*n*	Mean GHQ (*SE*)	*n*	Mean GHQ (*SE*)	*n*	Mean GHQ (*SE*)
Yes	18	20.1 (1.2)	27	16.6 (1.1)	42	15.8 (1.2)	130	11.3 (0.5)
No	34	16.7 (1.6)	546	9.3 (0.3)	134	13.6 (0.8)	2,702	6.0 (0.1)

Note. GHQ, General Health Questionnaire; *SE*, standard error.
Source: I. Levav, A. Ifrah, N. Geraisy, A. Grinshpoon, & R. Khwaled. (2007). Common mental disorders among Arab-Israelis: Findings from the Israel National Health Survey. *Israel Journal of Psychiatry and Related Sciences, 44*(2), 104–113.

when affected by any anxiety or affective disorder in the last 12 months: Jews, 8.6%; Palestinians, 3.8%. Among those respondents who had never sought such help, 5.8% of Jews and 7.5% of Palestinians nevertheless considered that they were in need of help. GHQ scores were higher among respondents who thought they needed help than among those who did not think they were in need of help and were consistently higher among Palestinian respondents (table 11.6).

SELF-APPRAISAL OF MENTAL HEALTH

Respondents were asked to rate their overall mental health from excellent to poor. The respective appraisals of mental health were reported as follows: excellent or very good (Palestinians, 61.2%, and Jewish Israelis, 72.8%); good (16% and 6.9%); fair (11.8% and 5.7%); and poor (4.2% and 1.2%). Women in both population groups were more likely than men to rate their mental health as poor. The difference between Palestinians and Jewish Israelis was statistically significant (Mann-Whitney, $p < .0001$).

SELF-APPRAISAL OF SOCIAL STATUS

Respondents rated their social status on a scale of 1 to 10 (lowest to highest) in relation to that of the population of Israel. Overall, the mean rating of the Palestinian respondents was 4.8 (*SE* 0.26), while among men, 5.1 (*SE* 0.48), and among women, 4.5 (*SE* 0.15). The mean rating of the Jewish Israeli respondents was significantly higher, overall and separately, for both genders: overall, 6.5 (*SE* 0.12), while among men, 6.8 (*SE* 0.21), and among women, 6.3 (*SE* 0.12).

General Discussion

Several constraints limited the examination of the common mental disorders among the Palestinian population in Israel. First, following the protocol of the WMH study, the Palestinian minority group was not oversampled (Demyttenaere et al., 2004). As a result, the relatively small number of cases in some cells ruled out more complex analyses, and differences that possibly existed did not reach statistical significance. Second, to increase the statistical power, Palestinians of Christian, Druze, and Muslim religious affiliations were grouped together, although they differ in many respects, as previously noted. A third limitation is that somatization disorders, which have been noted to be relatively frequent among Arab populations (Ghubash, 2001; Racy, 1980), but not by all authors (Al Lawati et al., 2000), were not addressed in this study. Last, the study was conducted during the second intifada, however, the differential impact of this conflict on the different Palestinian and Jewish Israeli groups was not specifically assessed.

Several strengths balanced out those limitations: the WMH Survey, of which this study was part, utilizes an identical system of case identification and diagnosis, thus enabling comparisons with Lebanon and Iraq, the two Arab countries that participated in the WMH study, and, eventually, with other countries. Our response rate was satisfactory, particularly among the Palestinian respondents (88%). Finally, we believe that the study met adequate standards of cultural sensitivity and awareness, taking into account, for instance, that the study of depressive affect necessitates identification of the linguistic patterns used by individuals to describe their emotional pattern when depressed (Amin, Hamdi, & Abou-Saleh, 2001).

Palestinians differed from Jewish Israelis in a number of parameters: they had higher scores of emotional distress, lower self-appraisal of mental health, and fewer requests for psychiatric help. The following factors, among others, may explain the higher emotional distress scores among Palestinian Israelis: response style might be imputed, as noted in a community-based study on the older adults (Shemesh et al., 2006). Palestinian respondents seem to more readily express and amplify complaints in contrast to their Jewish Israeli counterparts, as noted for each gender, educational level, and age group. Likely, the compounded social stress experienced by the Palestinian minority may have constituted an additional factor. Indeed, the Palestinian population, in addition to being more disadvantaged—which was subjectively acknowledged with regard to the self-appraisal of social status—is under the pressure of Westernization and the need to succeed in a developed country. In this dual process, Palestinian women are probably more affected than men owing to their subordinate status in a traditional, patriarchal society. Despite considerable health gains made by Palestinians, their status lags behind that of the Jewish Israeli majority (ICDC, 2005). This is analogous to other social fields where researchers have found that relative differences in income significantly affect happiness, even when absolute income is held constant (Blanchflower & Oswald, 2004).

Interestingly, the social stresses inherent in the minority status of Palestinians were not significantly associated with differential rates of common mental disorders. This lack of effect of social causation factors with regard to common mental disorders was similarly noted by Kessler, Foster, Saunders, and Stang (1995) but not by others (Skapinakis, Lewis, Araya, Jones, & Williams, 2005).

How does this study fare in relation to others conducted in Arab countries? Comparisons are hindered by both the rarity of community psychiatry surveys in the region (Ghubash, 2001) and by methodological issues, such as the use of different diagnostic instruments and the time period reported for the rates. The study in Al Ain, in the United Arab Emirates, used CIDI, but it reported lifetime rates (Ghubash, 2001), which are known to be unreliable. The aforementioned study in Dubai used the Present State Examination (PSE) (Ghubash et al., 1992), while in Lebanon the DIS-III was used for the same purpose (Weissman et al., 1996). It is only within the framework of the WMH Survey that Israel and Lebanon could compare prevalence rates.

Palestinian respondents sought less help from health services than their Jewish counterparts, possibly because of issues of stigma and/or less available culturally appropriate services. This pattern, however, was reversed with regard to the stated intention to consult when a disorder, affective or anxiety, was present. Importantly, studies have found that Palestinian women are more likely to make use of telephone counseling than men (Al-Krenawi, Graham, & Fakher-Aldin, 2003), although most mental health system users are men (Feinson, Handelsman, & Popper, 1992). This suggests that if the barriers of confidentiality and anonymity could be overcome, despite the widespread reservations toward mental health care, particularly among women, a greater proportion of those in need of care could make use of mental health services. Finally, although social and economic changes are taking place among Palestinians, the mental health system is still perceived as a Western development, which could conceivably act as a barrier to the use of mental health services in this population.

Despite major health gains, the social stresses of being a minority that is undergoing major social changes may explain the greater emotional distress among Palestinians. A combination of cultural and political factors, including the perceptions of mental disorder, psychiatric care, and stigma, as well as a lesser availability of culturally tailored services, may account for the marked treatment gap among Palestinians.

GIORA KAPLAN is Director of Research on Psychosocial Aspects of Health Unit at the Gertner Institute for Epidemiology and Health Policy Research, Tel Hashomer, Israel.

ITZHAK LEVAV is Affiliated Professor in the Department of Community Mental Health, Faculty of Social Welfare and Health Sciences, at the

University of Haifa, Israel. He is editor of *Psychiatric and Behavioral Disorders in Israel: From Epidemiology to Mental Health Action*, and editor (with Jutta Lindert) of *Violence and Mental Health: Its Manifold Faces*.

ORA NAKASH is a clinical psychologist and Professor in the School for Social Work at Smith College, Northampton, MA, and Adjunct Professor at the Baruch Ivcher School of Psychology at the Interdisciplinary Center in Herzliya, Israel.

Note

1. Acknowledgment: This chapter is based in part on I. Levav, A. Ifrah, N. Geraisy, A. Grinshpoon, and R. Khwaled. (2007). Common mental disorders among Arab-Israelis: Findings from the Israel national health survey. *Israel Journal of Psychiatry, 44*(2), pp. 104–113. The authors acknowledge with thanks the permission granted by *IJP*.

References

Al-Issa, I., & Al-Junun, A. (2002). *Mental illness in the Islamic world*. Madison, WI: International Universities Press.

Al-Krenawi, A. (1998). Family therapy with a multiparental/multispousal family. *Family Process, 37*(1), 65–81.

Al-Krenawi, A., & Graham, J. R. (1999). Gender and biomedical/traditional mental health utilization among the Bedouin-Arabs of the Negev. *Culture, Medicine and Psychiatry, 23*(2), 219–243.

Al-Krenawi, A., Graham, J. R., Dean, Y. Z., & Eltaiba, N. (2004). Cross-national study of attitudes towards seeking professional help: Jordan, United Arab Emirates (UAE) and Arabs in Israel. *International Journal of Social Psychiatry, 50*(2), 102–114.

Al-Krenawi, A., Graham, J. R., & Fakher-Aldin, M. (2003). Telephone counseling: A comparison of Arab and Jewish Israeli usage. *International Social Work, 46*(4), 495–509.

Al Lawati, J., Al Lawati, N., Al Siddiqui, M., Antony, S., Al Naamani, A., Martin, R., . . . Al Hussaini, A. (2000). Psychological morbidity in primary healthcare in Oman: A preliminary study. *Journal for Scientific Research: Medical Sciences, 2*, 105–110.

American Psychiatric Association. (2000). *Diagnostic and statistical manual of mental disorders* (4th ed., text rev.). Washington, DC: American Psychiatric Association.

Amin, Y., Hamdi, E., & Abou-Saleh, M. (2001). Depression in the Arab world. In A. Okasha & M. Mario (Eds.), *An Arab perspective* (pp. 89–122). Cairo: World Psychiatric Association, Scientific Book House.

Amir, M., Lewin-Epstein, N., Becker, G., & Buskila, D. (2002). Psychometric properties of the SF-12 in a primary care population in Israel [in Hebrew]. *Medical Care, 40*(10), 918–928.

Baer, L., Jacobs, D. G., Meszler-Reizes, J., Blais, M., Fava, M., Kessler, R. C., . . . Cukor, P. (1999). Development of a brief screening instrument: The HANDS. *Psychotherapy and Psychosomatics, 69*(1), 35–41.

Baron-Epel, O., Kaplan, G., & Moran, M. (2010). Perceived discrimination and health-related quality of life among Arabs and Jews in Israel: A population-based survey. *BMC Public Health, 10*(1), 282.

Baron-Epel, O., Kaplan, G., Weinstein, R., & Green, M. S. (2010). Extreme and acquiescence bias in a bi-ethnic population. *European Journal of Public Health, 20*(5), 543–548.

Blanchflower, D. G., & Oswald, A. J. (2004). Well-being over time in Britain and the USA. *Journal of Public Economics, 88*(7), 1359–1386.

Cheung, G. W., & Rensvold, R. B. (2000). Assessing extreme and acquiescence response sets in cross-cultural research using structural equations modeling. *Journal of Cross-Cultural Psychology, 31*(2), 187–212.

Demyttenaere, K., Bruffaerts, R., Posada-Villa, J., Gasquet, I., Kovess, V., Lepine, J., . . . Morosini, P. (2004). Prevalence, severity, and unmet need for treatment of mental disorders in the World Health Organization world mental health surveys. *JAMA, 291*(21), 2581–2590.

Department of Information and Evaluation. (2004). *Mental health in Israel. Statistical annual 2003* [in Hebrew]. Jerusalem: Israel Ministry of Health.

Elnekave, E., & Gross, R. (2004). The healthcare experiences of Arab Israeli women in a reformed healthcare system. *Health Policy, 69*(1), 101–116.

El-Rufaie, O., & Daradkeh, T. (1996). Validation of the Arabic versions of the thirty- and twelve-item general health questionnaires in primary care patients. *British Journal of Psychiatry, 169*(5), 662–664.

Feinson, M. C., Handelsman, M., & Popper, M. (1992). *Utilization of public ambulatory mental health services in Israel: A focus on age and gender patterns.* Jerusalem: JDC-Brookdale Institute of Gerontology and Adult Human Development in Israel; Israel Ministry of Health.

Ghubash, R. (2001). Epidemiological studies in the Arab world. In A. Okasha & M. Maj (Eds.), *An Arab perspective.* Cairo: World Psychiatric Association, Scientific Book House.

Ghubash, R., Hamdi, E., & Bebbington, P. (1992). The Dubai community psychiatric survey: I. Prevalence and socio-demographic correlates. *Social Psychiatry and Psychiatric Epidemiology, 27*(2), 53–61.

Ghubash, R., Hamdi, E., & Bebbington, P. (1994). The Dubai community psychiatric survey: Acculturation and the prevalence of psychiatric disorder. *Psychological Medicine, 24*(01), 121–131.

Gross, R., Glasser, S., Elisha, D., Tishby, O., Madar, J. D., Levitan, G., . . . Ponizovsky, A. (2014). Validation of the Hebrew and Arabic versions of the outcome questionnaire (OQ-45). *Israel Journal of Psychiatry and Related Sciences, 52*(1), 33–39.

Israel Center for Disease Control [ICDC]. (2005). *The health status of the Arab population in Israel* [in Hebrew]. Jerusalem: Israel Ministry of Health.

Israel Center for Disease Control [ICDC]. (2006). *Israeli national health interview survey (INHIS-1): Selected findings, publication 249* [in Hebrew]. Jerusalem: Israel Ministry of Health.

Kadri, N., & Moussaoui, D. (2001). Women's mental health in the Arab world. In A. Okasha & M. Maj (Eds.), *An Arab perspective* (pp. 189–206). Cairo: World Psychiatric Association, Scientific Book House.

Kaplan, G., Glasser, S., Murad, H., Atamna, A., Alpert, G., Goldbourt, U., & Kalter-Leibovici, O. (2010). Depression among Arabs and Jews in Israel: A population-based study. *Social Psychiatry and Psychiatric Epidemiology, 45*(10), 931–939.

Kessler, R. C., Foster, C. L., Saunders, W. B., & Stang, P. E. (1995). Social consequences of psychiatric disorders, I: Educational attainment. *American Journal of Psychiatry, 152*(7), 1026–1032.

Kessler, R. C., & Üstün, T. B. (2004). The world mental health (WMH) survey initiative version of the World Health Organization (WHO) composite international diagnostic interview (CIDI). *International Journal of Methods in Psychiatric Research, 13*(2), 93–121.

Kohn, R., Saxena, S., Levav, I., & Saraceno, B. (2004). The treatment gap in mental health care. *Bulletin of the World Health Organization, 82*(11), 858–866.

Krieger, N., Smith, K., Naishadham, D., Hartman, C., & Barbeau, E. M. (2005). Experiences of discrimination: Validity and reliability of a self-report measure for population health research on racism and health. *Social Science & Medicine, 61*(7), 1576–1596.

Levav, I., Ifrah, A., Geraisy, N., Grinshpoon, A., & Khwaled, R. (2007). Common mental disorders among Arab-Israelis: Findings from the Israel national health survey. *Israel Journal of Psychiatry and Related Sciences, 44*(2), 104–113.

Racy, J. (1980). Somatization in Saudi Women: A therapeutic challenge. *British Journal of Psychiatry, 137*(3), 212–216.

Saif Al Dawla, A. (2001). Social factors affecting women's mental health in the Arab region. In A. Okasha & M. Maj (Eds.), *An Arab perspective* (pp. 207–223). Cairo: World Psychiatric Association, Scientific Book House.

Sellers, R. M., Caldwell, C. H., Schmeelk-Cone, K. H., & Zimmerman, M. A. (2003). Racial identity, racial discrimination, perceived stress, and psychological distress among African American young adults. *Journal of Health and Social Behavior, 44*(3), 302–317.

Shemesh, A. A., Kohn, R., Blumstein, T., Geraisy, N., Novikov, I., & Levav, I. (2006). A community study on emotional distress among Arab and Jewish Israelis over the age of 60. *International Journal of Geriatric Psychiatry, 21*(1), 64–76.

Skapinakis, P., Lewis, G., Araya, R., Jones, K., & Williams, G. (2005). Mental health inequalities in Wales, UK: Multi-level investigation of the effect of area deprivation. *British Journal of Psychiatry, 186*(5), 417–422.

Smooha, S. (1999). The advances and limits of the Israelization of Israel's Palestinian citizens. In K. Abdel-Malek & D. C. Jacobson (Eds.), *Israeli and Palestinian identities in history and literature* (pp. 9–33). New York: St. Martin's.

Ware, J. E., Jr., Kosinski, M., & Keller, S. D. (1996). A 12-item short-form health survey: Construction of scales and preliminary tests of reliability and validity. *Medical Care, 34*(3), 220–233.

Weissman, M. M., Bland, R. C., Canino, G. J., Faravelli, C., Greenwald, S., Hwu, H.-G., . . . Lellouch, J. (1996). Cross-national epidemiology of major depression and bipolar disorder. *JAMA, 276*(4), 293–299.

12

PSYCHIATRIC HOSPITALIZATIONS AMONG PALESTINIAN CITIZENS IN ISRAEL

A Historical Cohort Study

Ido Lurie and Anat Fleischman

ACCORDING TO THE WORLD LITERATURE, ETHNIC MINORITIES ARE at higher risk of mental disorders (World Health Organization, 2012), with higher burden of disease, including severe mental illness (Boydell et al., 2001; Bresnahan et al., 2007; Fearon et al., 2006), depression (Missinne & Bracke, 2012; Williams et al., 2007), and PTSD (Roberts, Gilman, Breslau, Breslau, & Koenen, 2011). Moreover, the course of illness among minorities is affected because it is more chronic and severe (Williams et al., 2007). Additionally, ethnic minorities may not benefit from an equal level of care: they have less access to mental health services and are more likely to receive poorer quality care when treated (Satcher, 2001). Minorities also underuse both outpatient mental health services (Alegría et al., 2002; Neighbors et al., 2007) and inpatient services (Cook, Manning, & Alegría, 2013; Horvitz-Lennon, McGuire, Alegría, & Frank, 2009). Seemingly, psychiatric hospitalizations are often used as a proxy for symptomatic exacerbation (Levine, Lurie, Kohn, & Levav, 2011) and together with particularly early rehospitalization may serve as an indicator for the quality of inpatient and community services (Lyons et al., 1997).

In the original study reported on in this chapter, we aimed to map the patterns of psychiatric hospitalizations in the Palestinian population in Israel and compare those patterns to those of the Jewish population using a historical cohort study.

Method

We extracted the information from the National Psychiatric Case Register (NPCR) run by the Israel Ministry of Health and from the Israel Central Bureau of Statistics (Israel CBS). The NPCR cumulatively enters all admissions and discharges to psychiatric inpatient facilities (including psychiatric hospitals, day units, and psychiatric units in general hospitals) using a unique identification number (Levav et al., 2007). The study population comprised all Palestinian groups—including Muslims (n = 6,256), Christians (n = 864), and Druze (n = 849)—and Jews (n = 48,511) admitted to these facilities between 2000 and 2013.

The NPCR records multiple pieces of information, such as gender, religious affiliation, address, birth date, date of death, years of education, and marital status at time of admission. In addition, it includes hospitalization dates, number of admissions, accumulated length of stay, days in the community prior to hospitalization, and legal status of admission (voluntary or involuntary according to court or district psychiatrist [DP] order). It also records information about suicide attempts and substance (drug or alcohol) use during the two months preceding admission and death during hospitalization (all causes and suicide, in and outside the hospital). Lastly, it includes diagnoses on admission and discharge for each hospitalization, assigned by a board-certified psychiatrist at the facility. The diagnoses are recorded according to the *ICD-10*, while those made according to earlier classifications have been updated.

For this study, psychiatric diagnoses were grouped as follows: organic brain disorders (F00–F09), drug and alcohol use disorders (F10–F19), non-affective psychotic disorders (including schizophrenia) (F20–F29), affective disorders (F30–F39), neurotic disorders (F40–F48), and personality disorders (F60–F69). The category "Other disorders" included all other F and Z codes (clinical diagnoses and factors influencing health status, respectively). Specific diagnoses were also grouped as follows: schizophrenia (F20); bipolar affective disorder (F30–F31), depression (F32–F33), and PTSD (F43.1); and OCD (F42).

Only hospitalizations of persons over the age of 15 were included in our analysis. We excluded persons who died during the follow-up period in calculating the current age of the cohort. We estimated the socioeconomic status (SES) according to the residential status area, which is a neighborhood-based measure (Weiser et al., 2007). This value is derived from household census data based on number of persons per room, electrical appliances (e.g., air conditioning), and per capita income (Israel CBS, 1995). The residential status was obtained by linking patients' addresses with the census track and the ranking of the neighborhood as determined by the Israel CBS. Our study represented 10 crude SES clusters.

Statistical Analysis

The four national religious groups were compared regarding sociodemographic and clinical data. Continuous variables were compared using analysis of variance. Dichotomous variables were compared using the chi-squared (χ^2) test. Twelve-month incidence rates were calculated by new admissions per 100,000 population. Logistic regression was used to calculate incidence rate ratios and 95% confidence interval (CI) between groups. Survival from first to second hospitalization was estimated using the Kaplan-Meier method, and groups were compared using the logrank test. A univariate Cox proportional hazards regression model was used to investigate factors that might have influenced the risk for rehospitalization. In the third stage, a multivariate Cox proportional hazards regression model was used to determine an association between the variable and time to rehospitalization, adjusting to variables that were significant (0.05) at the second stage of analysis. All tests were two-tailed. Statistical analysis was performed using SPSS Statistics 22.0.

Ethical Issues

The study was approved by the institutional review board of Abarbanel Mental Health Center, affiliated with Tel Aviv University, and the Israel Ministry of Health's Legal and Ethical Clearance Board. Confidentiality was strictly assured since the coauthor (A. Fleischman) who analyzed the data had no access to the identity of the persons linked by the databases.

Results

The total number of persons aged 15 and over who were hospitalized in psychiatric facilities between 2000 and 2013 was 56,480. The majority of persons hospitalized in all groups were men (57.6%), and for Muslims and Druze, this was a significantly more frequent occurrence compared to Christians and Jews ($p < 0.05$ for all comparisons). Muslims and Druze were significantly younger in the study cohort than Jews and Christians ($p < 0.05$ for all comparisons). There was no significant age difference between Jews and Christians ($p = 0.99$) and between Muslims and Druze ($p = 0.97$). Women in this cohort were generally older than men, without statistically significant differences among the three Palestinian groups.

Christians had more years of education compared to Muslims ($p < 0.001$) and Druze ($p = 0.01$). The SES cluster was lowest among Muslims and significantly higher in Jews compared to Muslims, Christians, and Druze ($p < 0.05$ for all comparisons). There was no statistically significant difference between men and women in the educational level and in SES clusters in all population groups.

The mean time of follow-up (in years) did not reveal a statistically significant difference between men and women or among the four population groups. The mean age at first admission for all men in the cohort was 37.0 ± 17.7, and for women, 41.5 ± 20.3. For both men and women, Muslims and Druze were hospitalized at a significantly younger age compared to Jews and Christians ($p < 0.05$ for all comparisons), with no significant difference between Jews and Christians ($p = 0.2$). The sociodemographic and clinical characteristics of the study's groups are shown in table 12.1a and table 12.1b.

The mean number of hospitalizations for this cohort was 2.8 ± 3.7 for men and 2.4 ± 3.1 for women ($p < 0.05$). The mean number of hospitalizations during the follow-up period was significantly higher in Muslims compared to Jews and Christians for both men and women (2.9 ± 4.1 vs. 2.6 ± 3.4 and 2.5 ± 2.9, respectively;

Table 12.1a. Psychiatric Hospitalizations, 2000–2013: Sociodemographic Characteristics of the Study Groups

	Jews (*n* = 48,511)		Muslims (*n* = 6,256)		Christians (*n* = 864)		Druze (*n* = 849)	
	Men	**Women**	**Men**	**Women**	**Men**	**Women**	**Men**	**Women**
Demographic data								
Gender (%)	55.7	44.3	69.3	30.7	59.8	40.2	59.8	40.2
Age (in years, mean ±SD) (excluding dead)	41.8 ± 15.7	45.8 ± 18.2	38.6 ± 11.6	39.3 ± 12.6	42.5 ± 13.1	45.2 ± 15.4	38.8 ± 10.9	40.1 ± 11.8
	(23,470)	(18,619)	(4,100)	(1,854)	(459)	(301)	(614)	(197)
Ever married (%)	71.4	82.8	71.9	81.6	71.4	85.6	71.6	84.4
Immigrants (%)	38.8	45.4	5.9	8.2	44.1	52.4	8.1	11.2
Education (in years, mean ±SD)	11.1 ± 2.7	11.5 ± 2.9	9.3 ± 3.0	9.5 ± 3.2	10.8 ± 3.3	11.0 ± 2.7	10.3 ± 2.3	9.9 ± 3.2
1–6	4.5	4.0	14.5	15.7	9.2	7.3	7.1	17.9
7–12	82.1	78.2	80.4	77.9	75.6	78.7	91.1	75.0
13+	13.4	17.8	5.1	6.4	15.3	14.0	1.8	7.1
SES cluster (mean ±SD)	5.7 ± 1.7	5.9 ± 1.7	3.2 ± 1.7	3.3 ± 1.6	5.1 ± 1.8	5.2 ± 1.9	3.4 ± 1.0	3.5 ± 1.0
SES tertiles (%)								
Lower tertile	4.5	4.3	61.2	57.9	21.4	20.1	65.0	60.3
Middle tertile	53.5	51.0	31.4	34.1	45.9	42.3	34.3	38.2
Upper tertile	42.0	44.8	7.4	8.0	32.7	37.5	0.6	1.5
Mean follow-up (in years, mean ±SD)	6.8 ± 4.2	6.9 ± 4.1	6.8 ± 4.0	7.1 ± 4.1	7.0 ± 4.1	6.9 ± 4.3	6.8 ± 3.6	6.5 ± 4.0

Note. SD, standard deviation; SES, socioeconomic status.

Source: Adapted from National Psychiatric Case Register, Israel Ministry of Health, and Israel Central Bureau of Statistics.

Table 12.1b. Psychiatric Hospitalizations, 2000–2013: Clinical Characteristics of the Study Groups

	Jews (n = 48,511)		Muslims (n = 6,256)		Christians (n = 864)		Druze (n = 849)	
	Men	Women	Men	Women	Men	Women	Men	Women
Age at first admission (in years, mean ±SD)	37.9 ± 18.5	42.3 ± 20.7	32.4 ± 11.9	32.6 ± 12.8	37.0 ± 14.8	40.9 ± 17.4	32.5 ± 11.5	34.2 ± 12.3
Age at first admission, schizophrenia (in years, mean ±SD)	30.9 ± 12.7	38.1 ± 16.2	29.8 ± 10.1	33.2 ± 11.8	31.6 ± 10.5	41.1 ± 15.9	28.9 ± 9.7	30.7 ± 11.7
No. of hospitalizations (mean ±SD)	2.7 ± 3.6	2.4 ± 3.0	3.0 ± 4.0	2.8 ± 4.4	2.8 ± 3.3	2.0 ± 2.1	2.7 ± 3.7	2.3 ± 3.0
Cumulative days of hospitalization	134.2 ± 271.9	110.8 ± 206.7	102.6 ± 247.7	70.0 ± 166.0	142.1 ± 311.8	79.2 ± 160.3	94.2 ± 191.7	86.6 ± 153.9
Mean days per admission	47.8 ± 93.1	46.8 ± 79.4	29.5 ± 71.3	23.7 ± 51.5	44.5 ± 102.2	37.4 ± 54.3	30.1 ± 43.8	39.9 ± 95.6
Mean days in the community in between admissions	525.4 ± 650.5	545.1 ± 694.7	509.3 ± 615.3	486.8 ± 280.3	616.79 ± 791.9	630.9 ± 846.4	533.1 ± 643.1	448.1 ± 591.6
Any involuntary admission by district psychiatrist order (%)	34.9	30.6	33.5	30.2	35.8	32.6	22.2	22.4
Any involuntary admission by court order (%)	11.8	1.6	22.3	2.9	17.8	1.4	12.9	1.0

Any substance use (%)	31.5	13.0	34.0	6.7	40.0	15.3	25.6	4.9
Any suicide attempt (%)	21.7	24.9	20.0	29.7	25.0	31.4	29.7	26.3
Psychiatric diagnosis at last discharge (%)								
Organic mental disorders	7.5	8.1	5.0	3.7	7.0	5.8	6.7	2.4
Disorders/substance use	7.1	2.0	8.9	1.2	11.0	3.7	5.4	0.5
Disorders/alcohol use	2.4	0.6	2.2	0.3	5.6	2.3	1.9	0.0
Psychotic disorders	40.6	33.4	41.3	38.6	44.9	43.5	32.0	40.0
Schizophrenia	26.6	17.9	26.6	19.7	31.1	24.2	22.7	21.0
Mood disorders	16.9	26.8	6.6	16.1	10.8	22.2	8.4	27.8
Depression	9.3	17.0	3.7	11.7	7.5	15.6	6.4	23.4
Bipolar disorder	7.1	8.9	2.4	3.9	2.7	6.3	1.9	3.9
Neurotic disorders	10.4	10.4	11.7	18.6	10.4	12.7	27.2	18.5
PTSD	1.7	0.9	2.7	1.1	1.2	1.2	11.0	4.4
OCD	1.1	1.0	0.3	1.2	0.8	1.4	0.6	0.5
Personality disorders	5.5	8.8	7.1	11.0	4.3	7.5	7.6	4.4
Other disorders	11.9	10.4	19.4	10.9	11.6	4.6	12.7	6.3

Note. SD, standard deviation; PTSD, posttraumatic stress disorder; OCD, obsessive-compulsive disorder.

Source: Adapted from National Psychiatric Case Register, Israel Ministry of Health, and Israel Central Bureau of Statistics.

$p < 0.05$ for all comparisons). There was no significant difference between Muslims and Druze (2.9 ± 4.1 vs. 2.6 ± 3.5, respectively; $p = 0.12$).

The cumulative days in hospital were 129.4 ± 268.4 for men and 106.8 ± 203.1 for women ($p < 0.05$). The cumulative days were significantly higher in men than women in Muslims and Christians ($p < 0.05$ for all comparisons). Regarding mean days per admission, there was no significant difference between men and women (45.1 ± 90 and 44.8 ± 77.7, respectively; $p = 0.65$). Mean days per admission was significantly higher in Jews compared to Muslims and Druze ($p < 0.05$). The mean days per admission for Christians was significantly higher than for Muslims ($p < 0.05$).

Involuntary admissions by order of the DP were significantly lower among the Druze compared to all other groups ($p < 0.05$). Muslim men were hospitalized 1.8 times more often than Druze men under DP order; 1.5 times more often for Muslim women. Compared to the Druze, Jewish men were hospitalized 1.9 times more often under DP order; 1.5 times more often for Jewish women. Involuntary admissions by court order were significantly higher among Muslim men compared to men in all other groups ($p < 0.05$). Muslim men were hospitalized 2.2 times more often under court order compared to Jewish men, 1.3 times more often than Christian men, and 1.9 times more often than Druze men. Muslim women were involuntarily hospitalized by court order 1.8 times more often than Jewish women (2.9 vs. 1.6). Muslim men were involuntarily hospitalized 1.2 times more often than women.

For all four population groups, the proportion of substance use reported on admission (during the two months preceding admission) was significantly higher in men compared to women ($p < 0.05$ for all comparisons). The proportion of substance use among Christian men was higher compared to all other groups—1.5, 1.3, and 1.9 times more often than Jewish, Muslim, and Druze men, respectively. The proportion of substance use among Christian women was higher compared to Muslim women (2.5 times more) and Druze women (3.5 times more). There was no significant difference between Christian women and Jewish women.

For all population groups, except for the Druze, there were significantly more suicide attempts prior to the hospitalization among women compared to men ($p < 0.05$). In the Druze population group, there was no difference comparing men and women (29.7% vs. 26.3%, respectively; $p = 0.37$). Druze men had significantly more suicide attempts prior to their hospitalization compared to Muslim (odds ratio [OR] = 1.7) and Jewish (OR = 1.5) men. There was no significant difference between Druze men and Christian men.

The distribution of diagnoses is outlined in table 12.1b. Schizophrenia was diagnosed in men more often than women among Muslims (OR = 1.5), Christians (OR = 1.4), and Jews (OR = 1.7), but not among the Druze. Among all four groups, more disorders as a result of substance use were found in men compared to women (OR for Jews, 3.7; Muslims, 8.1; Christians, 3.2; and Druze, 11.7). For all population groups, women were diagnosed with depression significantly more often than men (OR = 2.0 for Jews, OR = 3.5 for Muslims, OR = 2.3 for Christians, and OR = 4.5 for Druze). PTSD was diagnosed in the Druze more often than in other groups

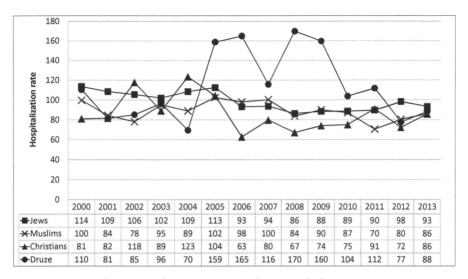

Figure 12.1. Hospitalization rate for men per 100,000 by national religious group, 2000–2013. *Source:* Adapted from National Psychiatric Case Register, Israel Ministry of Health, and Israel Central Bureau of Statistics.

	2000	2001	2002	2003	2004	2005	2006	2007	2008	2009	2010	2011	2012	2013
■ Jews	114	109	106	102	109	113	93	94	86	88	89	90	98	93
✕ Muslims	100	84	78	95	89	102	98	100	84	90	87	70	80	86
▲ Christians	81	82	118	89	123	104	63	80	67	74	75	91	72	86
● Druze	110	81	85	96	70	159	165	116	170	160	104	112	77	88

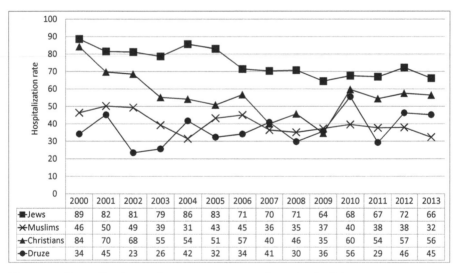

Figure 12.2. Hospitalization rate for women per 100,000 by national religious group, 2000–2013. *Source:* Based on data from National Psychiatric Case Register, Israel Ministry of Health, and Israel Central Bureau of Statistics.

	2000	2001	2002	2003	2004	2005	2006	2007	2008	2009	2010	2011	2012	2013
■ Jews	89	82	81	79	86	83	71	70	71	64	68	67	72	66
✕ Muslims	46	50	49	39	31	43	45	36	35	37	40	38	38	32
▲ Christians	84	70	68	55	54	51	57	40	46	35	60	54	57	56
● Druze	34	45	23	26	42	32	34	41	30	36	56	29	46	45

(OR = 7.4 compared to Jews, 4.6 compared to Muslims, and 8.9 compared to Christians).

The hospitalization trends between 2000 and 2013 for Jews, Muslims, Christians, and Druze are shown in figure 12.1 and figure 12.2 for men and women, respectively. Overall, there was a decrease in the hospitalization rate for men and

Table 12.2. Incidence Rate Ratios of Psychiatric Hospitalizations by National Religious Groups, 2000–2013*

Variable	Men		Women	
	Rate Ratio	95% CI	Rate Ratio	95% CI
Jews	1 (ref)	—	1 (ref)	—
Muslims	0.90	0.93–0.87	0.54	0.56–0.51
Christians	0.87	0.95–0.80	0.76	0.84–0.68
Druze	1.16	1.25–1.07	0.51	0.58–0.44

Note. CI, confidence interval.
* $p < 0.001$ for all comparisons.
Source: Adapted from National Psychiatric Case Register, Israel Ministry of Health, and Israel Central Bureau of Statistics.

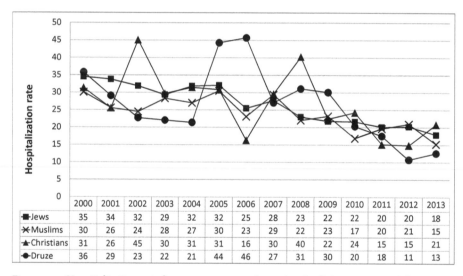

Figure 12.3. Hospitalization rate for men per 100,000 by national religious group with last discharge diagnosis of schizophrenia, 2000–2013. *Source:* Based on data from from National Psychiatric Case Register, Israel Ministry of Health, and Israel Central Bureau of Statistics.

women. In contrast, for Druze women, the rate increased from 34 per 100,000 in 2000 to 45 per 100,000 in 2013. The rate of hospitalizations was lower in all the Palestinian population groups compared to the Jewish population, for both men and women, except for Druze men. Rate ratios are presented in table 12.2.

The hospitalization trends between 2000 and 2013 for Jews, Muslims, Christians, and Druze who received their last discharge diagnosis of schizophrenia are shown in figure 12.3 and figure 12.4, for men and women, respectively.

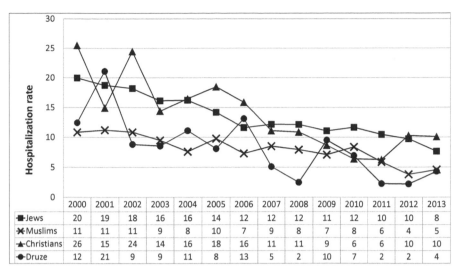

	2000	2001	2002	2003	2004	2005	2006	2007	2008	2009	2010	2011	2012	2013
■ Jews	20	19	18	16	16	14	12	12	12	11	12	10	10	8
✖ Muslims	11	11	11	9	8	10	7	9	8	7	8	6	4	5
▲ Christians	26	15	24	14	16	18	16	11	11	9	6	6	10	10
● Druze	12	21	9	9	11	8	13	5	2	10	7	2	2	4

Figure 12.4. Hospitalization rate for women per 100,000 by national religious group with last discharge diagnosis of schizophrenia, 2000–2013. *Source:* Based on data from National Psychiatric Case Register, Israel Ministry of Health, and Israel Central Bureau of Statistics.

Of the cohort, 43.9% of the patients had more than one hospitalization (range 2–79). Time to rehospitalization (measuring survival in the community) from the first (index) to the second hospitalization is presented in figure 12.5 and figure 12.6 for men and women, respectively. The time to rehospitalization was different between Jews and Muslims for both men and women (2,982 vs. 2,789 days and 3,108 vs. 2,968 days, respectively). Jews and Druze differed only among men (2,982 vs. 2,752 days) and Muslims and Christians only among women (2,968 vs. 3,329 days).

The results of bivariate and multivariate Cox models with time to rehospitalization are presented in table 12.3.

There was a significant difference between Muslims and Jews in the bivariate Cox model that was no longer significant after controlling for other sociodemographic and clinical variables. Being a man was significantly correlated with shorter time to rehospitalization (hazard ratio [HR] = 1.15, 95% CI, 1.11–1.20, $p < 0.01$). Discharge diagnosis of schizophrenia, substance use, suicide attempt in the two months prior to the hospitalization, involuntary hospitalization, and longer duration of index hospitalization were all significantly associated with shorter time to rehospitalization (HR = 1.74, 95% CI, 1.67–1.81; HR = 1.52, 95% CI, 1.46–1.58; HR = 1.77, 95% CI, 1.81–1.84; HR = 1.79, 95% CI, 1.71–1.84; HR = 1.26, 95% CI, 1.21–1.30, respectively; $p < 0.01$ for all comparisons). Compared to a higher level of education (more than 12 years of education), a lower level of education was significantly associated with shorter time to rehospitalization for both persons with 0–6 and 7–12 years of education in the bivariate model (HR = 1.20, 95% CI, 1.14–1.27, $p < 0.01$;

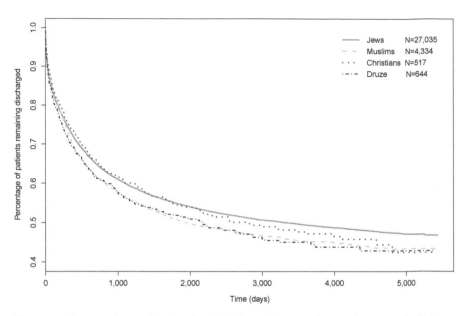

Figure 12.5. Time to rehospitalization after index hospitalization, for men, by national religious group (in days). *Source:* Based on data from from National Psychiatric Case Register, Israel Ministry of Health, and Israel Central Bureau of Statistics.

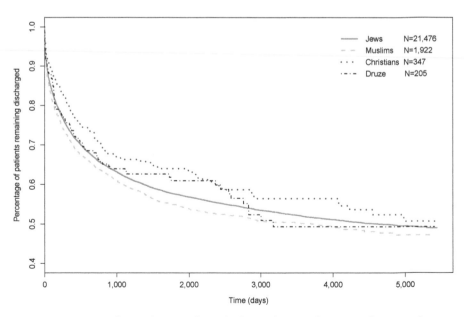

Figure 12.6. Time to rehospitalization after index hospitalization, for women, by national religious group (in days). *Source:* Based on data from National Psychiatric Case Register, Israel Ministry of Health, and Israel Central Bureau of Statistics.

Table 12.3. Bivariate and Multivariate Cox Models with Time to Rehospitalization (Days)

Variable	Bivariate model			Multivariate model[a]		
	Hazard Ratio	95% CI	*P*	Hazard Ratio	95% CI	*P*
Religion						
Muslims vs. Jews	1.11	1.07–1.15	< 0.001	1.10	0.98–1.12	< 0.18
Druze vs. Jews	1.10	1.00–1.21	< 0.06	1.10	0.95–1.23	< 0.22
Christians vs. Jews	0.96	0.86–1.06	< 0.38	0.80	0.70–0.92	< 0.01
Gender (men vs. women)	1.08	1.06–1.11	< 0.01	1.15	1.11–1.20	< 0.01
Schizophrenia vs. other diagnoses	2.10	2.00–2.11	< 0.01	1.74	1.67–1.81	< 0.01
Substance use	1.88	1.83–1.93	< 0.01	1.52	1.46–1.58	< 0.01
Suicide attempt	1.83	1.80–1.88	< 0.01	1.77	1.81–1.84	< 0.01
Involuntary index hospitalization	1.89	1.84–1.93	< 0.01	1.79	1.71–1.84	< 0.01
Length of hospitalization >14 days	1.24	1.21–1.27	< 0.01	1.26	1.21–1.30	< 0.01
Education						
0–6 years vs. 13+ years	1.20	1.14–1.27	< 0.01	1.08	1.02–1.14	< 0.01
7–12 years vs. 13+ years	1.15	1.06–1.14	< 0.01	1.02	0.94–1.11	< 0.65
SES cluster						
Middle tertile vs. upper tertile	1.13	1.08–1.18	< 0.01	1.14	1.06–1.23	< 0.01
Lower tertile vs. upper tertile	1.06	1.03–1.09	< 0.01	1.10	1.01–1.09	< 0.01

Note. CI, confidence interval; SES, socioeconomic status.
[a] Controlling for all the variables presented in the multivariate model.
Source: Adapted from National Psychiatric Case Register, Israel Ministry of Health, and Israel Central Bureau of Statistics.

HR = 1.15, 95% CI, 1.06–1.14, p = 0.01, respectively). In the multivariate model, only the lowest level of education (0–12 years) was significantly associated with shorter time to rehospitalization (HR = 1.08, 95% CI, 1.02–1.14, p < 0.01). Both lower and middle tertiles of SES were significantly associated with shorter time to rehospitalization (HR = 1.10, 95% CI, 1.01–1.09; HR = 1.14, 95% CI, 1.06–1.23, respectively; p < 0.01).

Discussion

All citizens and residents in Israel have free access to psychiatric hospitalization and are entitled to equal levels of treatment. However, significant differences in patterns of hospitalizations were found between the Palestinian and Jewish populations and among groups within the Palestinian population. Muslims were hospitalized more often (measured by mean number of admissions during the follow-up period) than

Jews and Christians, but not more often compared to Druze. Muslims in our study spent fewer days in the hospital per admission (compared to Jews and Christians) and were involuntarily hospitalized more often than the other groups (about half of all admissions), specifically by court order, both for men and women. This finding is similar to previous studies about the likelihood of involuntary admission among ethnic minorities (Anderson, Flora, Archie, Morgan, & McKenzie, 2014; Bhui et al., 2003; Davies, Thornicroft, Leese, Higgingbotham, & Phelan, 1996), which indicate a different pathway to care.

Women's utilization of psychiatric inpatient services was lower compared to men: they had a lower mean number of hospitalizations and fewer cumulative days in hospital. On average, Muslim women had the lowest mean days per admission while Christian women had the lowest mean number of hospitalizations. Only among the Druze were women hospitalized for more days per admission compared to men.

The rate of hospitalizations of persons with schizophrenia was lower for women compared to men in all four population groups. Although this may indicate a more favorable course and better prognosis for women with schizophrenia (Riecher-Rössler & Häfner, 2000), it may also indicate a different use of mental health services (as discussed later in this section).

Between 2000 and 2013, we found an overall decrease in hospitalization trends for all population groups. This trend was salient for persons with schizophrenia. These changes may be at least partly related to the structural reform in the Israeli mental health system (Grinshpoon, Shereshevsky, Levinson, & Ponizovsky, 2003; Haver, Kotler, & Baruch, 2003; Swartz, Kilian, Twesigye, Attah, & Chiliza, 2014) that resulted in the reduction of psychiatric hospital beds from 1.35 per 1,000 population in 1992 (total: 7,036 beds) to 0.44 per 1,000 in 2011 (total: 3,231 beds) (Department of Information and Evaluation, 2002, 2012).

Understanding the utilization of inpatient psychiatric services may pose a complex issue. Psychiatric hospitalization may serve as a proxy variable for symptomatic exacerbation in severe mental illnesses (Levine et al., 2011). However, hospitalization is also affected by other factors, including patients' help-seeking behavior; the support of the close social network (e.g., family relatives, spouse); cultural values, perceptions and beliefs; and the accessibility and quality of service provision in the community. Our results regarding hospitalizations concur with other studies that the Palestinian population underutilizes mental health services (Savaya, 1998). Several factors may explain this gap. First, this may be attributed to cultural and religious factors. The general attitude of the Palestinian population toward psychiatry and mental health professionals is negative and may be even suspicious (Savaya, 1998). Palestinian persons seek help for their emotional distress within the circle of family or traditional healers within their community ("the cultural canon"), which is preferred over "the professional" or "Western medicine" (Al-Krenawi, 2002 p. 9; Al-Krenawi & Graham, 2000). Palestinian people may view mental health experts as those who disregard religious values that can help the healing process (Al-Krenawi & Graham, 2000).

These views may have a political aspect as well, specific to the Israeli context. The mental health services may be identified with the state of Israel and its institutions, which may be viewed as part of the colonial regime. Hospitalization in state institutions may be perceived as coercive and even harmful (Al-Krenawi & Levav, 2009).

Additionally, stigma linked to mental health and psychiatric diagnoses constitute another barrier to service. In Palestinian society, stigma may influence one's life, especially among women. Psychiatric diagnosis may lead to social exclusion and marginalization, harming the marital prospects of the person with the diagnosis and his or her relatives. Stigma may lead to separation or divorce, which has economic, mental, and familial implications (Al-Krenawi & Graham, 1998). As a consequence, the person and his or her family may deny the need for intervention and treatment, may underutilize mental health services, or may use the service only in emergencies.

Hebrew language proficiency may also be involved in the lower use of mental health services among the Palestinian population in Israel. According to the Israel CBS's social survey (Struch, Shereshevsky, Naon, Daniel, & Fischman, 2009), 23% of the Palestinian population experienced difficulties in receiving general medical services because of the level of Hebrew language proficiency compared to 13% of the Jewish population. This gap may be even more complex in addressing mental health issues.

Interestingly, although Palestinian culture condemns suicide and suicidal behavior is considered a sin (Al-Krenawi & Graham, 2000; Al-Sabaie, 1989), there were no differences in suicide attempts prior to the hospitalization between the Palestinian and Jewish groups. However, completed suicide during hospitalization occurred only among Jews (78 cases).

Although inequality gaps of mental health utilization patterns still exist between the Palestinian and Jewish populations, with due caution, the data may indicate a trend toward closing these gaps in the past decade. This trend may resemble progress in other health outcomes in the Palestinian population in Israel: these include decreasing infant mortality (Tarabeia et al., 2004) and increased life expectancy at birth (Myers-JDC-Brookdale Institute, 2012).

Limitations

Although the data from the NPHR for this cohort is complete, this study has several limitations. It is retrospective and based only on registry data. No personal interviews were held with service users to learn about the barriers to treatment and attitudes toward psychiatric institutions. The method used for SES clustering was necessarily rather crude because we only had address information regarding the name of town or village and not neighborhood. This method may not identify lower- versus upper-SES neighborhoods. We did not relate to mixed Jewish and Palestinian towns, as well as to the rural versus urban settings.

Conclusions

When conceptualizing and optimizing mental health services for the Palestinian population in Israel, these data should be taken into account. The Palestinian population is a heterogeneous population with diverse needs and patterns of mental health service use among Muslims, Christians, and Druze and with differences between men and women. Although the trend is toward closing the gap, accessibility of services still needs to improve. As every person has the right to enjoy the highest standard of mental and physical health and to be treated in a humane and respectful manner (UN General Assembly, 2007), our results may help clinicians and policy makers plan appropriate mental health services delivered to this large minority group in the Israeli society.

IDO LURIE is a psychiatrist and Director of the Adult Psychiatric Clinic/ Shalvata Mental Health Center of the Clalit Health Service Fund, Israel. He is also Lecturer in the Department of Psychiatry of the Sackler School of Medicine, Tel Aviv University, Israel.

ANAT FLEISCHMAN is Director of Addiction Treatment Services and Dual Diagnosis Unit at Yaffo Community Mental Health Center, Israel, and Clinical Instructor in the Department of Psychiatry of Sackler Faculty of Medicine, Tel Aviv University, Israel.

References

Alegría, M., Canino, G., Ríos, R., Vera, M., Calderón, J., Rusch, D., & Ortega, A. N. (2002). Mental health care for Latinos: Inequalities in use of specialty mental health services among Latinos, African Americans, and non-Latino whites. *Psychiatric Services, 53*(12), 1547–1555.

Al-Krenawi, A. (2002). Mental health service utilization among the Arabs in Israel. *Social Work in Health Care, 35*(1–2), 577–589.

Al-Krenawi, A., & Graham, J. R. (1998). Divorce among Muslim Arab women in Israel. *Journal of Divorce & Remarriage, 29*(3–4), 103–119.

Al-Krenawi, A., & Graham, J. R. (2000). Culturally sensitive social work practice with Arab clients in mental health settings. *Health & Social Work, 25*(1), 9–22.

Al-Krenawi, A., & Levav, I. (2009). The epidemiology of mental health disorders among Arabs in Israel. In I. Levav (Ed.), *Psychiatric and behavioral disorders in Israel* (pp. 75–87). Jerusalem: Gefen.

Al-Sabaie, A. (1989). Psychiatry in Saudi Arabia: Cultural perspectives. *Transcultural Psychiatric Research Review, 26*(4), 245–262.

Anderson, K., Flora, N., Archie, S., Morgan, C., & McKenzie, K. (2014). A meta-analysis of ethnic differences in pathways to care at the first episode of psychosis. *Acta Psychiatrica Scandinavica, 130*(4), 257–268.

Bhui, K., Stansfeld, S., Hull, S., Priebe, S., Mole, F., & Feder, G. (2003). Ethnic variations in pathways to and use of specialist mental health services in the UK. *British Journal of Psychiatry, 182*(2), 105–116.

Boydell, J., Van Os, J., McKenzie, K., Allardyce, J., Goel, R., McCreadie, R. G., & Murray, R. M. (2001). Incidence of schizophrenia in ethnic minorities in London: Ecological study into interactions with environment. *British Medical Journal, 323*, 1–4.

Bresnahan, M., Begg, M. D., Brown, A., Schaefer, C., Sohler, N., Insel, B., . . . Susser, E. (2007). Race and risk of schizophrenia in a US birth cohort: Another example of health disparity? *International Journal of Epidemiology, 36*(4), 751–758.

Cook, B., Manning, W., & Alegría, M. (2013). Measuring disparities across the distribution of mental health care expenditures. *Journal of Mental Health Policy and Economics, 16*(1), 3–12.

Davies, S., Thornicroft, G., Leese, M., Higgingbotham, A., & Phelan, M. (1996). Ethnic differences in risk of compulsory psychiatric admission among representative cases of psychosis in London. *British Medical Journal, 312*, 533–537.

Department of Information and Evaluation. (2002). *Mental health in Israel. Statistical annual 2002.* Jerusalem: Israel Ministry of Health.

Department of Information and Evaluation. (2012). *Mental health in Israel. Statistical annual 2012.* Jerusalem: Israel Ministry of Health.

Fearon, P., Kirkbride, J. B., Morgan, C., Dazzan, P., Morgan, K., Lloyd, T., . . . Holloway, J. (2006). Incidence of schizophrenia and other psychoses in ethnic minority groups: Results from the MRC AESOP study. *Psychological Medicine, 36*(11), 1541–1550.

Grinshpoon, A., Shereshevsky, Y., Levinson, D., & Ponizovsky, A. (2003). Should patients with chronic psychiatric disorders remain in hospital? Results from a service inquiry/discussion. *Israel Journal of Psychiatry and Related Sciences, 40*(4), 268–273.

Haver, E., Kotler, M., & Baruch, Y. (2003). Special editorial: The structural reform of mental health services. *Israel Journal of Psychiatry and Related Sciences, 40*(4), 235–239.

Horvitz-Lennon, M., McGuire, T. G., Alegría, M., & Frank, R. G. (2009). Racial and ethnic disparities in the treatment of a Medicaid population with schizophrenia. *Health Services Research, 44*(6), 2106–2122.

Israel Central Bureau of Statistics [Israel CBS]. (1995). *Demographic characteristics of the population in localities and statistical areas.* Jerusalem: Israel Ministry of the Interior.

Levav, I., Lipshitz, I., Novikov, I., Pugachova, I., Kohn, R., Barchana, M., . . . Werner, H. (2007). Cancer risk among parents and siblings of patients with schizophrenia. *British Journal of Psychiatry, 190*(2), 156–161.

Levine, S. Z., Lurie, I., Kohn, R., & Levav, I. (2011). Trajectories of the course of schizophrenia: From progressive deterioration to amelioration over three decades. *Schizophrenia Research, 126*(1), 184–191.

Lyons, J. S., O'Mahoney, M. T., Miller, S. I., Neme, J., Kabat, J., & Miller, F. (1997). Predicting readmission to the psychiatric hospital in a managed care environment: Implications for quality indicators. *American Journal of Psychiatry, 154*(3), 337–340.

Missinne, S., & Bracke, P. (2012). Depressive symptoms among immigrants and ethnic minorities: A population based study in 23 European countries. *Social Psychiatry and Psychiatric Epidemiology, 47*(1), 97–109.

Myers-JDC-Brookdale Institute. (2012). *The Arab population in Israel: Facts and figures 2012.* Retrieved from http://www.iataskforce.org/sites/default/files/resource/resource-1114.pdf.

Neighbors, H. W., Caldwell, C., Williams, D. R., Nesse, R., Taylor, R. J., Bullard, K. M., . . . Jackson, J. S. (2007). Race, ethnicity, and the use of services for mental disorders: Results from the national survey of American life. *Archives of General Psychiatry, 64*(4), 485–494.

Riecher-Rössler, A., & Häfner, H. (2000). Gender aspects in schizophrenia: Bridging the border between social and biological psychiatry. *Acta Psychiatrica Scandinavica, 102*(407), 58–62.

Roberts, A. L., Gilman, S. E., Breslau, J., Breslau, N., & Koenen, K. C. (2011). Race/ethnic differences in exposure to traumatic events, development of post-traumatic stress disorder, and treatment-seeking for post-traumatic stress disorder in the United States. *Psychological Medicine, 41*(1), 71–83.

Satcher, D. (2001). *Mental health: Culture, race, and ethnicity. A supplement to mental health: A report of the surgeon general.* Rockville, MD: US Department of Health and Human Services.

Savaya, R. (1998). The under-use of psychological services by Israeli Arabs: An examination of the roles of negative attitudes and the use of alternative sources of help. *International Social Work, 41*(2), 195–209.

Struch, N., Shereshevsky, Y., Naon, D., Daniel, N., & Fischman, N. (2009). People with severe mental disorders in Israel: An integrated view of the service systems [in Hebrew]. Jerusalem: Myers-JDC-Brookdale Institute. Retrieved from http://brookdaleheb.jdc.org.il /_Uploads/PublicationsFiles/549-09-SevereMentalDisorders-REP-HEB.pdf.

Swartz, L., Kilian, S., Twesigye, J., Attah, D., & Chiliza, B. (2014). Language, culture, and task shifting—An emerging challenge for global mental health. *Global Health Action, 7*(23433), 1–4.

Tarabeia, J., Amitai, Y., Green, M., Halpern, G. J., Blau, S., Ifrah, A., . . . Jaber, L. (2004). Differences in infant mortality rates between Jews and Arabs in Israel, 1975–2000. *Israel Medical Association Journal, 6*(7), 403–407.

UN General Assembly. (2007). *Resolution 61/106: Convention on the rights of persons with disabilities.* Geneva: United Nations. Retrieved from http://www.refworld.org/docid /45f973632.html.

Weiser, M., Van Os, J., Reichenberg, A., Rabinowitz, J., Nahon, D., Kravitz, E., . . . Noy, S. (2007). Social and cognitive functioning, urbanicity and risk for schizophrenia. *British Journal of Psychiatry, 191*(4), 320–324.

Williams, D. R., Gonzalez, H. M., Neighbors, H., Nesse, R., Abelson, J. M., Sweetman, J., & Jackson, J. S. (2007). Prevalence and distribution of major depressive disorder in African Americans, Caribbean blacks, and non-Hispanic whites: Results from the national survey of American life. *Archives of General Psychiatry, 64*(3), 305–315.

World Health Organization. (2012). Risks to mental health: An overview of vulnerabilities and risk factors. Retrieved from http://www.who.int/mental_health/mhgap/risks_to_mental _health_EN_27_08_12.pdf.

13

SMOKING AMONG PALESTINIAN CITIZENS IN ISRAEL

Lital Keinan-Boker and Yael Bar-Zeev

Smoking, an addictive habit, is one of the most common forms of recreational drug use. Currently, there are more than a billion smokers worldwide, 80% of whom live in low- and middle-income countries. Overall, smoking rates for men are higher than for women. For example, in 2009, in the WHO Western Pacific Region, 51% of men aged 15 and over smoked some form of tobacco. Their rates were the highest in the world. Smoking among women was highest in the WHO European Region at 22% (World Health Organization [WHO], 2009).

The adverse effects of tobacco smoking on health have been known for many years. In 1964 the US Surgeon General appointed an expert committee to review and evaluate all data concerning the impact of tobacco exposure on health. The report published by that committee was the first in a chain of reports released by the US Surgeon General in the last 50-plus years. These detailed reports compile up-to-date scientific data and provide international consensus regarding the role of active as well as secondhand smoke in disease causation (US Department of Health and Human Services [US HHS], 2014). According to the data gathered through the years, active smoking is causally associated with chronic diseases such as cardiovascular disease, chronic obstructive pulmonary disease, diabetes, autoimmune diseases such as rheumatoid arthritis, many types of cancer (oropharynx, larynx, lung, esophagus, pancreas, colon and rectum, kidney, bladder, bone marrow, cervix), infectious diseases (e.g., pneumonia), and overall diminished health. It also affects fertility in both men and women and may cause congenital defects and lower birth weight in the case of maternal smoking during pregnancy (HSS, 2014). Importantly as well, environmental tobacco smoke (ETS) has been causally associated with cardiovascular disease and lung cancer in adults; with adverse reproductive effects in women; and with sudden infant death syndrome, ear and respiratory tract infections, other respiratory symptoms, and impaired lung function in children

(HSS, 2014). The US Surgeon General reports on smoking build a scientific foundation to support tobacco control programs and interventions (HSS, 2014). Indeed, tobacco control was the main focus of the 2013 WHO report on the global tobacco epidemic (WHO, 2013).

Even though the smoking habit crosses socioeconomic, gender, race, and ethnicity boundaries, it is not equally distributed. Thus, observed differences in morbidity and mortality between ethnic groups have often been explained by different lifestyles and health practices, smoking included, in addition to genetic factors (Kim, Ziedonis, & Chen, 2007; Kurian & Cardarelli, 2007; Liu et al., 2010). It is important, therefore, to study smoking patterns, particularly in specific population groups, as such data assist in identifying high-risk groups and tailoring specific interventions and control programs.

This chapter describes the prevalence and trends of tobacco use in the largest minority in Israel, the Palestinians, and the health outcomes that may be associated with smoking, as well as facilitating factors for smoking initiation and barriers for smoking cessation and the levels of exposure to ETS. To that end, we conducted a literature search and tracked updated publications, periodical reports, and other relevant data sources.

Tobacco Use among Palestinian Citizens in Israel: Prevalence and Time Trends

In 2015 the Palestinian population in Israel numbered 1,57,800 and comprised 20.8% of the total country population (Israel Central Bureau of Statistics [Israel CBS], 2016). This minority group is composed of Muslims (82.5%), Christians (9.0%), and Druze (8.5%) (Gharrah, 2013). Around 52% of the Palestinians reside in the Galilee, in the north of Israel, and another 16% (mostly Bedouins) live in the Negev area to the south. These groups are younger than the Jewish population: currently, 34% of the Palestinians are 0–14 years old (27% among Jewish Israelis) and only 4% are 65 years old and over (13% among Jewish Israelis) (Israel CBS, 2016). These data are relevant when studying the onset and distribution of the smoking habit.

Smoking prevalence among adults in Israel is mainly determined through health surveys where participants self-report on their lifestyle and habits. The surveys conducted by the Israel CBS and the Israel Ministry of Health are the primary sources of the data.

The CBS's social survey is an ongoing telephone survey that has been conducted since 2002. The study questionnaire includes a basic core (about 200 questions), the results of which provide updated information regarding the living conditions and welfare of all groups of the population, and a set of additional questions on ad hoc subjects (Israel CBS, 2018). The Israel Ministry of Health collects periodic data on smoking through its biannual telephone survey of knowledge, attitudes, and practices (KAP) of health behaviors (about 3,000–4,000 participants) and the INHIS, conducted every three or four years (about 10,000 participants). These national surveys are carried out on representative samples of the total Israeli population, and they enable the assessment of the prevalence of smoking and its trends.

Active Smoking

IN ADULTS

The 2010 social survey focused on health and health behaviors (N = 7,542; response rate, 73%) of individuals over the age of 20, 1,208 of them Palestinians (16%) (Israel CBS, 2010). According to the findings, 24.1% of Palestinians and 23.6% of Jews reported current smoking of at least one cigarette daily, and 6.7% and 18.6%, respectively, reported past smoking. The age at smoking initiation among current smokers appeared to be younger among Palestinians; 30.4% started before age 15 (20.3% among Jews) and most (75.1%) started before they were 19 (66.1% among Jews). Additionally, quantities smoked were larger among Palestinians—79.9% of the current smokers smoked 11 or more cigarettes a day (25.3% smoked more than 20 cigarettes a day), and 8.0% smoked 1–5 cigarettes daily. The proportion of Jews smoking 11 or more cigarettes a day was 52.7% (11.7% smoked more than 20 cigarettes a day), and 21.3% smoked 1–5 cigarettes daily (Israel CBS, 2010; Gharrah, 2013). Unfortunately, data regarding subgroups of the Palestinian population are scarce and usually not based on representative samples owing to small numbers.

In the 2010 KAP survey, conducted in 2010–2012 on a sample aged 21 and over (N = 4,935; 44.5% of them Palestinians, n = 2,196), current smoking was defined as a positive answer to the question, "Do you smoke daily or occasionally?" The results indicated that 24.3% of the Palestinian citizens in Israel and 19.8% of the Jewish Israeli citizens were categorized as current smokers. In both population groups, smoking rates were higher among males than among females, but among Palestinian citizens in Israel this gap was larger: smoking was reported by 43.4% and 6.5% of the Palestinian males and females, respectively, and by 23.9% and 16.0% of the Jewish males and females, respectively. A newer KAP survey, carried out in 2013 and using the same study tool, showed a slight reduction in smoking prevalence: 22.5% of the Palestinian citizens in Israel and 17.9% of the Jewish Israeli citizens were categorized as current smokers. Smoking rates were higher among males than among females in both population groups, and smoking prevalence was 39.2% and 5.9% in the Palestinian males and females, respectively, and 21.4% and 14.6% in the Jewish males and females, respectively (Israel Center for Disease Control [ICDC], 2017a). A more recent survey, the INHIS-III study of 2013–2015, reported active smoking prevalence of 43.9% in Palestinian males, 6.7% in Palestinian females, 22.1% in Jewish males, and 15.0% in Jewish females (ICDC, 2017c). Figure 13.1 presents the smoking prevalence rates in the total Israeli population aged 18 and over in 2016 by population group and gender (Public Health Services, 2017).

Among Palestinian males in Israel, smoking prevalence rates were highest in the 18–34 age group and then dropped among older age groups: 35–49, 50–64,

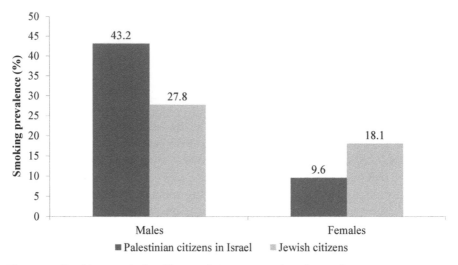

Figure 13.1. Smoking rates in Israel by population group and gender, aged 18+ years, 2016, (percent). *Source:* Public Health Services. (2017). *The minister of health report on smoking 2016* [in Hebrew]. Retrieved from https://www.health.gov.il/PublicationsFiles/smoking_2016.pdf.

65 and over. In Jewish Israeli males, smoking rates were highest in the 18–34 and 35–49 age groups and then decreased. Among Palestinian females in Israel, smoking prevalence rates, although quite low, tended to increase with age. In Jewish Israeli females, smoking prevalence rates were highest in the 18–34 age group but lower in the other age groups (fig. 13.2a and fig. 13.2b) (Public Health Services, 2017).

Almost a quarter (23.6%) of current smokers among Palestinian males in Israel reported smoking more than 20 cigarettes a day (14.8% among Jewish Israeli males) while 25.5% reported smoking less than 10 cigarettes a day (36.1% among Jewish Israeli males). In female Palestinian smokers in Israel, almost half (48.4%) reported smoking less than 10 cigarettes a day (40.8% among Jewish Israeli females) while 10.9% smoked more than 20 cigarettes a day (4.6% among Jewish Israeli females) (table 13.1) (Public Health Services, 2017). As for age at smoking initiation, the median age is similar in Palestinian males and Jewish females (18) but younger in Jewish males (17) and older in Palestinian females (21), while the mean age is lowest (18.1) among Jewish males and highest in Palestinian females (25.0) (table 13.2) (Public Health Services, 2017).

Smoking rates in both Palestinian and Jewish males tend to decrease with higher education (0–10 years of education: 48.9% and 27.7% in Palestinians and Jews, respectively; and 13+ years of education: 36.3% and 21.1% in Palestinians and Jews, respectively). In Palestinian females, the highest and lowest rates of current smoking were observed in the 0–10 and 11–12 years of formal education levels, respectively. In Jewish females, the highest and lowest rates were observed in the

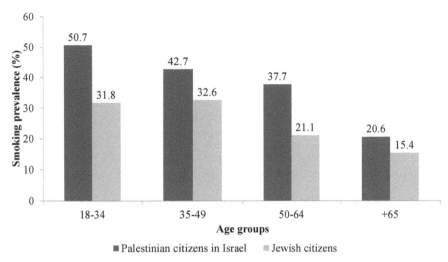

Figure 13.2a. Smoking rates for males in Israel by population group and age group, 2016 (percent). *Source:* Public Health Services. (2017). *The minister of health report on smoking 2016* [in Hebrew]. Retrieved from https://www.health.gov.il/PublicationsFiles/smoking_2016.pdf.

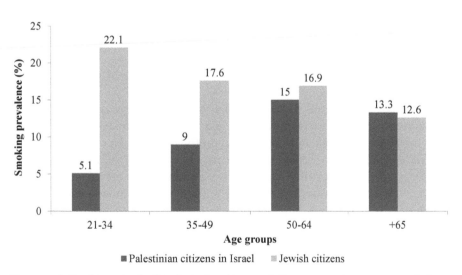

Figure 13.2b. Smoking rates for females in Israel by population group and age group, aged 18+ years, 2016 (percent). *Source:* Public Health Services. (2017). *The minister of health report on smoking 2016* [in Hebrew]. Retrieved from https://www.health.gov.il/PublicationsFiles/smoking_2016.pdf.

Table 13.1. Number of Cigarettes Smoked Daily by Population Group and Gender, 2016

Number of cigarettes smoked/day	Males		Females	
	Palestinian Israelis (%)	Jewish Israelis (%)	Palestinian Israelis (%)	Jewish Israelis (%)
Less than 10	25.5	36.1	48.4	40.8
Between 10 and 20	51.0	49.1	40.6	54.6
More than 20	23.6	14.8	10.9	4.6

Source: Public Health Services. (2017). *The Minister of Health report on smoking 2016*
[in Hebrew]. Retrieved from https://www.health.gov.il/PublicationsFiles/smoking_2016.pdf.

Table 13.2. Age of Cigarette Smoking Commencement by Population Group and Gender, 2016

Gender		Mean age in years	Median age in years
Males	Palestinian Israelis	19.4	18
	Jewish Israelis	18.1	17
Females	Palestinian Israelis	25.0	21
	Jewish Israelis	19.5	18

Source: Public Health Services. (2017). *The Mminister ofHealth report on smoking 2016*
[in Hebrew]. Retrieved from https://www.health.gov.il/PublicationsFiles/smoking_2016.pdf.

0–10 and 13+ years of formal education levels, respectively (fig. 13.3a, fig. 13.3b) (Public Health Services, 2017).

Trends of smoking in Israel are calculated based on results of different surveys through the years and are shown in figure 13.4. Unfortunately, data for Palestinians have only been available since 1996. Based on the available data, smoking rates in Palestinian males decreased between the mid-1990s (50%) and mid-2000s (40%) and then stabilized. In Palestinian females, smoking rates showed some decrease between the mid-1990s (12%) and the beginning of the 2000s (6%) and have been stable (5%–8%) since then. Smoking rates in the Jewish population have shown a constant decrease until recently (fig. 13.4) (Public Health Services, 2017).

Baron-Epel, Keinan-Boker, Weinstein, and Shohat (2010) looked more closely into these trends. They used data from the KAP (2000, 2002, 2004, 2006, 2008) and the INHIS-I (2003–2004) surveys for the years 2000–2008 and compared the trends of smoking in adult Palestinian men and Jewish men and women. The results indicated that from 2000 through 2008, an increase in smoking rates of about 6.5% was observed in Palestinian men aged 21–64, both educated and less educated. In Jewish men of the same age group, smoking declined during this period by 3.5%, mostly because of a reduction of smoking among educated respondents, and a similar trend was observed for Jewish women (Baron-Epel et al., 2010).

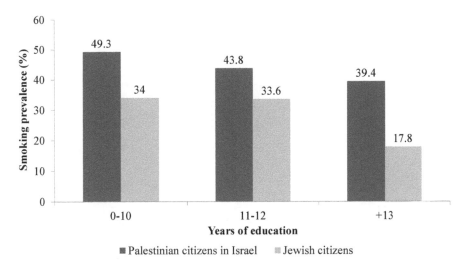

Figure 13.3a. Smoking rates for males in Israel by population group and education, aged 18+ years, 2016 (percent). *Source:* Public Health Services. (2017). *The minister of health report on smoking 2016* [in Hebrew]. Retrieved from https://www.health.gov.il/PublicationsFiles/smoking _2016.pdf.

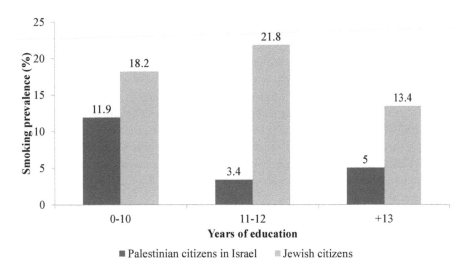

Figure 13.3b. Smoking rates for females in Israel by population group and education, aged 18+ years, 2016 (percent). *Source:* Public Health Services. (2017). *The minister of health report on smoking 2016* [in Hebrew]. Retrieved from https://www.health.gov.il/PublicationsFiles/smoking _2016.pdf.

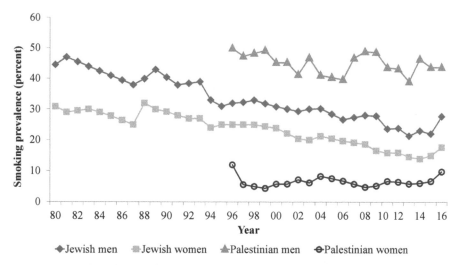

Figure 13.4. Trends in the prevalence of smoking for Israelis aged 18+ by population group and gender, 1980–2016 (percent). *Source:* Public Health Services. (2017). *The minister of health report on smoking 2016* [in Hebrew]. Retrieved from https://www.health.gov.il/PublicationsFiles /smoking_2016.pdf.

IN PREGNANT WOMEN

The Israel Ministry of Health conducted a survey in Mother and Child Health Clinics throughout Israel, in which the nursing staff interviewed 1,613 pregnant women and mothers of newborn infants with respect to folic acid supplementation utilization, smoking habits, onset of prenatal care, and demographic characteristics. Overall, 12.8% of the women who smoked had smoked either in the three months preceding their current pregnancy and/or during their pregnancy. However, smoking prevalence was much greater among the Jewish women (17.3%) than the Palestinian women (3.0%) ($p < 0.001$). The prevalence of smoking for the duration of the pregnancy was 1.8% among Palestinian women and 8.0% among Jewish women (Fisher et al., 2005).

IN ADOLESCENTS

The habit of smoking usually develops in adolescence and may be associated with youth violence (Molcho, Harel, & Dina, 2004); thus, it is important to record smoking prevalence in this age group. Health Behavior in School-aged Children (HBSC) is a multinational research program of the WHO that links together research institutes and other universities in 46 countries in Europe and North America. The Israeli branch was established in 1993 and has conducted six surveys in representative samples of sixth- (aged 11–12), eighth- (aged 13–14), and tenth- (aged 15–16) grade students (Harel-Fisch et al., 2011). The 2014 survey results indicated that 20.6% and

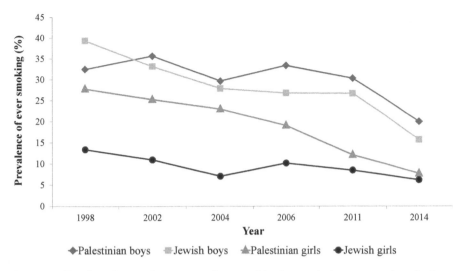

Figure 13.5. Trends in the prevalence rates of ever smoking by population group and gender in Israeli schoolchildren aged 12–16, 1998–2014 (percent). *Source:* Public Health Services. (2017). *The minister of health report on smoking 2016* [in Hebrew]. Retrieved from https://www.health .gov.il/PublicationsFiles/smoking_2016.pdf.

6.5% of Palestinian male and female students, respectively, and 14.9% and 6.9% of Jewish male and female students, respectively, had tried cigarettes or other forms of tobacco smoking. The time trends since 1998 show a decrease among Palestinian girls (13.4% in 1998, 6.5% in 2014), Jewish boys (39.4% in 1998, 14.9% in 2014), and Jewish girls (27.8% in 1998, 6.9% in 2014); among Palestinian boys, the trend was stable (32.5% in 1998, 30.3% in 2011) and decreased only recently (20.6% in 2014) (fig. 13.5) (Public Health Services, 2017).

When smoking at least once a week is considered, the prevalence is higher in boys compared to girls and in older compared to younger adolescents. The subgroup with the highest prevalence (32.1%) is tenth-grade Palestinian boys, and the one with the lowest rate (1.2%) is the subgroup of sixth-grade Jewish girls (fig. 13.6) (Public Health Services, 2017). As for smoking at least once a day, the reported rates were higher in Palestinians (8.3%; 12.2% in boys and 4.4% in girls) compared to Jews (3.8%; 5.5% in boys and 2.0% in girls) and higher in the tenth grade (8.5%; 12.6% in Palestinians and 7.0% in Jews) compared to the sixth grade (3.7%; 6.7% in Palestinians, 1.9% in Jews) (Public Health Services, 2017).

In a cross-sectional national study done on a representative sample of 13- to 14-year-old schoolchildren, Palestinians reported daily smoking more often than Jews (1.9% vs. 1.6%, $p > 0.05$), but the difference was statistically insignificant. Jews reported occasional smoking more often than Palestinians (5.1% and 3.6%, $p = 0.01$) (Graif, German, Ifrah, Livne, & Shohat, 2013).

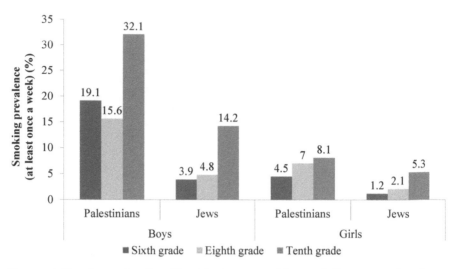

Figure 13.6. Prevalence rates of smoking at least once a week by population group and gender in Israeli schoolchildren aged 12–16, 2014 (percent). *Source:* Public Health Services. (2017). *The minister of health report on smoking 2016* [in Hebrew]. Retrieved from https://www.health.gov.il /PublicationsFiles/smoking_2016.pdf.

In a smaller study, based on 326 15- to 18-year-old schoolchildren residing in the town of Tayibe in Israel, a third (36.2%) of the sample smoked cigarettes (48.0% prevalence rate in boys and 23.3% in girls) (Korn & Magnezi, 2008). Interestingly, Azaiza, Shoham, Bar-Hamburger, and Abu-Asbeh (2009), who studied the prevalence of psychoactive drug use in 476 12- to 18-year-old Palestinian school dropouts also reported that tobacco was used by 30% of the participants.

Water-pipe (hookah, narghile, shisha) smoking has been practiced for more than 400 years in the Arabian Peninsula and in Turkey, India, Pakistan, and other countries. In recent years, this habit has gained popularity among youth globally. It is considered a trendy social activity, and awareness of the adverse health effects associated with it is low. However, hookah smokers are exposed to tobacco's toxic metabolites in higher concentrations than cigarette smokers because the tobacco doses used in hookahs are usually larger than the standardized tobacco content of cigarettes. Also, hookahs include no filters. The health impacts associated with hookah smoking are similar to those associated with cigarette smoking including addiction. In addition, infections may spread by sharing hookahs (e.g., *helicobacter pylori*), and elevated heart rate and blood pressure following hookah smoking have also been reported (Knishkowy & Amitai, 2005). Recently, Elias et al. (2012) suggested that adolescent hookah smoking may significantly affect driving behavior and increase the risk of being involved in road accidents (Elias et al., 2012).

The HBSC survey included questions regarding hookah smoking. Smoking a hookah was reported by 30.8% of Palestinians (41.5% prevalence rate in boys and

20.0% in girls) and 16.1% of Jews (21.1% in boys and 11.1% in girls). The highest rates were reported in tenth-grade Palestinian (54.8%) and Jewish (41.9%) boys and the lowest, in sixth-grade (2.8%) and eighth-grade (6.5%) Jewish girls. Time trends from 2002 through 2014 indicated a decrease in hookah smoking in both population groups and genders (Public Health Services, 2017). Smoking a hookah at least once a week was reported by 18.2% of Palestinians (26.5% prevalence rate in boys and 10.0% in girls), and 5.8% of Jews (8.3% in boys and 3.3% in girls). The highest rates were reported in tenth-grade (33.9%), eighth-grade (20.6%), and sixth-grade (24.9%) Palestinian boys and the lowest, in sixth-grade (0.6%) and eighth-grade (1.8%) Jewish girls. Time trends from 2002 through 2014 indicated an increase in hookah smoking among Palestinian boys and Jewish girls and a slight decrease among Palestinian girls and Jewish boys (Public Health Services, 2017). As for daily hookah smoking, it was reported by 8.0% of Palestinians (12.1% prevalence rate in boys and 3.9% in girls) and 2.2% of Jews (3.5% in boys and 1.0% in girls). The highest rates were reported in tenth-grade Palestinian boys (18.0%) and the lowest, in sixth-grade (0.4%) and eighth-grade (0.9%) Jewish girls (Public Health Services, 2017).

Among Tayibe high-school children, about a third (37.1%) of the sample had smoked a hookah (55.0% prevalence rate in boys and 17.4% in girls) (Korn & Magnezi, 2008).

ETS (Secondhand Smoke, Passive Smoking)

IN ADULTS

The 2010 CBS social survey also investigated exposure to ETS. Of the respondents, 82% of the Palestinians and 69.3% of the Jews reported being exposed to others' smoking in their surroundings in the month preceding the survey (Israel CBS, 2010; Gharrah, 2013). The exposure took place at work (prevalence rates of 55.4% and 39.8% in Palestinians and Jews, respectively) and at home (39.7% in Palestinians, 18.7% in Jews) but mostly elsewhere (67.9% in Palestinians and 54.3% in Jews). Palestinians were more likely than Jews to report high (23.8% vs. 16.6%, respectively) or moderate (23.6% vs. 18.7%, respectively) exposure to ETS (Israel CBS, 2010).

The KAP 2013 questionnaire included a question about exposure to ETS during the month preceding the interview. Exposure to ETS among nonsmokers was reported by 50.2% of the Palestinian males, 30.8% of the Jewish males, 52.8% of the Palestinian females, and 29.9% of the Jewish females (fig. 13.7). Most exposed Israeli Jews (males and females) indicated open (35.8% and 43.1%, respectively) and closed (43.5% and 37.9%, respectively) public spaces as their main exposure location, while Palestinian males indicated closed public spaces as their main exposure source (42.3%); Palestinian females were mostly exposed (65.7%) at home (ICDC, 2017a).

Preliminary findings from a biomonitoring study (using urinary cotinine levels) indicated that the exposure to ETS in the nonsmoking adult population in Israel is widespread and high. This particular study recorded no significant

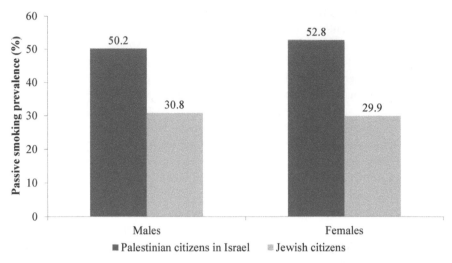

Figure 13.7. Environmental tobacco smoking (passive smoking) in the month preceding the interview in nonsmokers by population group and gender, aged 21+ years, 2013 (percent). *Source:* Israel Center for Disease Control. (2017a). *Health knowledge, attitudes and behaviors, 2013* [in Hebrew]. Publication No. 361. Jerusalem: Israel Ministry of Health.

difference between the Jewish and Palestinian subgroups, probably because of its small sample size (Levine et al., 2013).

IN ADOLESCENTS

The MABAT surveys are a series of studies conducted by the Israel Ministry of Health to assess the health and nutritional status of the general Israeli population. The MABAT youth survey was carried out in 2003–2004 on a representative sample of about 6,000 12- to 18-year-old Israeli schoolchildren. On the basis of the survey results, Noach et al. (2012) reported on the exposure of this age group to ETS. The results indicated that 85.6% of the participants were exposed to ETS: 40.0% at home, 31.4% at school, 73.3% at entertainment venues, and 16.3% at other locations. Lower paternal education and active smoking were associated with higher exposure. Palestinians were less likely to report exposure to ETS at school and entertainment venues and more frequently reported exposure at home compared to Jews. Secular Palestinians were less exposed than were religious Palestinians; the opposite was true among Jews (Noach et al., 2012).

Smoking Outcomes

Tobacco use is associated with severe health effects and high mortality rates. It is estimated that tobacco is responsible for the deaths of nearly six million people worldwide each year. More than five million of these deaths are the result of direct tobacco use while more than 600,000 are the result of nonsmokers being exposed to ETS (HSS, 2014; WHO, 2009).

Data on the incidence and prevalence of chronic diseases in Israel are available from national registries such as the Israel National Cancer Registry (INCR), national cross-sectional surveys such as the INHIS survey, designated surveys focusing on certain conditions such as asthma in schoolchildren or acute coronary syndromes, and recently also from the computerized databases of the HMOs that provide health insurance to all Israeli citizens and legal residents. Mortality data are available from the Israeli Death Causes Registry and the Israel CBS. We present some data on outcomes known to be associated with smoking or ETS among Palestinian citizens in Israel in the following discussion.

Chronic Diseases

CHRONIC OBSTRUCTIVE PULMONARY DISEASE (COPD)

Unfortunately, no data were found regarding the prevalence of COPD in the different population groups in Israel, even though this chronic disease is closely related to smoking. As for mortality from the disease, the rates (age-adjusted, per 100,000) for 2014 were higher in Palestinians compared to Jews: 13.4 and 8.8 in Palestinian and Jewish males, respectively, and 7.9 and 6.0 in Palestinian and Jewish females, respectively. Interestingly, mortality rates from pneumonia, which are often affected by active smoking, are higher in Palestinian males (10.4) compared to Jewish males (7.2) and similar in Palestinian and Jewish females (4.3) (ICDC, 2017b).

ASTHMA

The INHIS-II survey, performed by the Israel Ministry of Health in 2007–2010 on a representative sample (N = 10,331) of the population (aged 21 and over), collected information on the prevalence of certain chronic conditions, asthma included. The prevalence of asthma, based on self-report of a physician diagnosis of the disease, was lower in Palestinians compared to Jews and lower in males compared to females: the age-adjusted rate (per 100,000) in Palestinian males was 3.7; in Jewish males, 5.6; in Palestinian females, 4.0; and in Jewish females, 6.7 (ICDC, 2014). Similarly, the prevalence of asthma (age-adjusted, per 100,000) in the INHIS-III survey (2013–2015) was 4.6 and 8.9 in Palestinian and Jewish males, and 6.2 and 6.8 in Palestinian and Jewish females (ICDC, 2017c). Mortality from asthma has been decreasing in recent decades in both population groups and among both genders; however, mortality rates are higher in Palestinians compared to Jews.

As for adolescents, asthma prevalence in Palestinian youth (aged 13–14), based on repeated national surveys, was 4.9% in 1997, 4.5% in 2003, and 7.0% in 2009. Despite the recent increase, these rates were lower than the rates reported for Jews (7.8%, 7.2%, and 7.2%, respectively) (Graif et al., 2013; Romano-Zelekha et al., 2007).

HEART DISEASES

The INHIS-II survey findings with respect to heart diseases indicated that 8.2% of Palestinian males reported having been diagnosed by a physician with heart disease compared to 10.6% of Jewish males, and 5.9% reported being diagnosed with ischemic heart disease compared to 7.8% of the Jewish males. The corresponding rates for females were 7.2% and 7.1% in Palestinian and Jewish females, respectively, for heart disease; and 2.6% and 4.4% in Palestinian and Jewish females, respectively, for ischemic heart disease (ICDC, 2014). In the INHIS-III survey (2013–2015), the prevalence (age-adjusted, per 100,000) of self-reported physician-diagnosed ischemic heart disease was 5.7 and 6.4 in Palestinian and Jewish males and 3.5 and 3.1 in Palestinian and Jewish females (ICDC, 2017c).

Mortality from acute myocardial infarction and other ischemic heart disease is higher in Palestinians compared to Jews. Age-adjusted mortality rates per 100,000 in 2014 were 49.6, 30.2, 23.9, and 14.9 for Palestinian males, Jewish males, Palestinian females, and Jewish females, respectively (Israel CBS, 2016).

Salameh et al. (2008) examined risk factors for coronary artery disease among Jewish and Palestinian women in Jerusalem and reported that although the Palestinian patients were younger and smoked less compared to the Jewish patients, they were more likely to have a more extended disease and a worse outcome. Higher prevalence of other risk factors may have accounted for that (Salameh et al., 2008). Palestinian and Jewish women undergoing cardiac catheterization in Jerusalem also differed in their exposure to smoking: Palestinian patients were less likely to be active smokers but more likely to be exposed to ETS compared to Jewish patients (Jabara, Namouz, Kark, & Lotan, 2007).

CEREBROVASCULAR ACCIDENT (CVA), OR STROKE

Prevalence of a physician-diagnosed CVA, according to the INHIS-II survey findings, was lower in Palestinians compared to Jews: age-adjusted rates per 100,000 were 2.1 in Palestinian males, 4.2 in Jewish males, 1.4 in Palestinian females, and 2.1 in Jewish females (ICDC, 2014). In the INHIS-III survey, rates were similar in Palestinian (2.1) and Jewish (2.0) males but lower in Palestinian (0.8) compared to Jewish (1.4) females (ICDC, 2017c). However, mortality rates for CVA were higher in Palestinians compared to Jews: in 2014 the age-adjusted rates (per 100,000) were 24.4, 14.5, 19.1, and 11.4 for Palestinian males, Jewish males, Palestinian females, and Jewish females, respectively (Israel CBS, 2016).

CANCER

Data on cancer incidence are available from the INCR. This database was established in 1960 and has received reports on all cancer cases since 1982 by law with a high completeness rate (97% for solid tumors) (Fishler, Keinan-Boker, & Ifrah, 2017).

Based on the INCR database, cancer incidence rates among Palestinians are generally lower than the rates among Jews. In 2014 the age-standardized incidence rates (ASRs) (per 100,000) for all-site invasive cancer were 195.7 in Palestinian males, 243.6 in Jewish males, 167.6 in Palestinian females, and 257.9 in Jewish females. However, leukemia rates are almost similar in Palestinians and Jews, and lung cancer rates are higher in Palestinian males compared to Jewish males. The ASRs (per 100,000) for leukemia in 2014 were 8.0, 9.4, 5.4, and 5.3 in Palestinian and Jewish males and in Palestinian and Jewish females, respectively, and the ASR for lung cancer was 49.2 in Palestinian males and 28.6 in Jewish males (Israel National Cancer Registry, 2017). The five leading incident cancer types and the five leading death-causing cancer types in the Palestinian and Jewish population groups in 2014 are presented in table 13.3 and table 13.4, respectively.

Table 13.3. Percentage of New Invasive Cancer Cases Diagnosed in 2014 by Cancer Site, Population Group, and Gender

Palestinian males		Jewish males		Palestinian females		Jewish females	
Site	%	Site	%	Site	%	Site	%
Lung	19.9	Prostate	19.5	Breast	33.3	Breast	32.4
Colorectal	12.4	Colorectal	13.2	Colorectal	11.1	Colorectal	11.1
Prostate	11.2	Lung	11.1	Thyroid	7.4	Lung	6.7
NHL	6.0	Bladder	6.1	Endometrial	5.8	Thyroid	5.7
Bladder	5.4	NHL	6.0	NHL	5.7	Endometrial	5.5

Note. NHL, non-Hodgkin lymphoma.
Source: Adapted from Israel National Cancer Registry. (2017). Retrieved from https://www.health.gov.il/PublicationsFiles/cancer2014m.pdf

Table 13.4. Percentage of Cancer Mortality in 2014 by Cancer Site, Population Group, and Gender

Arab males		Jewish males		Palestinian females		Jewish females	
Site	%	Site	%	Site	%	Site	%
Lung	36.0	Lung	21.3	Breast	21.8	Breast	18.7
Colorectal	7.6	Colorectal	12.2	Colorectal	12.2	Lung	12.6
Pancreas	6.3	Prostate	8.5	Lung	8.5	Colorectal	11.1
Leukemia	5.8	Pancreas	8.2	Leukemia	5.5	Pancreas	8.9
Prostate	5.0	Bladder	5.5	Pancreas	4.8	Ovary	5.4

Source: Adapted from Israel National Cancer Registry. (2017). Retrieved from https://www.health.gov.il/PublicationsFiles/cancer2014m.pdf

Causes of Death

Mortality causes in Palestinian and Jewish males are quite similar, but mortality rates in Palestinian males are generally slightly higher than those of Jewish males. In 2011 the five leading causes of death in Palestinian males (age-adjusted rates per 100,000) were cancer (159.1) followed by heart diseases (126.1), diabetes (54.2), external causes (50.5), and CVA (49.0) (ICDC, 2014). In 2014 the five leading causes (of total mortality) were quite similar: cancer (21.4%), heart diseases (14.7%), external causes (10.2%), diabetes (6.5%), and COPD (4.8%) (ICDC, 2017b). The five leading causes of mortality in Jewish males in 2011 were cancer (147.9), heart diseases (97.6), external causes (32.0), CVA (31.0), and infectious diseases (28.1) (ICDC, 2014), while in 2014 cancer was the leading cause of death (26.4% of the total mortality), followed by heart diseases (16.3%), CVA (5.4%), infectious diseases (5.3%), and diabetes (5.1%) (ICDC, 2017b).

Mortality causes in Palestinian and Jewish females are quite similar, but mortality rates in Palestinian females are generally slightly higher than those of Jewish females, excluding cancer, influenza, and pneumonia. In 2011 the five leading causes of death (age-adjusted rates per 100,000) in Palestinian females were heart diseases (92.9), cancer (81.7), diabetes (56.9), CVA (39.9), and renal diseases (28.7) (ICDC, 2014). In 2014 the five leading causes of death (of total mortality) were slightly different: cancer (19.4%), heart diseases (14.7%), diabetes (9.8%), CVA (6.2%), and infectious diseases (5.0%) (ICDC, 2014). The five leading causes of mortality in Jewish females in 2011 were cancer (117.2), heart diseases (72.7), CVA (28.4), diabetes (23.2), and infectious diseases (22.4) (ICDC, 2014). The same was also true in 2014: cancer (26.0% of the total mortality), heart diseases (16.2%), CVA (6.0%), diabetes (5.6%), and infectious diseases (5.5%) (ICDC, 2017b).

The infant (aged 0–1) mortality rate in 2014 (per 1,000 live births) was 6.0 among Palestinians and 2.2 among Jews. Although these rates have been decreasing in recent decades, the gap between Palestinians and Jews remains (ICDC, 2017b). The main cause of infant death in Palestinians in 2009–2011 was congenital malformations, followed by perinatal causes (mostly immaturity). In Jews the leading cause was perinatal causes (mostly immaturity), followed by congenital malformations (ICDC, 2014).

Public Health Policies for Primary and Secondary Prevention of Smoking

The WHO Framework Convention on Tobacco Control (WHO FCTC) came into force on February 27, 2005, and has been ratified by 177 countries (WHO, 2005). The FCTC contains articles concerning the different strategies recommended, such as price and tax measures to reduce the demand for tobacco; protection from exposure to tobacco smoke; regulation of the contents of tobacco products; regulation of tobacco product disclosures; packaging and labeling of tobacco products; education, communication, training, and public awareness; tobacco advertising, promotion, and sponsorship; and demand reduction measures concerning tobacco dependence and cessation. The combined efforts focusing on these different strategies have brought about a large decline in smoking rates around the world (WHO, 2005).

Israel ratified the FCTC on August 2005 (WHO, 2005) and has been working to advance and implement various policies to reduce tobacco use. In May 2011, the Israeli government approved a national program that aimed to reduce tobacco use and its ill effects (Government Secretariat, 2011). This national program was based on the recommendations made by a public committee nominated to work on this subject (Israel Ministry of Health, 2010). Part of this committee's recommendations focused on the Palestinian population in Israel, specifically Palestinian men, because of the high smoking rates that characterize this particular population subgroup. As data on this subgroup was scarce, the Israel Ministry of Health decided to appoint a specific committee focusing on the Palestinian population and to allocate funds for further research. Consequently, a large epidemiological study focusing on the reasons for smoking initiation and barriers to cessation among Palestinian men has been carried out by researchers from Ben-Gurion University of the Negev, funded by the Israel Ministry of Health (Kalter-Leibovici et al., 2016).

In general, it is evident that the rate of ETS is higher in the Palestinian population in Israel (compared to the Jewish population). Banning smoking in public places is one of the most effective strategies to reduce involuntary smoking and to eliminate its ill effects (Hopkins et al., 2001; Vasselli et al., 2008). In Israel, a law banning smoking in public places was enacted in 1983 and amended many times in the following years. An amendment that came into effect in July 2012 included for the first time a ban on smoking in open spaces such as railway and bus platforms and outside swimming pools and their surroundings (Israel Ministry of Health, 2012). The latest addition (in 2018) referred to a smoking ban in hospitals, clinics and their open-air surroundings. These laws allow local authorities to issue high fines both to the owners of the public place and to the smokers themselves. However, they are not well enforced. Local authorities seldom perform inspections or impose financial penalties (Baron-Epel, Satran, Cohen, Drach-Zehavi, & Hovell, 2012). The law also requires local authorities to annually report on their law enforcement; however, many do not comply with this requirement. In the 2012 annual report to the Knesset, only 31 local authorities (of 256 local authorities) reported on the number of fines imposed for smoking in public places, and none of these were from the Palestinian local authorities. In total, 4,839 fines were issued in those 31 local authorities in 2012 (MoH, 2013). This is indeed a relatively small number of fines, implying a low level of law enforcement in Israel, especially by Palestinian local authorities.

Israel has implemented some successful strategies to reduce smoking. In 2010 it introduced smoking cessation technologies, including free group behavioral therapy, combined with subsidization of pharmacological treatment for all smokers interested in cessation, into the mandatory basket of medical services provided by Israeli HMOs to all citizens and legal residents by the NHI Law. Since then, a vast rise of 425% in the number of smokers attending smoking cessation groups has been documented (up from 6,000 to over 25,000 attendees in 2016) (Public Health Services, 2017). All HMOs offer groups that are conducted in Arabic and provide smoking cessation consultants from the Palestinian population, but there are no data concerning differential usage of this technology by the Palestinian smoking population (Public Health Services, 2017). However, a recent study identified that only 40% of Palestinian men reported ever receiving a physician's advice to quit smoking (Daoud et al., 2016) and that most of them (62%) were not ready to consider quitting (precontemplation state in the "stages of change") (Daoud et al., 2015). In 2015 another technology was added to the basket of health services in order to facilitate smoking cessation: subsidized nicotine replacement therapy for smokers who wished to quit but were unable to use prescription drugs (Public Health Services, 2017).

Health promotion programs in Israel are not always culturally sensitive to the Palestinian population. Culturally sensitive programs should take into account a wide range of factors, including, for example, differences in language, knowledge, values, customs, health beliefs, religion and religiosity, and family roles, among others (Rosen, Elroy, Ecker, & Isma'il, 2008). A study conducted by the Brookdale Institute in Israel on this issue (Rosen et al., 2008) indicated that many of the programs addressing smoking do not pay sufficient attention to specific factors influencing the high rate of smoking in the male Palestinian population, such as the high levels of stress and the limited enforcement of antismoking legislation in Palestinian areas. Furthermore, the printed health promotion materials being used need to be adapted. Although in general, the quality of the material was found to be high, several components needed improvement. Some of the Arabic in the materials was not sufficiently clear or precise, and the materials required a high level of health literacy. The materials included pictures and illustrations that did not reflect the Palestinian sector. In addition, no use was made of relevant sayings from the Qur'an when these could play a helpful role (Rosen et al., 2008).

Factors Associated with Smoking Initiation and Barriers to Smoking Cessation

As previously eluded to, religiosity has an impact on smoking status in the Palestinian population. Today, tobacco smoking is perceived to be lawful in Islamic law but discouraged (because of its harmful effects on smokers and their surroundings) (Ghouri, Atcha, & Sheikh, 2006). Religious rulings alone are unlikely to have a great impact on rates of smoking but could help if they are part of a more comprehensive approach to tackling smoking within this population (Ghouri et al., 2006).

Few studies regarding smoking commencement have been conducted specifically among the Palestinian population in Israel. A study carried out on high-school children in the Jerusalem district (Meijer, Branski, & Kerem, 2001) disclosed that a significant proportion of Palestinian students regarded smoking as a way to distinguish themselves from the crowd. Half the Palestinian female smokers in this study viewed other smoking children as "courageous." This was in contrast to "peer pressure," and "to be more accepted by the group," which were more common reasons for smoking initiation in the Jewish study participants (Meijer et al., 2001, p. 506).

The study that focused on high school students in the northern town of Tayibe (Korn & Magnezi, 2008) found that self-perception of low academic achievement and active smokers among household members were strong determinants in increasing the probability of smoking by the youngster, particularly with respect to hookah smoking. This study also showed that students from a secular and conservative background are more likely than students from a religious background to experiment with cigarette and hookah smoking (Korn & Magnezi, 2008).

Interestingly, in a study of adult smokers focusing on factors that influence the age of smoking initiation in different ethnic groups (Baron-Epel & Haviv-Messika, 2004), it was found that the absence of active smoking of certain household members (neither mother nor sibling smoking) did not affect the age of smoking initiation in the Palestinian participants. Paternal smoking seemed to be associated with the age of smoking initiation, but the results did not reach statistical significance (Baron-Epel & Haviv-Messika, 2004). In a study on smoking in American Palestinian youth (Kulwicki & Hill Rice, 2003), factors affecting smoking initiation were poor school performance, having a family member that smoked, peer pressure, and low parental education (Kulwicki & Hill Rice, 2003).

Discussion

In this chapter, we describe the current smoking status of the Palestinian citizens in Israel. The results indicate that smoking rates in Palestinian males are the highest, while in Palestinian females smoking rates are the lowest in Israel, creating a unique population group where about half the men actively smoke while women, mostly nonsmokers, and children are heavily exposed to ETS.

Overall, smoking prevalence in 2014 among Palestinian citizens in Israel (23.1%) was similar and at times even higher than prevalence rates in other Arab and Muslim countries (table 13.5) (WHO, 2015).

While health surveys on representative population samples are the most practical information sources for smoking prevalence rates, their limitations should be kept in mind. Baron-Epel, Haviv-Messika, Green, and Kalutzki (2004) compared self-reported smoking in Jews and Palestinians in Israel. They used data from the first MABAT (health and nutrition) survey conducted in 1999–2001 on a sample of 3,239 25- to 64-year-old responders by means of a face-to-face interview and from the 2000 KAP survey conducted on a sample of 4,713 participants in the same age group interviewed by telephone. While for Jews (males and females), no significant differences in smoking rates were observed between face-to-face and telephone

Table 13.5. Smoking Prevalence, Aged 15+, by Gender in Selected Countries, 2015 (Percent)

Country	Males	Females
Bahrain	48.8	7.6
Egypt	49.9	0.3
Iran	21.5	0.7
Israel[a]		
Palestinian citizens	43.9	9.8
Jewish citizens	27.8	17.7
Jordan	70.2	10.7
Lebanon	45.4	31.0
Morocco	45.4	1.4
Saudi Arabia	27.9	2.9
Turkey	39.5	12.4

[a] Israeli data adapted from Public Health Services. (2017). *The minister of health report on smoking 2016* [in Hebrew]. Retrieved from https://www.health.gov.il/PublicationsFiles /smoking_2016.pdf.
Source: World Health Organization. (2015). *Global health observatory (GHO) data: Prevalence of tobacco smoking.* Retrieved from http://www.who.int/gho/tobacco/use/en/.

interviews, a substantial difference between the two methods of data collection was recorded in the Palestinian population, where respondents were more likely to report being a smoker in the face-to-face interviews. This was especially apparent among Palestinian women (Baron-Epel et al., 2004).

The high smoking levels of the Palestinians in Israel are partially reflected in their morbidity and mortality status. Although cancer rates are generally lower in Palestinians compared to Jews, Palestinian males present the highest levels of lung cancer incidence. Likewise, mortality rates from COPD are higher in Palestinians compared to Jews.

In this chapter, we have also summarized the primary and secondary prevention strategies applied for smoking cessation and noncommencement in Israel in general and among Palestinians in particular. In contrast to the Jewish population, smoking rates in Palestinian men have not decreased, regardless of their educational level (Baron-Epel et al., 2010). Social and cultural factors may explain this— for example, smoking is considered a positive social norm in Palestinian society, and these positive norms prevent smoking cessation and form an environment, both physical and social, that supports smoking. Going against the norm in a more collective and traditional society may be more difficult than in a more individual-istic society (Baron-Epel et al., 2010).

Young Palestinian male adolescents form a high-risk group for both cigarette and hookah smoking initiation. This, too, may be rooted in the characteristics of Palestinian society in Israel, where the family is the strongest social unit (WHO, 2013). Hence, young individuals may be strongly influenced by smokers in their families and adopt this acceptable social behavior even if detrimental to their health, also out of a need to have a strong sense of belonging to the family (Kulwicki & Hill Rice, 2003). Smoking may be therefore perceived as a process of negative socialization in which the family and many key social figures—that is, role models such as teachers and doctors—who smoke are imitated (Kulwicki & Hill Rice, 2003). We are, therefore, in need of better-tailored interventions specifically targeting Palestinian society in general, and Palestinian teenagers in particular, to change smoking rates in this population group.

Conclusions and Recommendations

The WHO's well-accepted definition of "health" from 1946—a state of complete physical, mental, and social well-being and not merely the absence of disease or infirmity—dictates a broader and more novel approach to health promotion and improvement. However, many sectors of the specialized and nonspecialized health and mental health agents in Israel have limited or no knowledge about the full spectrum of health-related issues among Palestinians in Israel. Since active and passive tobacco use, in the form of cigarettes or hookahs and their secondhand smoke, is prevalent in this community, it is important to systematically gather the relevant data and create a sound evidence base that, in turn, will enable the tailoring of appropriate, culture-sensitive interventions and may in the long run also assist in improving the health of this community in all respects.

LITAL KEINAN-BOKER is Deputy Director of the Israel Center for Disease Control, Ministry of Health, Israel. She is Associate Professor of Epidemiology at the School of Public Health at the University of Haifa, Israel.

YAEL BAR-ZEEV is Director of the Center for Smoking Cessation and Prevention at Ben-Gurion University, Israel.

References

Azaiza, F., Shoham, M., Bar-Hamburger, R., & Abu-Asbeh, K. (2009). Psychoactive substance use among Arab adolescent school dropouts in Israel: A phenomenon and its implications. *Health & Social Care in the Community, 17*(1), 27–35.

Baron-Epel, O., & Haviv-Messika, A. (2004). Factors associated with age of smoking initiation in adult populations from different ethnic backgrounds. *European Journal of Public Health, 14*(3), 301–305.

Baron-Epel, O., Haviv-Messika, A., Green, M. S., & Kalutzki, D. N. (2004). Ethnic differences in reported smoking behaviors in face-to-face and telephone interviews. *European Journal of Epidemiology, 19*(7), 679–686.

Baron-Epel, O., Keinan-Boker, L., Weinstein, R., & Shohat, T. (2010). Persistent high rates of smoking among Israeli Arab males with concomitant decrease in rate among Jews. *Israel Medical Association Journal, 12*(2), 732–737.

Baron-Epel, O., Satran, C., Cohen, V., Drach-Zehavi, A., & Hovell, M. F. (2012). Challenges for the smoking ban in Israeli pubs and bars: Analysis guided by the behavioral ecological model. *Israel Journal of Health Policy Research, 1*(1), 28.

Daoud N., Hayek S., Biderman A., Mashal A., Bar-Zeev Y., & Kalter-Leibovici O. (2016). Receiving family physician's advice and the "stages of change" in smoking cessation among Arab minority men in Israel. *Family Practice, 33*(6), 626–632.

Daoud N., Hayek S., Sheikh Muhammad A., Abu-Saad K., Osman A., Thrasher, J. F., & Kalter-Leibovici, O. (2015). Stages of change of the readiness to quit smoking among a random sample of minority Arab male smokers in Israel. *BMC Public Health*, 15, 672.

Elias, W., Assy, N., Elias, I., Toledo, T., Yassin, M., & Bowirrat, A. (2012). The detrimental danger of water-pipe (hookah) transcends the hazardous consequences of general health to the driving behavior. *Journal of Translational Medicine, 10*(1), 126.

Fisher, N., Amitai, Y., Haringman, M., Meiraz, H., Baram, N., & Leventhal, A. (2005). The prevalence of smoking among pregnant and postpartum women in Israel: A national survey and review. *Health Policy, 73*(1), 1–9.

Fishler, Y., Keinan-Boker, L., & Ifrah, A. (Eds.). (2017). *The Israel national cancer registry: Completeness and timeliness of the data* [in Hebrew]. Publication No. 365. Jerusalem: Israel Center for Disease Control.

Gharrah, R. (2013). *Arab society in Israel.* Vol. 6: *Population, society, economy* [in Hebrew]. Jerusalem: Van Leer Jerusalem Institute, Hakibbutz Hameuchad.

Ghouri, N., Atcha, M., & Sheikh, A. (2006). Influence of Islam on smoking among Muslims. *British Medical Journal, 332*(7536), 291–294.

Government Secretariat. (2011). *A national program to decrease smoking and its hazardous effects* [in Hebrew]. Decision No. 3247 of the 32nd Israeli Government. Retrieved from http://www.pmo.gov.il/Secretary/GovDecisions/2011/Pages/des3247.aspx.

Graif, Y., German, L., Ifrah, A., Livne, I., & Shohat, T. (2013). Dose-response association between smoking and atopic eczema: Results from a large cross-sectional study in adolescents. *Dermatology, 226*(3), 195–199.

Harel-Fisch, Y., Walsh, S., Boniel-Nissim, M., Dzhalovsky, A., Amit, S., & Habib, J. (2011). *Health behaviors in school-aged children (HBSC): A World Health Organization cross-national study* [in Hebrew]. Israel: Bar Ilan University. Retrieved from https://hbsc.biu.ac.il/books.html.

Hopkins, D. P., Briss, P. A., Ricard, C. J., Husten, C., Carande-Kulis, V. G., Fielding, J. E., . . . the Task Force on Community Preventive Services. (2001). Reviews of evidence regarding interventions to reduce tobacco use and exposure to environmental tobacco smoke. *American Journal of Preventative Medicine, 20*(Suppl. 2), 16–66.

Israel Center for Disease Control [ICDC]. (2014). *Health 2013* [in Hebrew]. Publication No. 354. Jerusalem: Israel Ministry of Health.

Israel Center for Disease Control [ICDC]. (2017a). *Health knowledge, attitudes and behaviors, 2013* [in Hebrew]. Publication No. 361. Jerusalem: Israel Ministry of Health.

Israel Center for Disease Control [ICDC]. (2017b). *Highlights of health in Israel 2016* [in Hebrew]. Publication No. 371. Jerusalem: Israel Ministry of Health.

Israel Center for Disease Control [ICDC]. (2017c). *Israel national health interview survey 3, 2013–2015* [in Hebrew]. Retrieved from https://www.health.gov.il/publicationsfiles/inhis _3main_findings.pdf.

Israel Central Bureau of Statistics [Israel CBS]. (2010). *Social survey 2010* [in Hebrew]. Publication no. 1477. Retrieved from http://www.cbs.gov.il/webpub/pub/text_page.html ?publ=6&CYear=2010&CMonth=1.

Israel Central Bureau of Statistics [Israel CBS]. (2016). *Annual data, 2016*. Retrieved from https:// www.cbs.gov.il/en/publications/Pages/2016/Statistical-Abstract-of-Israel-2016-No-67.aspx.

Israel Central Bureau of Statistics [Israel CBS] (2018). *The Social Survey*. Retrieved from http:// surveys.cbs.gov.il/Survey/.

Israel Ministry of Health. (2010). *Report of the public committee on reducing tobacco use in Israel* [in Hebrew]. Retrieved from https://www.health.gov.il/PublicationsFiles/smoke2011 _30052012.pdf.

Israel Ministry of Health. (2012). *Extension of ordinance on prevention of smoking in public places*. Retrieved from http://www.health.gov.il/English/News_and_Events /Spokespersons_Messages/Pages/29042012_1.aspx.

Israel Ministry of Health. (2013). *The minister of health report to the parliament on smoking in Israel* [in Hebrew]. Retrieved from https://www.health.gov.il/PublicationsFiles/smoking _2014.pdf.

Israel National Cancer Registry. (2017). *Report on cancer incidence and mortality in 2014* [in Hebrew]. Retrieved from https://www.health.gov.il/PublicationsFiles/cancer2014 _01022017.pdf.

Jabara, R., Namouz, S., Kark, J. D., & Lotan, C. (2007). Risk characteristics of Arab and Jewish women with coronary heart disease in Jerusalem. *Israel Medical Association Journal, 9*(4), 316–320.

Kalter-Leibovici, O., Chetrit, A., Avni, S., Averbuch, E., Novikov, I., & Daoud, N. (2016). Social characteristics associated with disparities in smoking rates in Israel. *Israel Journal of Health Policy Research, 5*(1), 36–47.

Kim, S. S., Ziedonis, D., & Chen, K. (2007). Tobacco use and dependence in Asian American and Pacific Islander adolescents: A review of the literature. *Journal of Ethnicity in Substance Abuse, 6*(3–4), 113–142.

Knishkowy, B., & Amitai, Y. (2005). Water-pipe (narghile) smoking: An emerging health risk behavior. *Pediatrics, 116*(1), e113–e119. Retrieved from https://doi.org/10.1542/peds.2004-2173.

Korn, L., & Magnezi, R. (2008). Cigarette and nargila (water pipe) use among Israeli Arab high school students: Prevalence and determinants of tobacco smoking. *Scientific World Journal, 8*, 517–525.

Kulwicki, A., & Hill Rice, V. (2003). Arab American adolescent perceptions and experiences with smoking. *Public Health Nursing, 20*(3), 177–183.

Kurian, A. K., & Cardarelli, K. M. (2007). Racial and ethnic differences in cardiovascular disease risk factors: A systematic review. *Ethnicity and Disease, 17*(1), 143–152.

Levine, H., Berman, T., Goldsmith, R., Göen, T., Spungen, J., Novack, L., . . . Grotto, I. (2013). Exposure to tobacco smoke based on urinary cotinine levels among Israeli smoking and nonsmoking adults: A cross-sectional analysis of the first Israeli human biomonitoring study. *BMC Public Health, 13*(1), 1241.

Liu, R., So, L., Mohan, S., Khan, N., King, K., & Quan, H. (2010). Cardiovascular risk factors in ethnic populations within Canada: Results from national cross-sectional surveys. *Open Medicine, 4*(3), e143–e153. Retrieved from https://www.ncbi.nlm.nih.gov/pmc/articles /PMC3090103/.

Meijer, B., Branski, D., & Kerem, E. (2001). Ethnic differences in cigarette smoking among adolescents: A comparison of Jews and Arabs in Jerusalem. *Israel Medical Association Journal, 3*(7), 504–507.

Molcho, M., Harel, Y., & Dina, L. O. (2004). Substance use and youth violence. A study among 6th and 10th grade Israeli school children. *International Journal of Adolescent Medicine and Health, 16*(3), 239–252.

Noach, M. B., Steinberg, D. M., Rier, D. A., Goldsmith, R., Shimony, T., & Rosen, L. J. (2012). Ethnic differences in patterns of secondhand smoke exposure among adolescents in Israel. *Nicotine & Tobacco Research, 14*(6), 648–656.

Public Health Services. (2017). *The minister of health report on smoking 2016* [in Hebrew]. Retrieved from https://www.health.gov.il/PublicationsFiles/smoking_2016.pdf.

Romano-Zelekha, O., Graif, Y., Garty, B.-Z., Livne, I., Green, M. S., & Shohat, T. (2007). Trends in the prevalence of asthma symptoms and allergic diseases in Israeli adolescents: Results from a national survey 2003 and comparison with 1997. *Journal of Asthma, 44*(5), 365–369.

Rosen, B., Elroy, I., Ecker, N., & Isma'il, S. (2008). *Health promotion activities in the Israeli Arab population: To what extent are they culturally appropriate and what can be done to make them more so?* Jeruslem: Myers-JDC-Brookdale Institute.

Salameh, S., Hochner-Celnikier, D., Chajek-Shaul, T., Manor, O., & Bursztyn, M. (2008). Ethnic gap in coronary artery disease: Comparison of the extent, severity, and risk factors in Arab and Jewish middle-aged women. *Journal of the Cardiometabolic Syndrome, 3*(1), 26–29.

US Department of Health and Human Services [US HHS]. (2014). *The health consequences of smoking—50 years of progress: A report of the surgeon general.* Rockville, MD: US Department of Health and Human Services. Retrieved from http://www.surgeongeneral .gov/library/reports/50-years-of-progress/50-years-of-progress-by-section.html.

Vasselli, S., Papini, P., Gaelone, D., Spizzichino, L., De Campora, E., Gnavi, R., . . . Laurendi, G. (2008). Reduction incidence of myocardial infarction associated with a national legislative ban on smoking. *Minerva Cardioangiologica, 56*(2), 197–203.

World Health Organization [WHO]. (2005). *WHO framework convention on tobacco control.* Retrieved from http://apps.who.int/iris/bitstream/10665/42811/1/9241591013.pdf.

World Health Organization [WHO]. (2009). *Global health observatory (GHO) data: Prevalence of tobacco use, 2009.* Retrieved June 20, 2017, from: http://www.who.int/gho/tobacco /use/en/.

World Health Organization [WHO]. (2013). *WHO report on the global tobacco epidemic, 2013. Enforcing bans on tobacco advertising, promotion and sponsorship.* Retrieved from http:// apps.who.int/iris/bitstream/10665/85380/1/9789241505871_eng.pdf?ua=1.

World Health Organization [WHO]. (2015). *Global health observatory (GHO) data: Prevalence of tobacco smoking.* Retrieved from http://www.who.int/gho/tobacco/use/en/.

PART IV

VIOLENT BEHAVIOR AND MENTAL HEALTH AMONG PALESTINIAN CITIZENS IN ISRAEL

14

CHILD ABUSE AND NEGLECT AMONG PALESTINIAN CITIZENS IN ISRAEL

Haneen Elias and Raghda Alnabilsy

THIS CHAPTER DEALS WITH THE PROBLEM OF CHILD abuse and neglect among Palestinian boys and girls in Israel. We examine its incidence, risk factors, consequences, as well as patterns of coping and help seeking based on the available research literature. The discussion of the problem focuses on the sociocultural and political context of Palestinian society in Israel as an indigenous minority with unique characteristics. This minority can be distinguished from the majority society in its culture, traditions, language, heritage, and customs. The Palestinian minority is not typical because it is not a group of voluntary immigrants or refugees but rather an indigenous ethnic-national group that has become a minority in its own land (Harel, 2002).

In recent decades, extensive research has been conducted on the incidence and prevalence of children and adolescents who have been exposed to violence in their families of origin in multiple countries (Euser et al., 2013; Fallon et al., 2013; Leventhal, Martin, & Gaither, 2012). In contrast, empirical knowledge about the extent of the problem in Palestinian societies is still limited (Haj-Yahia & Ben-Arieh, 2000). Likewise, empirical knowledge about the consequences of the problem, strategies for coping, and responses available to victims and their families is also lacking.

Importantly as well, most of the intervention programs that have been developed to deal with the problem in Israel are based on Western approaches (Shalhoub-Kevorkian, 2000), as are the Israeli child protection laws (Al-Krenawi & Graham, 2000). This implies that the majority group formulates the policies, the patterns of action, and the intervention programs for child protection according to its values (Jamal, 2005). As a result, it is difficult to examine and understand the problem in the specific context of the indigenous minority, as well as to adapt interventions to the needs and values of Palestinian society in Israel. Against this background, the aims of the chapter are to discuss the problem of child abuse and neglect, with emphasis on the cultural and social context of Palestinian society as a minority group born in Israel, and to shed light on the political relevance of the Palestinian social context in Israel to the problem definition, its incidence, risk factors, and ways of coping.

Definition of the Problem

The World Health Organization (WHO) defined child maltreatment at a 1999 conference, referring to its prevention: "Child abuse or maltreatment constitutes all forms of physical and/or emotional ill-treatment, sexual abuse, neglect or negligent treatment or commercial or other exploitation, resulting in actual or potential harm to the child's health, survival, development or dignity in the context of a relationship of responsibility, trust or power" (Krug, Mercy, Dahlberg, & Zwi, 2002, p. 59). The definition relates to a broad range of acts of abuse. This chapter focuses on child abuse and neglect by parents, family members, and/or those who are responsible for the children in the family.

The literature relates to four general types of maltreatment and abuse:

1. Physical abuse is defined as severe and ongoing intentional abuse of children through the use of physical force against body organs using a tool or instrument that inflicts various wounds on the children (Boyer & Kadman, 2007). Physical abuse has been categorized in terms of the severity of the damage inflicted: mild wounds (scratches, bruises), moderate wounds (several wounds, a single fracture, or mild burns), and severe wounds (multiple wounds, deep and pervasive burns, abdominal damage, damage to the central nervous system (Antonoly, 2007).

2. Sexual abuse is defined in the *DSM-IV* (American Psychiatric Association, 1994) as using the minor to gratify the sexual desires typically by an adult or adolescent. Sexual abuse has been divided into three main types: rape (nonconsensual intercourse, forced intercourse using threats, forced intercourse using abuse, sodomy, and indecent acts), sexual exploitation (exploiting the minor to engage in a sexual act through bribery or to produce child pornography), and incest (sexual abuse by a close relative). These acts can be committed separately or concurrently against a given victim (Lev-Weisel, 2007).

3. Emotional abuse occurs when the responsible adult fails to provide an appropriate, supportive environment for children, which affects the child's health and emotional development. Abusive acts include restricting the child's movement, belittling, scorning, threatening, intimidating, discriminating against, and rejecting the child (Krug et al., 2002).

4. Neglect occurs when the responsible parent deprives the child of care in the areas of health, education, emotional development, and nutrition, as well as shelter and provision of secure living conditions for the child (Krug et al., 2002).

These definitions, mainly based on health aspects, relate to a broad range of acts of child and adolescent abuse, which raises two main issues. First, in light of the extensive catalog of abusive acts that are treated by multidisciplinary professionals (e.g., doctors, lawyers, psychologists, social workers, educators), a common definition of child abuse is needed that can be adopted in different sociocultural and sociopolitical contexts. Second, although these definitions provide good objective and universal descriptions of abuse, they lack a sensitive perspective that takes into account the extent that contexts can protect against or perpetuate the abuse. The relevant contexts are the culture of the family and the sociopolitical environment. The following paragraphs attempt to shed light on the context for defining the problem that, among other factors, determines the way it is dealt with.

Palestinian society in Israel is characterized by a collective sociocultural and political orientation (Haj-Yahia, 1999). Family interests and family commitments are given priority over individual commitments or the desire for self-fulfillment. Interpersonal relationships are characterized by inequality in terms of gender and age (Haj-Yahia & Sadan, 2007). In this context, the hierarchy of power and interpersonal relations is defined by gender and age, in that men and adults have more social, cultural, economic, and political power than women and children (Matsumoto, 1996). Thus, children have an inferior social status, which causes them to be dependent on the responsible adults. This dependence, which is reflected in obedient behavior, showing respect, and attempts to meet the expectations of adults, often requires victims of child abuse to keep the abuse secret and sometimes even to accept the abuse as part of the authority of adults to educate them. The choice of keeping the abuse secret to cope with the situation derives from the collectivist orientation of Palestinian society and reflects acceptance of that orientation and identification with it. This explanation has been supported by Haj-Yahia and Sadan (2007), who argued that members of collectivist societies derive their identity from the collective and believe that the good reputation and status of their family carries over to their own reputation as individuals.

Moreover, the social values that dictate collectivist relationships often perpetuate the victimization of abused children. For example, traditional Palestinian families believe that it is positive and desirable for extended family members, particularly grandparents and uncles, to be involved in raising children, providing for the children's needs, and promoting their development (Haj-Yahia, 1995). Instead, we argue that the multiple parent figures that bear responsibility for childcare and education can confuse the child and can even increase the chances of keeping abuse a secret within the family. This can also perpetuate the victimization of children and cause children to accept any abusive behavior by adults.

Another complication of the victimization experienced by Palestinian victims of child abuse in Israel is related to the inaccessibility and inflexibility of the therapeutic system, as reflected in the failure to adapt intervention programs for this population, as well as in the tension that ensues between the Western professional values that guide professionals in the intervention process and the collectivist cultural values (Abu-Baker & Dwairy, 2003). We assume that this tension creates an ongoing, unresolved conflict that harms the children and contributes to perpetuating their victimization. We therefore argue that Palestinian children in Israel not only experience direct victimization by the responsible perpetrator but also that their suffering, abuse, and victimization may be compounded.

The Incidence and Dimensions of the Problem

Haj-Yahia, Musleh, and Haj-Yahia (2002) conducted a survey among 1,640 Palestinian adolescents in Israel that clearly revealed that a high percentage of them had experienced psychological aggression and physical violence by their parents and siblings. The findings of that survey identified 10%–56% of Palestinian adolescents who had experienced psychological aggression by their fathers; 9%–53%, by their mothers; and 14%–56%, by their siblings (these widely varying rates resulted from the wide ranges of responses that were received on different types of abuse examined in that study). The most frequent form of psychological aggression by parents and siblings was heated argument with the adolescent, whereas threats with a knife, gun, stick, chair, or other lethal weapon were more rare. The findings also revealed that 0.5%–26% of the Palestinian adolescents had experienced physical violence by their fathers; 0.6%–26%, by their mothers; and 0.9%–33%, by their siblings. Furthermore, the findings revealed that assault, grabbing, and pushing were the most prevalent acts of physical violence, whereas the use of a knife, gun, or other lethal weapon was less prevalent. Notwithstanding this research evidence, the real incidence of abuse against Palestinian adolescents might be much higher than the reports indicate. This assumption is based on the understanding that adolescents might cover up their victimization because of shame, fear of revenge, or the desire to avoid arousing painful memories (Katar, 1998).

In 2013 Eisikovits and Lev-Weisel, of the Center for the Study of Society at the University of Haifa, conducted a comprehensive epidemiological survey that aimed to estimate the incidence of different forms of child maltreatment, neglect, and abuse, as well as to examine the factors that facilitate and inhibit exposure to abuse. The survey was conducted among a national sample of Jewish and Palestinian youth aged 12 (sixth grade), 14 (eighth grade), and 16 (tenth grade). The total sample consisted of 8,239 Jewish youth and 2,274 Palestinian youth. The main findings with regard to abuse of Jewish and Palestinian youth are presented next.

Almost half of the Jewish Israeli youth (48.5%) reported experiencing one or more types of abuse: boys were more likely to experience physical and emotional abuse, whereas girls were more likely to experience sexual abuse and family violence. Of the Jewish youth, 17.6% reported that they had been sexually abused; 14.1% had experienced physical abuse; 14.3%, physical neglect; and 27.8%, emotional abuse.

The survey findings on Palestinian youth in Israel revealed even more frequent abuse. They indicated that over two-thirds of the Palestinian youth (67.7%) reported experiencing one or more types of abuse. In addition, the findings indicated that Palestinian boys were more likely to experience physical and sexual abuse, whereas Palestinian girls were more likely to experience emotional abuse and be exposed to family violence. Furthermore, the findings showed that 22.3% of the Palestinian youth (boys and girls) reported that they had experienced sexual abuse, while 11.8% of them reported that they had experienced severe sexual abuse. About half of the youth who had been sexually abused (49.4%) reported that they had experienced sexual abuse more than once, and over half of those youth (54.7%) indicated that the abuse had continued during the last year. Two-thirds of the youth who had been sexually abused reported that the abuse had occurred within the family. Regarding physical abuse, 27.6% reported that they had experienced such abuse; 15.2% of them had been physically abused by an adult whom they knew, and 66.8% reported that the abuse had occurred within the family. The survey findings further indicated that 33.4% of the youth reported experiencing physical neglect, and about 30% of the youth reported that as a result of the neglect they had become sick. Of those youth, 59.7% had sought medical treatment. In addition, 40.1% of the children reported experiencing emotional abuse, while 22% had experienced emotional neglect (Eisikovits & Lev-Weisel, 2013).

It appears that in the dimensions of abuse that were examined in the preceding survey (sexual abuse, physical abuse, physical neglect, emotional abuse, and emotional neglect), the percentage of Palestinian youth who had experienced abuse was higher than the percentage of Jewish youth. This highlights the need for governmental ministries to formulate policies and invest appropriate resources to reduce the incidence of the problem in Palestinian society. The survey findings also reflect the difficult reality in which Jewish and Palestinian youth live in Israel but do not purport to explain the differential rates of abuse. An explanation of these differences could shed light on some of the risk factors of abuse among the Palestinian population in Israel as an indigenous minority group. The next section presents a comprehensive discussion of risk factors deriving from the reality of life among the Palestinian population of Israel that may shape and determine the severity of the problem.

Risk Factors

In this section, we examine sociopolitical, familial, and personal risk factors for child abuse and neglect.

Sociopolitical Risk Factors

To fully understand these sociopolitical risk factors, we first need to examine the status of Palestinian citizens in Israel. Al-Haj (2000) referred to the citizenship of Israeli Palestinians as a "double periphery." They are marginalized by both Israeli society and the Arab world. According to Rouhana (1997), Israel is a constitutionally ethnic country where there is a substantive contradiction between the democratic and ethnic components in its laws. Ghanem (2002) argued that the analysis of the civil status of Palestinian citizens in Israel indicates that they have civil and political rights as individuals, yet the state of Israel has a structure that gives preference to Jewish residents. The civil and social exclusion that Palestinian citizens in Israel experience creates inferior living conditions characterized by poverty, unemployment, inadequate housing conditions (Doyle, 1996), discrimination in employment conditions (Schtayner, 2013), and discrimination at the level and scope of services provided (Abu-Baker, 2007). All these factors were found to be related to increased risk for child abuse and neglect (Doyle, 1996). The following sections elaborate on the relationship between these risk factors and the problem of child abuse.

POVERTY

The Palestinian population in Israel has been poorer than the Jewish population since the establishment of the state in 1948. The poverty rate for Palestinian families has remained high and reached 54.3% in 2012. Other indexes, such as the depth and severity of poverty, have also revealed that levels of distress are higher among the Palestinian population than among the total poor population in Israel (Inwald, Heller, Barkali, & Gottlieb, 2012). Zielinski (2009) found that child abuse is related to socioeconomic status. According to Zielinski, compared with adults who did not experience abuse in childhood, those who experienced abuse are more likely to have lived in poverty as children and are more likely to be unemployed as adults. Living in poverty in urban areas was found to increase the chances of exposure to trauma (Gill & Page, 2006). At the same time, people who have experienced trauma and live in poverty are more likely to experience recurrent abuse (Klest, 2012). In addition, findings have revealed that the relationship between the experience of childhood trauma and the experience of victimization in adulthood is substantially more significant among people living in poor communities (Klest, 2012). Moreover, poverty was associated with consistently inferior psychological consequences (Santiago, Kaltman, & Miranda, 2013). Based on the findings of studies that have examined the relationship between poverty and child abuse and neglect, it can further be concluded that residents of poor Palestinian neighborhoods in Israel have a low quality of life; they lack material resources, and their subsistence needs are not provided for. In our view, living in the shadow of continuous deprivation can harm the ability of adults to endure the difficult conditions, so that they are not available to deal with their children's needs and even abuse their children. This argument is consistent with the conclusions of Haj-Yahia and Ben-Arieh (2000), as shown later in this discussion.

UNEMPLOYMENT

This is another risk factor for child abuse and neglect. Chronic unemployment of the head of the household and subsistence on a minimum wage in a family with a large number of children are factors that increase the dependence of Palestinian families to a greater extent than Jewish families on government transfer payments, especially from the NII. These factors also lead to the institutionalization of poverty in Palestinian society (Shihadeh, 2004).

DISCRIMINATION AT THE LEVEL OF SERVICES

Studies conducted over the years have shown that the Palestinian minority is discriminated against in several social arenas such as education, higher education, employment, and law enforcement (Ghanem, 2002; Rouhana, 1997; Smooha, 1998).

For example, inequality in health services is reflected in the poor quality of these services as well as in the lack of available and accessible services (McLeigh, 2013). Furthermore, the inferior level of education and welfare services has also posed a considerable burden for professionals. This has prevented them from early identification and treatment of individuals and families in serious situations such as child and adolescent abuse.

Family and Personal Risk Factors

The empirical literature that has examined the relationship between family and personal risk factors and child abuse in Palestinian society in Israel is limited. Generally, risk factors have been associated with sociodemographic characteristics of the parents that may predict abuse, such as father's age, parents' level of education, residential environment, and religious affiliation, and with the status of the child in the family and the parental role.

FATHER'S AGE

Haj-Yahia and Ben-Arieh (2000) found that the older the fathers were, the greater the likelihood of their using physical violence against their adolescent children.

PARENTS' LEVEL OF EDUCATION

The lower the fathers' level of education, the more they used psychological and physical violence against their adolescent children, while the lower the mothers' level of education, the more they used physical violence against their adolescent children. Additionally, the lower the parents' level of education, the more the siblings used physical violence and psychological aggression against each other (Haj-Yahia & Ben-Arieh, 2000).

RESIDENTIAL ENVIRONMENT

The findings indicated that in a smaller residential environment (rural and Bedouin areas), fathers, mothers, and siblings were more likely to use psychological and physical violence against the adolescents in the family (Haj-Yahia & Ben-Arieh, 2000).

RELIGIOUS AFFILIATION

The findings indicated that the experience of abuse correlated positively with religious affiliation (Muslim adolescents experienced more abuse than did Christian adolescents) (Haj-Yahia & Ben-Arieh, 2000).

STATUS OF THE CHILD IN THE FAMILY AND THE PARENTAL ROLE

Another aspect in examining the risk factors is the child's status with reference to the way he or she has been raised and educated and how he or she has developed.

Thus, we attempt to shed light on how the status of Palestinian children in the family, their process of socialization, and their rights and obligations constitute risk factors for child abuse. Parental roles are affected by the traditional orientation of the Palestinian family. The father is described as an authority figure that sets boundaries, establishes behavior codes, and enforces discipline, whereas the mother's role is to support, educate, and raise the children. Children are expected to obey their parents and fulfill their parents' expectations (Barakat, 1993). Those who fail to do so can be punished, and their parents can impose sanctions on them. In a study on patterns of punishment among Palestinian parents in Israel, Dwairy (1998) found that, for the most part, the need to exert authority is what determines how most parents act in the process of educating their children. In our view, this perspective emphasizes the inferior status of children in the family as well as their obligation to fulfill their parents' demands. Failure to do so gives the parents legitimization to hurt their children and to use physical force or verbal and psychological abuse as way of educating their children.

The review of these risk factors indicates that their causes are diverse and complex. Some of them relate to the policy of the establishment, which discriminates against the Palestinian minority in Israel in terms of planning as well as in terms of allocation of adequate resources and infrastructures for Palestinian localities. In other words, it can be argued that sociopolitical factors such as poverty, unemployment, and discrimination at the level of the services are significant factors for child abuse and for lowering the threshold for parental abuse against children. Moreover, factors relating to the status of parents and children within the family, which derive from the socialization process, are also significant factors for child abuse.

The Consequences of Child Abuse

Haj-Yahia et al. (2002) examined 1,640 Palestinian adolescents living in seven Palestinian villages and cities and in one mixed Jewish-Palestinian city in Israel. The study focused on the incidence of abuse of adolescents by parents and siblings, as well as the mental health consequences of abuse. The consequences for adolescents were examined according to hopelessness, psychological adjustment problems, and low self-esteem. The findings revealed that adolescents who had experienced physical violence by their fathers, mothers, and siblings reported high levels of hopelessness, psychological adjustment problems, and low self-esteem. Similar results were found for adolescents who had experienced psychological aggression by fathers and mothers. In addition, the results of that survey revealed that these three areas of mental health outcomes were particularly salient among adolescent girls and among families where the father was unemployed. The results further revealed that the larger the family was and the lower the father's level of education, the more the adolescents reported psychological adjustment problems and low self-esteem.

The literature has also addressed the consequences of sexual abuse against Palestinian girls (children and adolescents) in Israel. The honor of the Palestinian family as a patriarchal unit is associated with the honor of the male family members and is based on the existence of rules that apply mainly to women and dictate their behavior, activities, desires, and even their thoughts (Shalhoub-Kevorkian, 1998). The quality of families in Palestinian society is evaluated on the basis of their adherence to the principle of family honor, which is harmed whenever one of the rights of the family is violated, including cases of abuse against the women in the family (Almuaqat, 2006). Damage to family honor entails serious social consequences such as social labeling and shame. These factors often lead to murder of women by family members or to women's suicide with the encouragement of family members in order to relieve the family of shame (Shalhoub-Kevorkian, 1998). In cases of sexual abuse, the victims often know that they are the ones who are sacrificed for the family honor (Almuaqat, 2006). Hence, they keep silent to maintain family honor, even when they compromise their own honor and neglect their physical and mental health.

The consequences of sexual abuse are also related to the extent to which the Palestinian girl preserves her hymen. The girl's sexuality is not perceived as belonging to her. Rather, it is perceived as belonging to the extended family and sometimes even to the *hamula*. Hence, she is obligated to preserve her sexual purity and her virginity until she marries (Abu-Baker, 2007). Thus, victims of sexual abuse in Palestinian society are more concerned about preserving their hymen than they are about their mental health because this is what usually determines their future (Abu-Baker & Dwairy, 2003). One of the consequences of losing virginity is the potential threat to the honor of the girl and her family and sometimes even to the girl's life (Almuaqat, 2006).

Other consequences of sexual abuse for girls relate to the shame and suffering experienced afterward. In a cultural context where concepts such as "shame," "honor," and "guilt" play a major role, the exposure of sexual abuse can have a negative impact on her mental state and even threaten the victim's life (Shalhoub-Kevorkian, 2003). Girls who experience sexual abuse and exploitation are victims in two ways: they are victims of the perpetrator and the crime, and they are victims of the general social response. This includes keeping silent and covering up the crime and the victimization; labeling and accusing the victim; normalizing the crime; and legal, therapeutic, social, and cultural prohibitions against treating the victims (Abu-Baker & Dwairy, 2003; Shalhoub-Kevorkian, 2003). Moreover, perpetrators are aware of the collective mentality and exploit it to their advantage when they commit the act. For example, they can threaten to publicly shame the victim as a means of dominating her. The threat generates psychological suffering over and above the suffering caused by the sexual abuse itself, as it causes the victim to feel a sense of forced loneliness because of the difficulty entailed in exposing the abuse (Abu-Baker, 2007; Shalhoub-Kevorkian, 2003). Thus, victims do not expose the abuse because they are afraid that they will be blamed by their families, that they will be scorned, and that they will be accused of failing to protect their bodies and of cooperating with the act of abuse (Abu-Baker, 2007).

The discussion of the consequences of sexual abuse raises two important issues: one relates to the dearth of research on the experience, characteristics, motives, and consequences of sexual abuse against boys in Palestinian society in Israel. In this connection, the following question arises: Does the lack of attention to the problem among boys derive from attempts to protect and preserve the values of the patriarchal society, which maintains the traditional perspective that sexual abuse is limited to girls? Or, alternatively, does the gender of researchers in Palestinian society dictate and affect their choice of the population they examine? The other issue is that in terms of the consequences of sexual abuse, the discussion in Western society focuses on the victim—that is, on the victim's experience of abuse and the personal consequences of abuse for the victim (e.g., Littleton, Grills-Taquechel, Buck, Rosman, & Dodd, 2013; Patrick & Maggs, 2010). In contrast, the discussion of the consequences of sexual abuse in Palestinian society focuses on the society and on the collectivist perspective. Based on that perspective, an attempt is made to shed light on the extent of the consequences experienced by the victim. To understand the experiences and status of the victims of sexual abuse, it is first necessary to understand the meaning of the collective, family honor, shame, and preservation of the hymen.

In general, it is important to expand the investigation and examine the consequences of child abuse in Palestinian society in Israel on several levels, based on an ecological model (Bronfenbrenner, 1979). The few studies that have been presented to date have mainly addressed the consequences of child abuse at the personal level while examining sociodemographic variables and attempting to understand the sociopolitical context of the problem. Thus, we argue that further research should be conducted among more diverse populations, including different age groups (infants, young children, and adolescents) as well as residents of different areas of Israel, and people who differ in terms of various sociodemographic characteristics such as social status, level of education, religion, and family size. It is also important that these studies examine the physical, cognitive, mental health, emotional, and behavioral consequences of child abuse and neglect.

In addition, we recommend examining the relevance of cultural and family values to the consequences of the problem for the victims and their families. For example, the values of maintaining family honor and keeping family secrets have a considerable impact on the responses of the victims as well as on the responses of the families and the surrounding community. We also recommend examining the problem at the macrolevel to gain insights into the consequences at the social and political levels. These studies should examine the relationship between child abuse in Palestinian society and mobilization of resources to identify and treat the problem while considering the policies for dealing with the problem in the relevant governmental institutions (e.g., welfare, education, justice, health). In addition, it is important to conduct research that will examine the relationship between the problem of child abuse and the emergence of social problems such as street violence, dropping out of school, use of addictive substances, and involvement in deviant behavior. To the best of our knowledge, no research has been conducted to date on the effect of child abuse on the emergence of social problems in Palestinian society in Israel. Based on the ecological perspective, it is also vital to conduct research on personal resilience among children who have experienced abuse in order to shed light on their experiences and understand how they develop in the shadow of abuse.

Strategies for Coping and Seeking Help

In this section, we deal with the ways that children and their families cope with the problem of abuse. First, we attempt to determine whether and to whom the victims and their families report the abuse. What coping strategies do they adopt to deal with the abuse? Lastly, we examine how the therapeutic systems deal with the Palestinian population as an indigenous minority group.

In the survey conducted by Eisikovits and Lev-Weisel (2013) among Jewish and Palestinian youth aged 12, 14, and 16, most of the Palestinian participants indicated that they preferred to report the abuse to one of their parents. Their preferences for reporting were as follows (in descending order): mother, father, friends, the school counselor or a teacher, a doctor or nurse, a social worker. The survey participants (those who had been abused and those who had not) indicated that the three factors that inhibit exposure of the perpetrator and reporting of the experience of abuse are shame, fear for themselves, and fear that their family will be harmed. In contrast, the three factors that facilitated reporting of exposure and reporting of the abuse were the desire to punish the perpetrator, a good relationship with an adult that the child trusts and can confide in, and a sense of injustice.

Abud-Halabi (2004) examined Palestinian parents' definitions of the phenomenon as well as different patterns of child abuse and neglect, in addition to examining their willingness to report these incidents to different family members, to welfare services, and to the police. The study was conducted among about 240 Palestinian parents in Israel, and the findings revealed that the parents were more willing to report incidents of sexual and physical abuse than they were to report cases of emotional abuse and neglect. The study also found that the parents' preferences for reporting were ranked as follows (in descending order): the nuclear family, the extended family, welfare services, the police. The findings also revealed that with regard to the relationship between cultural values and willingness of Palestinian parents to report incidents of child abuse and neglect, the more they endorsed traditional parent-child relations based on the dominant values in Palestinian society, the less willing they were to report cases of emotional abuse to nuclear family members and the less willing they were to report cases of sexual and physical abuse to welfare services and the police. The study also examined the relationship between sociodemographic variables and the parents' willingness to report cases of child abuse. It was found that fathers showed a greater tendency than mothers to report cases of emotional abuse to members of the nuclear or extended family, whereas no differences were found between fathers and mothers with regard to reporting physical violence. Moreover, no difference was found between Muslim and Christian parents in willingness to report cases of physical abuse to members of the nuclear family, members of the extended family, welfare services, and the police. Druze parents were more willing than Muslim and Christian parents to report cases of emotional child abuse to the aforementioned agents. They also showed a greater tendency than Muslim and Christian parents to report cases of neglect to authorities outside of the family (welfare services or the police). A significant positive relationship was also found between the parents' level of education and their willingness to report cases of neglect to nuclear family members as well as their willingness to report cases of emotional abuse to the police. Furthermore, it was found that employed parents showed more willingness than unemployed parents to acknowledge and report child abuse to the aforementioned agents. The study also examined predictors of willingness to report by a profile that had been constructed for the study. The findings revealed that Druze parents who had served in the army were more willing to report cases of child abuse than all others.

According to Shalhoub-Kevorkian (1998), failure to report child abuse to formal authorities can be attributed to the informal system of cultural and family control in Palestinian society, which has a strong influence. The social and cultural control is reflected in the expectation that members of Palestinian society should conform to the dominant behavior norms and values, which are mainly conservative and traditional (Abu-Baker & Dwairy, 2003). In cases of emotional, personal, and family distress, individuals first utilize all of the personal resources at their disposal. Afterward, they turn to the family system for assistance, and if this does not succeed they turn to the formal support system (D'Abate, 1994). Palestinian society does not trust formal services and service providers, especially police and other law enforcement agents, which are perceived as contentious, as breaking up families, and as representing the oppressive, discriminatory establishment (Haj-Yahia, 2003). In a similar vein, Abud-Halabi (2004) argued that avoidance of reporting to agents outside of the family such as the police and welfare services might be related to the political reality of the Palestinian citizens in Israel. Abud-Halabi also argued that opposition to using formal services reflects the main values of family privacy, family reputation, family solidarity, cohesion, support, and mutual dependence among family members.

Another issue elicited by the discussion of coping strategies relates to the way that the therapeutic systems deal with children in indigenous minority groups who are victims of abuse and neglect. Numerous studies have emphasized the difficulty and failure of the system in interventions with various minority populations (e.g., Bernard, 2001; Dylan, Regehr, & Alaggia, 2008). Munro (2004) argued that the reason for the failure is that in certain cases of child abuse and neglect among children in minority groups, the inflexibility and inaccessibility of therapeutic agencies fosters an accusatory environment. Therapists use uniform and general therapeutic standards for everyone and often have difficulty working with populations whose culture, color, ethnic background, and socioeconomic status are different (Lachman & Bernard, 2006). The prevailing therapeutic perspective of child abuse in Israel is Western/individualist and considers the state to be responsible for protecting citizens and providing solutions to victims, such as shelter and education as well as social and psychological treatment (Abu-Baker & Dwairy, 2003). This perspective is not appropriate in non-Western societies, such as the Palestinian society in Israel, which maintain a collective orientation and consider the family rather than the state to be responsible for the well-being and protection of children. This conflict between collectivist values and the Western therapeutic perspective might exacerbate the harm and pain to the victim (Dwairy, 1998).

The review of strategies for coping with child abuse in Palestinian society in Israel indicates that these strategies typify the status of indigenous minority groups. Studies conducted throughout the world have emphasized the lack of resources and knowledge needed to protect and treat indigenous minority groups when a violent incident occurs (e.g., Nancarrow, 2006). Moreover, studies conducted in Canada on indigenous groups have highlighted the double violation of basic human rights in various areas, such as in the treatment of child abuse. Social workers employed in social services do not receive sufficient training that relates to the context of indigenous families. Moreover, beliefs and values of social workers are influenced by Western European policies that are not necessarily consistent with the values of the local families and cultures (Blackstock, Prakash, Loxley, & Wien, 2005). The main conclusion deriving from this review is that the coping strategies of Palestinian victims of child abuse and their families in Israel are influenced by two main elements: one is the collectivist values that dictate the strategies used by individuals and families to cope with child abuse, and the second is the treating system, which has adopted a Western-oriented perspective that is not consistent with the values of Palestinian society in Israel. Moreover, there is an inequitable distribution of resources that is not adequate for helping Palestinian victims and their families cope with the problem of child abuse in Israel.

Conclusion

In this chapter, we attempt to shed light on the problem of child abuse and neglect in Palestinian society in Israel based on various aspects that include the definition of the problem and its incidence, risk factors for child abuse, its consequences, and strategies for coping and seeking help with the problem. Research has found that the range of incidence of child abuse is broad.

Our review highlights the need for governmental ministries to adopt policies and allocate adequate resources to reduce the incidence of child abuse and neglect in Palestinian society. The discussion indicates that the risk factors are diverse and complex and that they are related to various levels of individual and family life, as well as to the lives of the Palestinian population and its status as an indigenous minority in Israel. Poverty, unemployment, and discrimination in services are examples of sociopolitical risk factors that may account for the problem. Demographic variables such as father's age, parents' level of education, residential environment, religious affiliation, and factors related to the child's status can also explain the problem. At the same time, we recommend broadening the investigation of parenting styles and parent-child relations and examining their relationship to child abuse. Examination of the consequences of the problem also highlights the need to adopt an ecological perspective. Specifically, it is important to conduct research that will consider different age groups and residents of different areas (i.e., different types of localities) that have distinct sociodemographic characteristics. It is also important to examine various aspects of the consequences—such as physical, cognitive, psychological, emotional, and behavioral—and to emphasize how cultural values relate to the consequences of the abuse for the victims.

The discussion of coping strategies underscores two main issues. One is the lack of trust among the Palestinian population in the institutions and the external professional agents that provide interventions, as evidenced in the low rates of reporting abuse. The second issue relates to the Western-oriented services and professional interventions adopted by the majority group, which need to be better-suited to the sociocultural and sociopolitical contexts as well as the demands and needs of the Palestinian minority in Israel. This situation can widen the gaps between the available means and the problems that have to be addressed. In light of this reality, comprehensive research should be conducted on the needs of children who are victims of abuse and the needs of their families. In addition, an intervention model should be designed that is sensitive to the sociocultural context of Palestinian citizens in Israel.

HANEEN ELIAS is Researcher and Lecturer in the Department of Social Work at Ruppin Academic Center, Israel.

RAGHDA ALNABILSY is Researcher and Lecturer in the Department of Social Work at Ruppin Academic Center, Israel.

References

Abu-Baker, K. (2007). *Identifying child abuse and neglect: Introduction to intercultural Palestinian society* [in Hebrew]. Jerusalem: Ashalem.

Abu-Baker, K., & Dwairy, M. (2003). Cultural norms versus state law in treating incest: A suggested model for Palestinian families. *Child Abuse & Neglect, 27*(1), 109–123.

Abud-Halabi, Y. (2004). *Palestinian parents' definitions of different patterns of child abuse and neglect, and their willingness to report such cases to various entities in the family, social services, and the police* [in Hebrew] (Unpublished MA thesis). The Hebrew University of Jerusalem, Israel.

Al-Haj, M. (2000). Identity and orientation among Israeli Arabs: A situation of double periphery [in Hebrew]. In R. Gavison & D. Hacker (Eds.), *The Jewish-Arab rift in Israel: A reader* (pp. 13–33). Jerusalem: Israel Democracy Institute.

Al-Krenawi, A., & Graham, J. R. (2000). Culturally sensitive social work practice with Palestinian clients in mental health settings. *Health & Social Work, 25*(1), 9–22.

Almuaqat, P. (2006). *Sexual abuse within the family: Between reality and the law* [in Hebrew]. Jerusalem: Center for Gender Studies.

American Psychiatric Association. (1994). *Diagnostic and statistical manual of mental disorders* (4th ed.). Washington, DC: American Psychiatric Association.

Antonoly, E. (2007). Child physical abuse [in Hebrew]. In Y. Ben-Yehuda, Y. Horowitz, & D. Hovav (Eds.), *Child abuse and neglect in Israel* (pp. 396–434). Jerusalem: Ashalem.

Barakat, H. (1993). *The Palestinian world: Society, culture, and state*. Los Angeles: University of California Press.

Bernard, C. A. (2001). *Constructing lived experiences: Representations of black mothers in child sexual abuse discourses*. Aldershot, UK: Ashgate.

Blackstock, C., Prakash, T., Loxley, J., & Wien, F. (2005). *Wen:de: We are coming to the light of day*. Ottawa: First Nations Child and Family Caring Society of Canada.

Boyer, Y., & Kadman, Y. (2007). Between physical punishment to abuse: The commonalities outweigh the differences [in Hebrew]. In Y. Ben-Yehuda, Y. Horowitz, & D. Hovav (Eds.), *Child abuse and neglect in Israel* (pp. 673–780). Jerusalem: Ashalim.

Bronfenbrenner, U. (1979). *The ecology of human development: Experiments by design and nature*. Cambridge, MA: Harvard University Press.

D'Abate, D. (1994). The role of social network supports of Italian parents and children in their adjustment to separation and divorce. *Journal of Divorce & Remarriage, 20*(1–2), 161–187.

Doyle, C. (1996). Current issues in child protection: An overview of the debates in contemporary journals. *British Journal of Social Work, 26*(4), 565–576.

Dwairy, M. (1998). *Cross-cultural counseling: The Palestinian case*. New York: Haworth.

Dylan, A., Regehr, C., & Alaggia, R. (2008). And justice for all? Aboriginal victims of sexual violence. *Violence Against Women, 14*(6), 678–696.

Eisikovits, Z., & Lev-Weisel, R. (2013). *Abuse, neglect and violence against children and youth in Israel: Between frequency and the report. Epidemiology of child abuse among children in Israel* [in Hebrew]. Haifa: The Center of Society Research, University of Haifa.

Euser, S., Alink, L. R., Pannebakker, F., Vogels, T., Bakermans-Kranenburg, M. J., & Van IJzendoorn, M. H. (2013). The prevalence of child maltreatment in the Netherlands across a 5-year period. *Child Abuse & Neglect, 37*(10), 841–851.

Fallon, B., Ma, J., Allan, K., Pillhofer, M., Trocmé, N., & Jud, A. (2013). Opportunities for prevention and intervention with young children: Lessons from the Canadian incidence study of reported child abuse and neglect. *Child and Adolescent Psychiatry and Mental Health, 7*(1), 1–13.

Ghanem, A. (2002). The Palestinians in Israel: Political orientation and aspirations. *International Journal of Intercultural Relations, 26*(2), 135–152.

Gill, J. M., & Page, G. G. (2006). Psychiatric and physical health ramifications of traumatic events in women. *Issues in Mental Health Nursing, 27*(7), 711–734.

Haj-Yahia, M. M. (1995). Toward culturally sensitive intervention with Palestinian families in Israel. *Contemporary Family Therapy, 17*(4), 429–447.

Haj-Yahia, M. M. (1999). Violence against women in the social-cultural context of Palestinian society [in Hebrew]. In C. Rabin (Ed.), *On being different in Israel: Ethnicity and treatment* (pp. 219–242). Tel Aviv: Ramot, Tel Aviv University Press.

Haj-Yahia, M. M. (2003). Palestinian women's attitudes toward different patterns of coping with violence against women by partners [in Hebrew]. In E. Leshem & D. Roer-Strier (Eds.), *Cultural diversity as a challenge of human services* (pp. 195–228). Jerusalem: Magnes, The Hebrew University of Jerusalem Press.

Haj-Yahia, M. M., & Ben-Arieh, A. (2000). The incidence of Palestinian adolescents' exposure to violence in their families of origin and its sociodemographic correlates. *Child Abuse & Neglect, 24*(10), 1299–1315.

Haj-Yahia, M. M., Musleh, K., & Haj-Yahia, Y. M. (2002). The incidence of adolescent maltreatment in Palestinian society and some of its psychological effects. *Journal of Family Issues, 23*(8), 1032–1064.

Haj-Yahia, M. M., & Sadan, A. (2007). Battered women in collective societies: Issues of intervention and empowerment [in Hebrew]. *Society and Welfare, 27*, 423–451.

Harel, H. (2002). *Minority and identity: The relationship between exposure to Jewish society and devising a "self identity" and ethnic identity formation of Palestinian adolescents* [in Hebrew]. Tel Aviv: Tel Aviv University Press.

Inwald, M., Heller, A., Barkali, N., & Gottlieb, D. (2012). *Poverty and social gaps: Annual report* [in Hebrew]. Jerusalem: National Insurance Institution, Administration of Research and Planning.

Jamal, A. (2005). *Deliberations on collective rights and the national state.* Haifa: Mada al-Carmel: Arab Center for Applied Social Research.

Katar, S. (1998). *Domestic abuse.* Bethesda, MD: Austin & Winfield.

Klest, B. (2012). Childhood trauma, poverty, and adult victimization. *Psychological Trauma: Theory, Research, Practice, and Policy, 4*(3), 245–251.

Krug, E. G., Mercy, J. A., Dahlberg, L. L., & Zwi, A. B. (2002). World report on violence and health. *The Lancet, 360*, 1083–1088.

Lachman, P., & Bernard, C. (2006). Moving from blame to quality: How to respond to failures in child protective services. *Child Abuse & Neglect, 30*(9), 963–968.

Leventhal, J. M., Martin, K. D., & Gaither, J. R. (2012). Using US data to estimate the incidence of serious physical abuse in children. *Pediatrics, 129*(3), 458–464.

Lev-Weisel, R. (2007). Childhood sexual abuse, trauma, secondary traumatization and re-trauma [in Hebrew]. In Y. Ben-Yehuda, Y. Horowitz, & D. Hovav (Eds.), *Child abuse and neglect in Israel* (pp. 556–581). Jerusalem: Ashalim.

Littleton, H. L., Grills-Taquechel, A. E., Buck, K. S., Rosman, L., & Dodd, J. C. (2013). Health risk behavior and sexual assault among ethnically diverse women. *Psychology of Women Quarterly, 37*(1), 7–21.

Matsumoto, D. (1996). *Culture and psychology.* Pacific Grove, CA: Brooks/Cole.

McLeigh, J. D. (2013). Protecting children in the context of international migration. *Child Abuse & Neglect, 37*, 1056–1068.

Munro, E. (2004). The impact of child abuse inquiries since 1990. In N. Stanley & J. Manthorpe (Eds.), *The age of the inquiry: Learning and blaming in health and social care* (pp. 75–91). London: Routledge.

Nancarrow, H. (2006). In search of justice for domestic and family violence: Indigenous and non-indigenous Australian women's perspectives. *Theoretical Criminology, 10*(1), 87–106.

Patrick, M. E., & Maggs, J. L. (2010). Profiles of motivations for alcohol use and sexual behavior among first-year university students. *Journal of Adolescence, 33*(5), 755–765.

Rouhana, N. N. (1997). *Palestinian citizens in an ethnic Jewish state: Identities in conflict.* New Haven, CT: Yale University Press.

Santiago, C. D., Kaltman, S., & Miranda, J. (2013). Poverty and mental health: How do low-income adults and children fare in psychotherapy? *Journal of Clinical Psychology, 69*(2), 115–126.

Schtayner, T. (2013). *Breaking inequality: Dealing with employment discrimination against Palestinians in* Israel [in Hebrew]. Jerusalem: Israel Democracy Institute.

Shalhoub-Kevorkian, N. (1998). Response in case of sexual violence against a child in Palestinian society: Defense, silence, deterrence or punishment [in Hebrew]. *Criminal, 7*, 161–195.

Shalhoub-Kevorkian, N. (2000). The efficacy of Israeli law in preventing violence within Palestinian families living in Israel. *International Review of Victimology, 7*, 47–66.

Shalhoub-Kevorkian, N. (2003). Who is defended? Palestinians girls in Israel and child protection policy [in Hebrew]. In M. Hovev, L. Sabah, & M. Amir (Eds.), *Trends in criminology: Theory, policy and practice* (pp. 553–583). Jerusalem: The Hebrew University of Jerusalem.

Shihadeh, M. (2004). *Unemployment and exclusion: The Palestinian minority in Israel's labor markets* [in Hebrew]. Haifa: Mada al-Carmel: Arab Center for Applied Social Research.

Smooha, S. (1998). The implications of the transition to peace for Israeli society. *The Annals of the American Academy of Political and Social Science, 555*(1), 26–45.

Zielinski, D. S. (2009). Child maltreatment and adult socioeconomic well-being. *Child Abuse & Neglect, 33*(10), 666–678.

15

PALESTINIAN CHILDREN IN ISRAEL

*Involvement in School Violence as
Victims and Perpetrators*

Mona Khoury-Kassabri

SCHOOL VIOLENCE IS A MAJOR SUBJECT OF CONCERN for students, parents, school staff, and the general public, especially because of its adverse impact on students' physical and emotional well-being and academic performance (Khoury-Kassabri, Benbenishty, Astor, & Zeira, 2004; Mishna, 2012).

This chapter uses an ecological/contextual theory (Bronfenbrenner, 1979) to argue that to understand students' behavior, attention should be paid simultaneously to the child's individual characteristics and to the social context of the child's development (Kuppens, Grietens, Onghena, Michiels, & Subramanian, 2008). Thus, the first goal of this chapter is to understand children's involvement in both victimization and the perpetration of violence by integrating various factors at the individual level. The second goal is to identify the effects of the larger social and school contexts—school organization, the community in which the school is embedded, and the characteristics of the students' families, including their culture and country of residence.

As part of this theoretical approach in which school violence is viewed as a whole-school phenomenon, the chapter does not focus only on violence among students but also on students' use of violence toward teachers and on teachers' victimization of students. First, I present the theoretical basis and empirical findings regarding students' experiences of victimization and students' perpetration of violence against peers and teachers. This is followed by a discussion on students' victimization by school staff.

Students' Victimization by Peers and Students' Use of Violence toward Peers and Teachers

A considerable number of previous empirical studies of peer-to-peer violence have focused on direct, overt behavioral patterns, such as physical violence (e.g., hitting, kicking) and verbal violence (e.g., cursing, verbally humiliating, name-calling) (Benbenishty & Astor, 2005). More recent studies have demonstrated the importance of focusing on indirect forms of violence. Despite the slight differences among relational, indirect, and social forms of aggression (Coyne, Archer, & Eslea, 2006), they all relate to behaviors by which intentional harm is caused to others by damaging their social relationships or feelings of peer acceptance (Crick, Casas, & Mosher, 1997; Crick & Grotpeter, 1995; Ostrov & Keating, 2004). Excluding individuals from group activities, spreading rumors about them, and maliciously gossiping about them are some examples of this type of aggression.

This chapter relies on Benbenishty and Astor's (2005) definition of school violence as any behavior intended to harm, physically or emotionally, persons in school, and their property (as well as school property). I define victimization as a student's report that another student or staff member perpetrated school violence against him or her in the school or on the way to or from school. This broad definition includes verbal and social violence (such as curses, humiliation, social exclusion); threatening behaviors (direct, indirect, extortion, scary behavior); physical violence (such as pushes, kicks, punches, beating); stealing and damaging property; weapon use (carrying, threatening, using); and sexual harassment (Benbenishty & Astor, 2005, p. 16).

Besides peer-to-peer violence, this chapter also examines students' use of violence toward teachers. Little empirical or theoretical attention has been paid to teacher victimization as an aspect of school violence, although some studies have examined teachers' reports of victimization by their students (Akiba, LeTendre, Baker, & Goesling, 2002; Gottfredson, Gottfredson, Payne, & Gottfredson, 2005; Payne, Gottfredson, & Gottfredson, 2003). An examination of teachers' victimization is important because teachers who feel unsafe in the classroom might be limited in their ability to fulfill their duties (Wilson, 1980; Wolkind & Rutter, 1994). In this study, violent behavior of a student toward teachers includes several types of violent acts, such as cursing at or humiliating a teacher; threatening to hurt a teacher; biting, shoving, or hitting a teacher; using a chair or other implement to hurt a teacher; and destroying a teacher's personal belongings (Benbenishty & Astor, 2005; Khoury-Kassabri, 2012a).

Prevalence of School Violence

Studies among Israeli students have shown that their involvement in school violence as victims and perpetrators is relatively high (Benbenishty & Astor, 2005). Public schools in Israel are organized by the ethnic/cultural affiliation of the student's family, with Palestinian students and teachers almost exclusively in Israeli-Arab schools. In a study of 3,375 fourth- through sixth-grade students (63.7% Palestinian) in Israel, Khoury-Kassabri (2012b) found that more Palestinian than Jewish students had been both physically and indirectly victimized by peers in the month prior to the study (73.8% and 67.8% vs. 62.3% and 64.7%, respectively). However, these differences were not statistically significant. In contrast, Jewish Israeli students reported being verbally victimized by peers significantly more often than Palestinian students (83.4% vs. 68.8%, respectively). Among students in junior high and high school, it was found that Palestinian students reported being exposed to severe physical and indirect victimization to a greater extent than Jewish Israeli students, while the opposite was found with respect to verbal victimization. These differences were all statistically significant (Khoury-Kassabri, Astor, & Benbenishty, 2009).

With respect to perpetration, about one in two Palestinian students in Israel (52.5%) reported carrying out at least one aggressive act against a peer, and 20.0% reported acting aggressively toward a teacher at least once in the month prior to the study. Among Palestinian students in Israel, there were significantly more reports of violence against peers and teachers than among Jewish Israeli students (44.3% vs. 9.0%, respectively) (Khoury-Kassabri, 2012a).

The Consequences of Students' Violence and Victimization by Peers

Aggressive behavior toward students affects all members of the school—students and their families, teachers, and other school personnel. Most knowledge of such behavior as described in this chapter is based on international literature that has explored the effects of school violence on students and teachers, while little is known about this topic among Palestinian students in Israel. Future local studies should examine these effects.

Studies have shown that youth involvement in violence may lead to many psychological difficulties (McMahon & Washburn, 2003) and is associated with numerous negative outcomes, including greater academic and interpersonal difficulties, decreased physical health, and peer rejection (Coie, Lochman, Terry, & Hyman, 1992; Mishna, 2012; Schwartz, Gorman, Nakamoto, & McKay, 2006). Longitudinal studies have shown that perpetration and victimization of school violence are predictors of later depression (Ttofi, Farrington, Lösel, & Loeber, 2011a) and offending behaviors (Ttofi, Farrington, Lösel, & Loeber, 2011b).

Victims of violent crime suffer emotional pain, fear, vulnerability, and mistrust of others (Mishna, 2012). Studies have shown that victimized children are vulnerable to many types of psychological difficulty and distress. They tend to feel more anxious, depressed, lonely, and have lower self-esteem than nonvictims (Beaty & Alexeyev, 2008; Hawker & Boulton, 2000). Victimized children reported skipping school more often than others (Khoury-Kassabri, 2012b).

In addition, student involvement in aggressive behaviors on school grounds disrupts the learning environment; both students' ability to learn and teachers' ability to teach are jeopardized (Kingery, Coggeshall, & Alford, 1998; Mercy & Rosenberg, 1998). A substantial amount of teachers' attention is focused on achieving order and cooperation in class (Emmer & Hickman, 1991; Geving, 2007; Innes & Kitto, 1989). Consequently, many teachers feel overwhelmed by classroom behavioral problems and perceive aggression at school as a serious problem (Martin, Linfoot, & Stephenson, 1999).

Violence also comes with financial costs in lost productivity, as well as in emergency, medical, and social support costs in schools and in the community (Amodei & Scott, 2002). In addition, youth violence has many societal and financial costs both for individual victims and for the larger society (Limbos et al., 2007). Previous research in the United States has shown that a single case of serious and long-term youth crime could cost society up to five million US dollars (Cohen & Piquero, 2009).

Risk Factors for Peer-to-Peer Victimization and Perpetrating Violence toward Others

Using a multilevel analysis, Khoury-Kassabri and colleagues have sought to identify the individual and contextual factors that may explain students' involvement in school violence (Khoury-Kassabri, 2011, 2012a; Khoury-Kassabri, Benbenishty, & Astor, 2005; Khoury-Kassabri et al., 2004). The results of these studies among Jewish Israeli and Palestinian students in Israel revealed that at the individual level, gender was found to be a significant predictor of student involvement in violence. Consistent with many previous studies, it was found that boys are exposed more often than girls to verbal victimization and to moderate and severe physical victimization by peers (Khoury-Kassabri, 2011; Khoury-Kassabri et al., 2004). Boys also reported initiating aggression against peers and teachers more often than girls (Khoury-Kassabri, 2012a). A reverse trend regarding gender was found with respect to indirect victimization, which was reported more often by girls than boys (Attar-Schwartz & Khoury-Kassabri, 2008; Khoury-Kassabri, 2011; Landau, Björkqvist, Lagerspetz, Österman, & Gideon, 2002; Owens, Daly, & Slee, 2005).

It might be assumed that the greater involvement of girls than boys in indirect aggression is the result of girls' higher verbal ability, particularly speech production, which is relevant to this type of victimization (Bennett, Farrington, & Huesmann, 2005). In addition, Crick and Grotpeter (1995) argued that when aggressing, or attempting to cause harm to others, children do so in ways that are most likely to damage the social goals of the target. Thus, boys are likely to use direct physical and verbal forms of aggression—usually against other boys—that hinder the instrumentally oriented dominance goals that tend to be characteristic of boys (Block, 1983). Girls are more likely to use more covert, indirect aggression—usually against other girls—as a means of achieving such social goals as maintaining status, power, and popularity in peer groups (Crick, 1997; Crick et al., 1997; Leadbeater, Boone, Sangster, & Mathieson, 2006; Zahn-Waxler & Polanichka, 2004).

Khoury-Kassabri (2012a) also found that the gap between boys and girls in the perpetration of aggressive acts toward teachers is significantly larger among Palestinian students than among Jewish students. In a study of junior high and high school students, Khoury-Kassabri et al. (2005) found that this gap is also larger with respect to perpetrating violence toward peers. These results might be explained by cultural differences between both ethno-national groups. While much of the Jewish sector in Israel tends to be characterized by Western family values (Mikulincer, Weller, & Florian, 1993), the Palestinian population is largely characterized by traditional, patriarchal, and authoritarian family values (although some studies find considerable variation among Palestinian groups within Israel (Cohen, 2007; Haj-Yahia, 2000, 2002). In a traditional society, males are usually expected to be dominant, assertive, and active, whereas females are usually expected to be passive, submissive, and obedient (Haj-Yahia, 1995). Boys might, therefore, feel more justified in acting aggressively toward others, even toward teachers, while girls might be more reserved. Further examination of this interaction is required to fully understand what causes the noted gender differences.

With respect to age differences, in a study of primary school students, Khoury-Kassabri (2011) found that for both Jewish and Palestinian students in Israel, the younger the students are, the higher their reports of physical victimization by peers. Smith, Madsen, and Moody (1999) have presented several hypotheses for the decline in victimization with age that might explain these results. One theory is that younger children are outnumbered at school by older children who are in a position to victimize them. Additionally, as indicated by Khoury-Kassabri et al. (2005), older students may be able to protect themselves better than younger students and are therefore involved in fewer physically violent acts.

In a study of junior high and high school students, it was found that for both Jewish and Palestinian students in Israel, the younger the adolescents were, the higher their reports of involvement in violent acts toward peers (Khoury-Kassabri et al., 2005). These results might be attributed to other contextual factors that affect the age difference in violent behavior, such as dropout levels owing to expulsion and suspension that are more common among older adolescents, especially those involved in school misconduct and in problematic school behavior (Welsh, Greene, & Jenkins, 1999).

In addition to student characteristics, studies have examined the contextual factors that may contribute to the variation among schools in their levels of school violence. Khoury-Kassabri et al. (2004) used hierarchical linear modeling to examine the differences between Jewish and Palestinian schools in Israel in the relationships between school-level variables—SES of the school's neighborhood and of students' families, school size and class size, school level (junior high or high) and school climate—and students' victimization reports. Two of the study's significant findings are examined next.

In both Jewish and Arab Israeli schools, school policy—as representing school climate characteristics—and positive relationships between teachers and students were associated negatively with school victimization. In a study among Jewish and Palestinian students, Khoury-Kassabri (2008) found that perpetration of aggression against peers and teachers was lower when the students in the class perceived of their school as having a consistent, fair, and clear policy against violence.

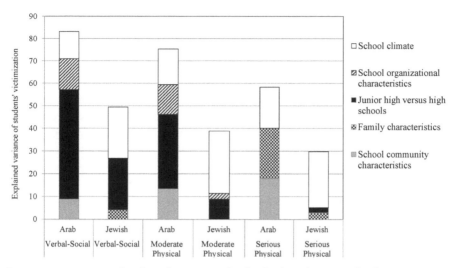

Figure 15.1. Proportion of explained variance in levels of violence between schools. *Source:* M. Khoury-Kassabri. (2008). *The relationship between teachers' self-efficacy and attitudes toward the use of violence and teachers' use of violence toward students* [in Hebrew]. Jerusalem: Hebrew University of Jerusalem.

Additionally, it was found that high levels of victimization were reported in Palestinian-Israeli schools characterized by high percentages of students from low SES families and schools in low SES neighborhoods. SES was found to make only a minor contribution to the explained variance in Jewish schools (fig. 15.1).

These findings support claims by many researchers and educators that positive school climate characteristics are associated with lower levels of school violence (Dupper & Meyer-Adams, 2002; Gottfredson et al., 2005; Payne et al., 2003; Schreck, Miller, & Gibson, 2003; Stewart, 2003). Positive student-teacher relationships were also found to be associated with lower levels of aggression (Khoury-Kassabri, 2008). Supportive relationships may reduce students' sense of alienation toward their school and give them a chance to develop positive relationships with adults who support, consult, and help them overcome their emotional and behavioral problems (Dwyer, Osher, & Hoffman, 2000). These findings emphasize the importance of warm, supportive, stable relationships between school personnel and students.

As mentioned earlier, the results of Khoury-Kassabri's (2008) study suggest that the SES of the child's environment does not always function as a risk factor for violent behavior. One way to explain this finding is to see the role of the school and its internal resources (such as a skilled professional staff and therapeutic resources) as protective factors that can mitigate the effects of the environment surrounding the school. Palestinian Israeli schools may have fewer internal resources than Jewish Israeli schools. The former students attend larger classes than Jewish Israeli students, and their schools tend to be less well-equipped than their Jewish counterparts (e.g., they tend to have fewer facilities, such as libraries, computers, and science laboratories). Moreover, Palestinian teachers in Israel receive less in-service training than Jewish teachers (Tatar & Horenczyk, 2003).

There may be many reasons why Palestinian schools in Israel have fewer internal resources. One of these could be the unequal distribution of public funds. Compared with the Jewish majority, the Palestinian minority in Israel receives less public funding for services such as education (Hareven, 2002; Kop, 2005). Furthermore, in Israel local municipalities are responsible for allocating a significant part of the resources dedicated to education. Thus, Palestinian Israeli localities with a weak economic base have fewer resources and fierce competition over priorities. Fewer resources for schools may negatively influence their ability to help at-risk children and schools, and therefore students and schools are affected more by their SES. The greater investment of resources in Jewish Israeli schools may enable them to create school environments that support and protect children from low SES and thus mitigate the impact of community SES on their behavior. This tentative interpretation requires empirical examination.

Student Victimization by School Staff

While student violence at school receives widespread attention, only limited notice has been taken of students' victimization by school staff (Hyman & Perone, 1998). Teachers' emotional maltreatment may be verbal or nonverbal, including name-calling, mocking of the student's appearance and (dis)abilities, humiliating the student in front of classmates, and engaging in discriminatory behavior against certain students (Benbenishty, Zeira, Astor, & Khoury-Kassabri, 2002).

Some forms of physical maltreatment may be regarded as intentional, and corporal punishment may be accepted. Hyman (1990) defined corporal punishment in school (committed by school staff) as the infliction of pain or confinement as a penalty for a student's offense. In many other instances, physical maltreatment by staff in school is not part of a harsh educational policy advocating corporal punishment. Rather, staff may react unofficially to infractions of discipline and provocation by using various degrees of force, such as pushing, shoving, slapping, pinching, punching, or kicking. Staff may also adopt punitive policies and practices that disregard and undermine students' rights (Hyman & Snook, 2000).

Frequency of Staff Maltreatment

Benbenishty, Zeira, Astor, et al. (2002) have examined the prevalence of student victimization by school staff in Israel (sexual harassment, emotional and physical maltreatment). They found that students in Israel reported high levels of maltreatment including corporal punishment, even though Israeli law bans corporal punishment in educational settings. Palestinian students in Israel reported significantly higher levels of staff maltreatment than Jewish students. A study among 7,205 Jewish students and 3,205 Palestinian students in junior high and high schools found that while 9.3% of the Jewish students reported having been physically victimized by school staff in the month prior to the study, 27.7% of the Palestinian students reported experiences of physical victimization. Sexual victimization was reported by 6.5% of Jewish students, and verbal victimization was reported by 23.0% compared to 14.9% and 32.5%, respectively, among Palestinian students in Israel (Benbenishty, Zeira, & Astor, 2002). A study among 3,215 Jewish (secular and religious students) and 2,257 Palestinian students in primary schools reported a similar trend. Physical victimization by school staff for Palestinian students was more than two times greater than those of Jewish children (38.3% vs. 16.8%, respectively), although the gap was smaller with respect to emotional victimization (32.2% vs. 28.0%, respectively) (Benbenishty, Zeira, Astor, et al., 2002).

Much of what is known about maltreatment by staff is based on self-reports of students about experiencing victimization by school teachers and other school personnel. Khoury-Kassabri's study (2008) of 532 Jewish (29%) and Palestinian (71%) first- through sixth-grade homeroom teachers across Israel was among the first to explore the subject from the teacher's perspective. This study found that higher levels of corporal punishment were reported by Palestinian teachers than by Jewish teachers.

Khoury-Kassabri's (2008) study findings concur with those of other studies. Approximately a quarter of the teachers (24.5%) reported using corporal punishment with a student at least once in the month prior to filling out the questionnaire used in the study. The vast majority of these reports were from Palestinian teachers (33.8% vs. 1.9% of the Jewish teachers). In addition, one in five Palestinian teachers in Israel reported using emotional violence toward a student in their classroom during the last month compared to 3% of Jewish Israeli teachers (Khoury-Kassabri, 2008).

Unfortunately, the use of violence by staff is not only experienced by school-aged children but is also in use among younger children. In a study of 86 Palestinian kindergarten teachers from the northern and central parts of Israel, Khoury-Kassabri, Attar-Schwartz, and Zur (2014) found that more than a quarter of these teachers (27.9%) indicated they were likely to use corporal punishment in cases of misbehaving children in their kindergarten class.

Consequences of Staff Maltreatment

These high rates of corporal punishment and emotional and verbal victimization by school personnel should concern parents, educators, professionals, and the public at large. Victimization by school staff may have a seriously adverse impact on children. Both teaching and nonteaching school staff are especially significant sources of physical and emotional support and protection for children. Younger students, in particular, turn to school personnel for aid and comfort when they are in need.

The adults in school are, or ideally should be, a child's immediate source of support when he or she is threatened or bullied. However, often students who are victimized fear the teacher rather than see him or her as a source of support; they may view the teacher as an aversive individual in their lives, someone to avoid (Benbenishty, Zeira, Astor, et al., 2002; Hyman, 1990).

Because they are unable to rely on teacher support, students subjected to ridicule, physical assault, isolation, verbal discrimination, and sexual harassment by school personnel are more likely to develop problems in school, aggressive behaviors, fearful reactions, somatic complaints, dependency, regression, and reexperiences of the trauma inflicted by the educator (Educator Induced Posttraumatic Stress Disorder [EIPTSD]((Hyman & Wise, 1979; Hyman, Zelikoff, & Clarke, 1988).

Aggressive and violent behavior against children by educators and school staff may also result in a strong "social learning" effect (Imbrogno, 2000, p. 131). Students may see these aggressive types of behavior as legitimate forms of social influence and conflict resolution. Thus, certain practices by the educational staff that were originally intended to curb student violence may actually increase the frequency and severity of violence by these students and their peers (Hyman & Perone, 1998; Hyman & Snook, 2000; Khoury-Kassabri, 2012a). Most previous research examining the contribution of staff violence on children's psychosocial outcomes focused on Western societies and has not included Palestinian children in Israel. The examination of such effects is pending.

Predictors of Staff Use of Violence toward Students

Khoury-Kassabri (2006) investigated the impact of student, family, and school factors on staff use of violence in schools. The goal of the study was to determine whether there are groups of children that are more vulnerable to maltreatment by staff and which school contexts are associated with more staff maltreatment of students.

With respect to gender difference, Jewish and Palestinian boys in Israel were more frequently emotionally, physically, or sexually victimized by school staff than girls (for similar results, see also Anderson & Payne, 1994; Gregory, 1995). The differences between boys' and girls' victimization are more pronounced with regard to physical maltreatment, and the gap is larger in Palestinian schools in Israel (fig. 15.2). Teachers may possibly maltreat boys more often because of a greater need to confront and punish them. Additionally, the differences between girls' and boys' reports of maltreatment, especially physical maltreatment, may reflect cultural values, especially in a traditional society that considers touching the female body to be inappropriate. These females may therefore be less exposed to physical maltreatment by teachers (Youssef, Attia, & Kamel, 1998).

With respect to school contextual factors, higher levels of emotional, physical, and sexual maltreatment by staff members were found in schools located in low SES communities and that had a large proportion of students from low SES families.

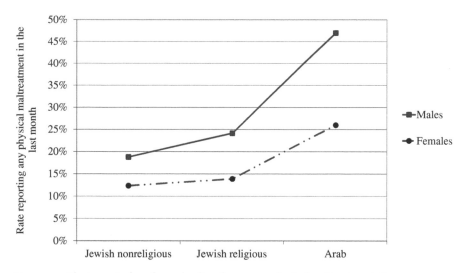

Figure 15.2. The impact of gender and cultural group on physical maltreatment. *Source:* M. Khoury-Kassabri. (2006). Student victimization by educational staff in Israel. *Child Abuse & Neglect, 30*(6), 691–707.

Parents who are economically disadvantaged may not feel involved and powerful enough in the school to speak out on behalf of their children, even when they are aware of maltreatment by school staff. In such cases, staff may feel that the parents are too stressed and powerless to question how their children are being treated by staff. Teachers may be more careful to avoid behaviors that may be questioned by involved, resourceful, and powerful parents.

In addition, students in Palestinian schools in Israel reported much more maltreatment by staff than students in Jewish Israeli schools, especially physical maltreatment, even after controlling for the SES of the school's community (fig. 15.3). Further studies are needed to disentangle the various factors responsible for this finding.

In an effort to understand these differences and the high level of Palestinian teachers' use of violence, Khoury-Kassabri (2012b) studied a large sample of homeroom teachers (382 homeroom teachers, 70.8% females) from 30 schools across Israel. Jewish teachers were also included in the study; however, as previously indicated, because of their low numbers in reporting using violence toward students, the study focused on Palestinian teachers. Self-administered questionnaires were completed, and respondents were kept anonymous. The study addressed teachers' efficacy beliefs in both academic and behavioral situations and explored the relationships of these beliefs with teachers' use of violent behavior. The findings (Khoury-Kassabri, 2012b) showed that teachers' use of physical and emotional violence was directly associated with teachers' belief in their efficacy to

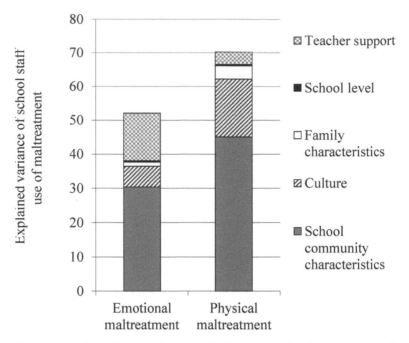

Figure 15.3. Explained variance between schools in students' maltreatment by staff. *Source:* M. Khoury-Kassabri. (2006). Student victimization by educational staff in Israel. *Child Abuse & Neglect, 30*(6), 691–707.

affect positive outcomes among their students. The greater the teachers' beliefs in their ability to deal with behavioral and emotional problems by bringing positive outcomes, the lower their reports of using emotional and physical violence toward their students.

However, teaching efficacy does not directly affect their use of physical and emotional violence. Instead, the effect of teaching efficacy is mediated by the teachers' attitudes toward the use of physical violence. The more the teachers believe that students can be taught, given their family background, SES, and school conditions (teaching efficacy), the lower their support for the use of physical violence with students and, as a result, the lower their actual use of both physical and emotional violence.

This sense of a teacher's ability to handle academic and behavioral difficulties without resorting to violence is critical when dealing with disadvantaged populations (Coleman & Karraker, 1997). In this regard, Palestinian teachers in Israel face an especially difficult task because of the inequalities of the educational system in the country and the conditions under which these teachers work (Tatar & Horenczyk, 2003). Personal efficacy is critical because in an environment of poverty and inequality, teachers may receive the message that their ability to be effective is reduced. An indication of this trend was found in the comparative study conducted by Khoury-Kassabri (2008) between Palestinian and Jewish teachers: self-efficacy was found to be significantly lower among Palestinian teachers. In addition, Palestinian teachers' approval of emotional and physical violence was significantly higher. Thus, teachers' beliefs in their efficacy and ability to bring about change in their students, despite the contextual circumstances, are crucial.

Conclusions

Research in Israel shows that Palestinian students and teachers experience high levels of victimization. This violence has many negative effects on the victims' physical, behavioral, emotional, and cognitive conditions (Daniels, Bradley, & Hays, 2007) and therefore urgently needs to be addressed.

The results of a number of studies indicate that school violence should be addressed from an ecological perspective (Barboza et al., 2009). It is important to refrain from focusing solely on the characteristics of students at risk of victimization or on the so-called troublemakers. Instead, it is essential to identify the cultural, structural, social, and school contexts in which victimization and perpetration is more prevalent. Furthermore, the study by Khoury-Kassabri et al. (2005) indicates that the effects of certain risk factors are not universal (such as the effects of SES in Jewish and Palestinian schools). Thus, assessments and interventions should be sensitive to social and cultural aspects that affect risk factors.

School climate characteristics were shown to be relevant to almost all aspects of school violence (Khoury-Kassabri et al., 2005). From a practice perspective, these results indicate that improving intraschool contexts, such as developing a comprehensive and consistent school policy and maintaining good student-teacher relationships, might be effective in reducing school violence in a wide range of contexts (Gottfredson et al., 2005; Payne et al., 2003).

Overall, the results of the presented studies strongly suggest that students in schools embedded in the most extremely impoverished neighborhoods require the highest levels of academic, social, and emotional attention and assistance.

The findings suggest that providing resources (such as well-trained school personnel; in-service training for school staff; the addition of therapeutic professionals such as social workers, counselors, and psychologists; and allocations for intervention programs) to schools to enhance the quality of the internal climate can create environments that could help protect students from the ill effects of the outer environment.

The results presented in this chapter point to the disturbing phenomenon of student victimization by school staff. The findings indicate that students who are exposed to more serious victimization by staff come from families and schools with fewer resources. Besides the need for allocating sufficient resources to these schools, this situation calls for empowering parents and children in economically disadvantaged areas to speak up, report maltreatment, and demand better care by teachers. Child and family advocates should pay special attention to establishing mechanisms to monitor and report inappropriate treatment of children by their educational staff (such as fair, open, and quick investigations of complaints made by children and consistently enforced sanctions taken against maltreating staff; encouraging teachers and other school personnel not to be part of the situation; and reporting child maltreatment by school personnel to the school principal and the Israel Ministry of Education). The main message should be that children have the right to be treated with respect and that any kind of mistreatment of children in the home or in schools is intolerable. It should also be emphasized that the use of physical punishment is considered an infraction of the rights of the child by the UN Convention on the Rights of the Child (Khoury-Kassabri & Straus, 2011).

The results presented in this chapter indicate that teachers who justify the use of violence toward students who have discipline problems and act violently toward others are more likely to use violence toward their students. Thus, to help students at risk of maltreatment, mental health practitioners and other professionals who work with parents, children, and school personnel should initiate a public campaign to raise awareness and change the attitudes and common beliefs of teachers and parents about the use of corporal punishment and the emotional abuse of children. Such a public campaign should emphasize the many negative effects of emotional and physical violence toward children.

In addition, irrespective of attitudes and ideologies, many teachers use corporal punishment because they lack the alternative skills and tools to deal with students, especially those engaged in repeated bullying or disruptive behavior (Benbenishty, 2003; Khoury-Kassabri, 2008). Hence, it is essential to support teachers, especially by providing more training and raising awareness regarding the negative effects of emotional and physical violence toward children, to help them cope effectively with difficult situations without resorting to violence. To achieve this goal, training opportunities for teachers in Israel and other countries need to be expanded. Khoury-Kassabri (2008) found that Palestinian teachers reported significantly more need for training about how to handle behavioral problems than Jewish teachers. It was also discovered that self-efficacy is significantly lower among Palestinian teachers than Jewish teachers. Therefore, more training is needed for them. This training program should pay more attention to factors that support the development of a strong sense of efficacy among teachers. More should be invested in developing teachers' beliefs about their abilities to teach and to handle the behavioral and emotional problems of their students.

Even though the focus of Khoury-Kassabri's (2010) study was not on the sociopolitical context of the Palestinian society in Israel, these aspects should not be overlooked. Palestinian citizens in Israel are a minority group characterized by higher rates of poverty and unemployment and much lower governmental expenditure of public funds for educational, health, and social services compared with the Jewish majority (Hareven, 2002). The results presented in this chapter have shown that a significant amount of the variance between school levels of staff violence toward students is attributed to the socioeconomic differences between Palestinians and Jews in Israel (Khoury-Kassabri, 2006).

In sum, the findings discussed in this chapter show that both teachers and students are exposed to high levels of violence. Interventions designed to deal with this problem should be directed to the entire school community (students, staff, and parents) rather than focusing only on violent teachers or students. This perspective captures the role of mental health practitioners who are concerned with reshaping the school environment rather than simply targeting individual students or teachers.

MONA KHOURY-KASSABRI is Professor in the School of Social Work and Social Welfare at the Hebrew University of Jerusalem, Israel.

References

Akiba, M., LeTendre, G. K., Baker, D. P., & Goesling, B. (2002). Student victimization: National and school system effects on school violence in 37 nations. *American Educational Research Journal, 39*(4), 829–853.

Amodei, N., & Scott, A. A. (2002). Psychologists' contribution to the prevention of youth violence. *Social Science Journal, 39*(4), 511–526.

Anderson, S., & Payne, M. A. (1994). Corporal punishment in elementary education: Views of Barbadian schoolchildren. *Child Abuse & Neglect, 18*(4), 377–386.

Attar-Schwartz, S., & Khoury-Kassabri, M. (2008). Indirect versus verbal forms of victimization at school: The contribution of student, family, and school variables. *Social Work Research, 32*(3), 159–170.

Barboza, G. E., Schiamberg, L. B., Oehmke, J., Korzeniewski, S. J., Post, L. A., & Heraux, C. G. (2009). Individual characteristics and the multiple contexts of adolescent bullying: An ecological perspective. *Journal of Youth and Adolescence, 38*(1), 101–121.

Beaty, L. A., & Alexeyev, E. B. (2008). The problem of school bullies: What the research tells us. *Adolescence, 43*(169), 1–11.

Benbenishty, R. (2003). *School violence in Israel.* Jerusalem: Hebrew University of Jerusalem. (Hebrew)

Benbenishty, R., & Astor, R. A. (2005). *School violence in context: Culture, neighborhood, family, school, and gender.* New York: Oxford University Press.

Benbenishty, R., Khoury-Kassabri, M., & Astor, R. A. (2006). *A national study of school violence in Israel: Implications for theory, practice, and policy* [in Hebrew]. Jerusalem: Ministry of Education.

Benbenishty, R., Zeira, A., & Astor, R. A. (2002). Children's reports of emotional, physical and sexual maltreatment by educational staff in Israel. *Child Abuse & Neglect, 26*(8), 763–782.

Benbenishty, R., Zeira, A., Astor, R. A., & Khoury-Kassabri, M. (2002). Maltreatment of primary school students by educational staff in Israel. *Child Abuse & Neglect, 26*(12), 1291–1309.

Bennett, S., Farrington, D. P., & Huesmann, L. R. (2005). Explaining gender differences in crime and violence: The importance of social cognitive skills. *Aggression and Violent Behavior, 10*(3), 263–288.

Block, J. H. (1983). Differential premises arising from differential socialization of the sexes: Some conjectures. *Child Development, 54*(6), 1335–1354.

Bronfenbrenner, U. (1979). Basic concepts. In U. Bronfenbrenner (Ed.), *The ecology of human development* (pp. 3–15). Cambridge, MA: Harvard University Press.

Cohen, A. (2007). An examination of the relationship between commitments and culture among five cultural groups of Israeli teachers. *Journal of Cross-Cultural Psychology, 38*(1), 34–49.

Cohen, M. A., & Piquero, A. R. (2009). New evidence on the monetary value of saving a high risk youth. *Journal of Quantitative Criminology, 25*(1), 25–49.

Coie, J. D., Lochman, J. E., Terry, R., & Hyman, C. (1992). Predicting early adolescent disorder from childhood aggression and peer rejection. *Journal of Consulting and Clinical Psychology, 60*(5), 783–792.

Coleman, P. K., & Karraker, K. H. (1997). Self-efficacy and parenting quality: Findings and future applications. *Developmental Review, 18*(1), 47–85.

Coyne, S. M., Archer, J., & Eslea, M. (2006). "We're not friends anymore! Unless . . .": The frequency and harmfulness of indirect, relational, and social aggression. *Aggressive Behavior, 32*(4), 294–307.

Crick, N. R. (1997). Engagement in gender normative versus nonnormative forms of aggression: Links to social–psychological adjustment. *Developmental Psychology, 33*(4), 610–617.

Crick, N. R., Casas, J. F., & Mosher, M. (1997). Relational and overt aggression in preschool. *Developmental Psychology, 33*(4), 579–588.

Crick, N. R., & Grotpeter, J. K. (1995). Relational aggression, gender, and social-psychological adjustment. *Child Development, 66*(3), 710–722.

Daniels, J. A., Bradley, M. C., & Hays, M. (2007). The impact of school violence on school personnel: Implications for psychologists. *Professional Psychology: Research and Practice, 38*(6), 652–659.

Dupper, D. R., & Meyer-Adams, N. (2002). Low-level violence a neglected aspect of school culture. *Urban Education, 37*(3), 350–364.

Dwyer, K. P., Osher, D., & Hoffman, C. C. (2000). Creating responsive schools: Contextualizing early warning, timely response. *Exceptional Children, 66*(3), 347–365.

Emmer, E. T., & Hickman, J. (1991). Teacher efficacy in classroom management and discipline. *Educational and Psychological Measurement, 51*(3), 755–765.

Geving, A. M. (2007). Identifying the types of student and teacher behaviours associated with teacher stress. *Teaching and Teacher Education, 23*(5), 624–640.

Gottfredson, G. D., Gottfredson, D. C., Payne, A. A., & Gottfredson, N. C. (2005). School climate predictors of school disorder: Results from a national study of delinquency prevention in schools. *Journal of Research in Crime and Delinquency, 42*(4), 412–444.

Gregory, J. F. (1995). The crime of punishment: Racial and gender disparities in the use of corporal punishment in US public schools. *Journal of Negro Education, 64*(4), 454–462.

Haj-Yahia, M. M. (1995). Toward culturally sensitive intervention with Arab families in Israel. *Contemporary Family Therapy, 17*(4), 429–447.

Haj-Yahia, M. M. (2000). Wife abuse and battering in the sociocultural context of Arab society. *Family Process, 39*(2), 237–255.

Haj-Yahia, M. M. (2002). Attitudes of Arab women toward different patterns of coping with wife abuse. *Journal of Interpersonal Violence, 17*(7), 721–745.

Hareven, A. (2002). Towards the year 2030: Can a civil society shared by Jews and Arabs evolve in Israel? *International Journal of Intercultural Relations, 26*(2), 153–168.

Hawker, D. S., & Boulton, M. J. (2000). Twenty years' research on peer victimization and psychosocial maladjustment: A meta-analytic review of cross-sectional studies. *Journal of Child Psychology and Psychiatry, 41*(4), 441–455.

Hyman, I. A. (1990). *Reading, writing, and the hickory stick*. Lexington, MA: Lexington Books.

Hyman, I. A., & Perone, D. C. (1998). The other side of school violence: Educator policies and practices that may contribute to student misbehavior. *Journal of School Psychology, 36*(1), 7–27.

Hyman, I. A., & Snook, P. A. (2000). Dangerous schools and what you can do about them. *Phi Delta Kappan, 81*(7), 489–501.

Hyman, I. A., & Wise, J. H. (1979). *Corporal punishment in American education.* Philadelphia: Temple University Press.

Hyman, I. A., Zelikoff, W., & Clarke, J. (1988). Psychological and physical abuse in the schools: A paradigm for understanding post-traumatic stress disorder in children and youth. *Journal of Traumatic Stress, 1*(2), 243–267.

Imbrogno, A. R. (2000). Corporal punishment in America's public schools and the UN convention on the rights of the child: A case for nonratification. *Journal of Law and Education, 29*(2), 125–147.

Innes, J., & Kitto, S. (1989). Neuroticism, self-consciousness and coping strategies, and occupational stress in high school teachers. *Personality and Individual Differences, 10*(3), 303–312.

Khoury-Kassabri, M. (2006). Student victimization by educational staff in Israel. *Child Abuse & Neglect, 30*(6), 691–707.

Khoury-Kassabri, M. (2008). *The relationship between teachers' self-efficacy and attitudes toward the use of violence and teachers' use of violence toward students* [in Hebrew]. Jerusalem: Hebrew University of Jerusalem.

Khoury-Kassabri, M. (2011). Student victimization by peers in elementary schools: Individual, teacher-class, and school-level predictors. *Child Abuse & Neglect, 35*(4), 273–282.

Khoury-Kassabri, M. (2012a). Perpetration of aggressive behaviors against peers and teachers as predicted by student and contextual factors. *Aggressive Behavior, 38*(4), 253–262.

Khoury-Kassabri, M. (2012b). The relationship between teacher self-efficacy and violence toward students as mediated by teacher's attitude. *Social Work Research, 36*(2), 127–139.

Khoury-Kassabri, M., Astor, R. A., & Benbenishty, R. (2009). Middle Eastern adolescents' perpetration of school violence against peers and teachers: A cross-cultural and ecological analysis. *Journal of Interpersonal Violence, 24*(1), 159–182.

Khoury-Kassabri, M., Attar-Schwartz, S., & Zur, H. (2014). The likelihood of using corporal punishment by kindergarten teachers: The role of parent-teacher partnership, attitudes, and religiosity. *Child Indicators Research, 7*(2), 369–386.

Khoury-Kassabri, M., Benbenishty, R., & Astor, R. A. (2005). The effects of school climate, socioeconomics, and cultural factors on student victimization in Israel. *Social Work Research, 29*(3), 165–180.

Khoury-Kassabri, M., Benbenishty, R., Astor, R. A., & Zeira, A. (2004). The contributions of community, family, and school variables to student victimization. *American Journal of Community Psychology, 34*(3–4), 187–204.

Khoury-Kassabri, M., & Straus, M. A. (2011). Discipline methods used by mothers: The contribution of ethnicity, socioeconomic status, and child's characteristics. *Child Indicators Research, 4*(1), 45–57.

Kingery, P. M., Coggeshall, M. B., & Alford, A. A. (1998). Violence at school: Recent evidence from four national surveys. *Psychology in the Schools, 35*(3), 247–258.

Kop, Y. (2005). *Israel's social services 2004.* Jerusalem: Taub Center for Social Policy Studies in Israel.(Hebrew)

Kuppens, S., Grietens, H., Onghena, P., Michiels, D., & Subramanian, S. (2008). Individual and classroom variables associated with relational aggression in elementary-school aged children: A multilevel analysis. *Journal of School Psychology, 46*(6), 639–660.

Landau, S. F., Björkqvist, K., Lagerspetz, K. M., Österman, K., & Gideon, L. (2002). The effect of religiosity and ethnic origin on direct and indirect aggression among males and females: Some Israeli findings. *Aggressive Behavior, 28*(4), 281–298.

Leadbeater, B. J., Boone, E. M., Sangster, N. A., & Mathieson, L. C. (2006). Sex differences in the personal costs and benefits of relational and physical aggression in high school. *Aggressive Behavior, 32*(4), 409–419.

Limbos, M. A., Chan, L. S., Warf, C., Schneir, A., Iverson, E., Shekelle, P., & Kipke, M. D. (2007). Effectiveness of interventions to prevent youth violence: A systematic review. *American Journal of Preventive Medicine, 33*(1), 65–74.

Martin, A. J., Linfoot, K., & Stephenson, J. (1999). How teachers respond to concerns about misbehavior in their classroom. *Psychology in the Schools, 36*(4), 347–358.

McMahon, S. D., & Washburn, J. J. (2003). Violence prevention: An evaluation of program effects with urban African American students. *Journal of Primary Prevention, 24*(1), 43–62.

Mercy, J. A., & Rosenberg, M. L. (1998). Preventing firearm violence in and around schools. In D. S. Elliot, B. A. Hamburg, & K. R. Williams (Eds.), *Violence in American schools: A new perspective* (pp. 159–187). New York: Cambridge University Press.

Mikulincer, M., Weller, A., & Florian, V. (1993). Sense of closeness to parents and family rules: A study of Arab and Jewish youth in Israel. *International Journal of Psychology, 28*(3), 323–335.

Mishna, F. (2012). *Bullying: A relationship-based guide to assessment, prevention, and intervention*. New York: Oxford University Press.

Ostrov, J. M., & Keating, C. F. (2004). Gender differences in preschool aggression during free play and structured interactions: An observational study. *Social Development, 13*(2), 255–277.

Owens, L., Daly, A., & Slee, P. (2005). Sex and age differences in victimisation and conflict resolution among adolescents in a south Australian school. *Aggressive Behavior, 31*(1), 1–12.

Payne, A. A., Gottfredson, D. C., & Gottfredson, G. D. (2003). Schools as communities: The relationships among communal school organization, student bonding, and school disorder. *Criminology, 41*(3), 749–778.

Schreck, C. J., Miller, J. M., & Gibson, C. L. (2003). Trouble in the school yard: A study of the risk factors of victimization at school. *Crime & Delinquency, 49*(3), 460–484.

Schwartz, D., Gorman, A. H., Nakamoto, J., & McKay, T. (2006). Popularity, social acceptance, and aggression in adolescent peer groups: Links with academic performance and school attendance. *Developmental Psychology, 42*(6), 1116–1127.

Smith, P. K., Madsen, K. C., & Moody, J. C. (1999). What causes the age decline in reports of being bullied at school? Towards a developmental analysis of risks of being bullied. *Educational Research, 41*(3), 267–285.

Stewart, E. A. (2003). School social bonds, school climate, and school misbehavior: A multilevel analysis. *Justice Quarterly, 20*(3), 575–604.

Tatar, M., & Horenczyk, G. (2003). Dilemmas and strategies in the counselling of Jewish and Palestinian Arab children in Israeli schools. *British Journal of Guidance & Counselling, 31*(4), 375–391.

Ttofi, M. M., Farrington, D. P., Lösel, F., & Loeber, R. (2011a). Do the victims of school bullies tend to become depressed later in life? A systematic review and meta-analysis of longitudinal studies. *Journal of Aggression, Conflict, and Peace Research, 3*(2), 63–73.

Ttofi, M. M., Farrington, D. P., Lösel, F., & Loeber, R. (2011b). The predictive efficiency of school bullying versus later offending: A systematic/meta-analytic review of longitudinal studies. *Criminal Behaviour and Mental Health, 21*(2), 80–89.

Welsh, W. N., Greene, J. R., & Jenkins, P. H. (1999). School disorder: The influence of individual, institutional, and community factors. *Criminology, 37*(1), 73–116.

Wilson, H. (1980). Parental supervision: A neglected aspect of delinquency. *British Journal of Criminology, 20*(3), 203–235.

Wolkind, S., & Rutter, M. (1994). Sociocultural factors. In L. A. Hersov, M. Rutter, & E. Taylor (Eds.), *Child and adolescent psychiatry: Modern approaches* (pp. 83–100). Oxford, UK: Blackwell Scientific.

Youssef, R. M., Attia, M. S.-E.-D., & Kamel, M. I. (1998). Children experiencing violence II: Prevalence and determinants of corporal punishment in schools. *Child Abuse & Neglect, 22*(10), 975–985.

Zahn-Waxler, C., & Polanichka, N. (2004). All things interpersonal: Socialization and female aggression. In M. Pullataz & K. L. Bierman (Eds.), *Aggression, antisocial behavior, and violence among girls: A developmental perspective* (pp. 48–68). New York: Guilford.

16

INTIMATE PARTNER VIOLENCE AGAINST PALESTINIAN WOMEN IN ISRAEL AND THE RELEVANCE OF THE SOCIOCULTURAL AND SOCIOPOLITICAL CONTEXT

Raghda Alnabilsy and Haneen Elias

THIS CHAPTER DEALS WITH THE PROBLEM OF INTIMATE partner violence (IPV) against engaged and married Palestinian women in Israel. We present a definition of the problem and examine dimensions, consequences, and strategies for coping with it and consider the relevance of the sociocultural and sociopolitical context of Palestinian society in Israel. As we present the existing information, we also attempt to point out the knowledge that is still lacking in this field.

Notably, most of the information we have about the problem of violence against women has been collected from studies done in Western societies, which are substantially different from conservative and collectivist societies, such as the Palestinian society in Israel (Haj-Yahia, 2011; Haj-Yahia & Shhadi, 2005). In Western societies, the sociocultural context (e.g., the status of the family in society and in the life of the individual in particular; expectations of marriage and spousal relations; and the status of women in the private, family, and public domains) is significantly different from that of Palestinian citizens in Israel. This is also true of the sociopolitical context (e.g., the availability of health and welfare services, perception of the majority society and its institutions by the Palestinian minority, poverty and unemployment, and the national and civil status of Palestinian citizens in Israel). In addition, existing research on violence against women in the Arab world does not represent the unique political context of Palestinian women in Israel. Note here that the latter are part of an indigenous national minority living under Israeli rule since 1948, while women in Arab countries are part of their country's majority (Shalhoub-Kevorkian, 2004).

Definition of the Problem of Violence against Women

Violence against women takes place behind closed doors in the home. Although one of the most severe problems in the world, it is hidden and understated (Alnabilsy, 2013). IPV refers to physical, sexual, emotional, verbal, economic, spiritual, and/or social abuse on the part of one partner (typically the male) against the other (Iverson et al., 2013; Lawson, 2012; Walker, 2009). This definition is accepted among all or almost all mental health professionals. However, additional patterns of violence against Palestinian women are relevant to the sociocultural and sociopolitical context of Palestinian society in Israel (Haj-Yahia, 2000b; Shalhoub-Kevorkian, 2000, 2010). Shoham (2012) indicated that one of the main problems entailed in defining violence against Palestinian women in Israel relates to various social and cultural perceptions of women, particularly in the family. Indeed, cultural differences sometimes do not allow for a unified definition of domestic violence and violence against women in different societies, and a consensus cannot be reached.

Examination of the sociopolitical context of violence against Palestinian women in Israel indicates that these women have been exposed to violence based on gender, socioeconomic status, and nationality, as well as to political violence. Following the Nakba in 1948, Palestinian residents of Israel became an indigenous minority in a state with a Jewish majority (Ghanem, 2011). Palestinian women were harmed more than men by the political and economic crisis that affected the entire Palestinian society as a result of their relatively low social, economic, and political status. These women were required to absorb, contain, and cope with the crises, political traumas, and frustrations experienced by men in the Palestinian family and society (Shalhoub-Kevorkian & Daher-Nashif, 2013). In addition, then as today, women have had to bear responsibility for managing the household, educating and caring for the children, and maintaining the family unit. They were also expected to refrain from divorce and preserve the good reputation of their families and partners (Haj-Yahia, 2011; Shalhoub-Kevorkian & Daher-Nashif, 2013).

Curiously, only a few studies have addressed the characterization of violence as it is actually reported by Palestinian women in Israel in terms of the sociocultural and sociopolitical context of the Palestinian minority in Israel (Haj-Yahia, 2000b; Haj-Yahia & Shhadi, 2005; Shalhoub-Kevorkian, 2010). Haj-Yahia (2000b) interpreted various behaviors of Palestinian women who are victims of violence in the sociocultural context of Palestinian society, which is characterized by such values as maintaining the woman's honor vis-à-vis her children and enhancing her status as a mother; maintaining the woman's honor vis-à-vis the husband's family and enhancing her status in the extended family system; maintaining the family's privacy and preventing outsiders from knowing about or intervening in the situation; maintaining the good reputation of the woman, her sisters, and her daughters in the community and refraining from insulting them in public; and maintaining the woman's status as the parent who educates her children and manages the household. Harmful behaviors and verbal abuse by the woman's partner, such as insulting her in front of her children or family, undermining her maternal role in the presence of the children, and other behaviors were described by the victims as violent acts that harm them and their families.

In the professional literature on the definition of violence against Palestinian women in Israel, there is almost no mention of the experiences of the women as previously described. Alnabilsy (2013) examined the experiences of women in Israel who are victims of violence and live with their partners. The women participating in that study mentioned that they also experienced violence by the extended family as well as social violence by neighbors, friends, and acquaintances. In addition, the Palestinian women described their experience with unintended harm caused by services and social agencies when they sought assistance to deal with instances of IPV. Specifically, this harm is manifested by the agencies' lack of understanding and insensitivity to the context the victims live in, as well as by the provision of services ill-suited to the needs of the women and their children, by the social services' perception of the women as resistant. They are perceived so because they tend to fit the conditions of their lives to that of their husbands, on one hand, and refuse to accept the services offered to them by the social services, on the other. Moreover, these women usually have difficulty in dealing with these services because they are not fluent in Hebrew. We believe that further research and a new conceptualization of the problem of violence against Palestinian women is necessary to address all of the components of the problem in the context of the Palestinian family and society, as well as in the context of Israeli society as a whole. The definition of the problem of violence against Palestinian women in Israel is related to conservative, traditional social and cultural norms—specifically to nonegalitarian relations between men and women as well as to the patriarchal, collective character of Palestinian society (Haj-Yahia, 2011).

Therefore, future research should rely on a broad definition of violence against Palestinian women in Israel while examining the systems in the woman's environment that might be involved in harming her, as well as the social, cultural, and political context previously described. This new definition should include various types of violence by the woman's partner, family members, community, and formal and informal community agencies.

The Incidence of Violence against Palestinian Women in Israel

It is important to note the lack of research aimed at estimating the incidence of IPV against Palestinian women in Israel. The dearth of research evidence may emphasize the complexity of the problem, as reflected in attempts to hide it and in the lack of consensus regarding the different definitions of violence against women (Malley-Morrison & Hines, 2004; Shoham, 2012; Stover, 2005). In addition, there is a tendency in Palestinian society to downplay violent incidents in the family, to refrain from reporting them, and to avoid lodging complaints to formal agencies that are viewed, rightly or wrongly, as representing and serving the Israeli establishment. Thus, inaccurate estimates may also be partly because only cases that are reported and known to the welfare services and the police are documented. Moreover, there is no documentation relating to violence against women by people other than the intimate partner, such as other family members (Alnabilsy, 2013).

A summary of findings from two surveys that evaluated the incidence of IPV against women in Palestinian society are presented next. The first survey included 1,111 engaged women (Haj-Yahia, 2000a), and the second included 2,102 married women (Haj-Yahia, 2000b). In the first survey, the women were asked whether they had experienced verbal/psychological, physical, or sexual abuse by their partner during the engagement period. In the second, the women were asked whether they had experienced the same types of violence during the 12 months preceding the survey.

The first survey indicated that, with regard to verbal and psychological aggression, 48% of the engaged Palestinian women reported that their fiancé had yelled, threatened, or humiliated them; approximately 12% reported that their fiancé had insulted and sworn at them; and approximately 11% reported that their fiancé had scorned, ignored, or belittled them. The engaged women were also presented with 12 acts that measured their experience with physical aggression: 10% reported that their fiancé had forcefully pushed or grabbed them; about 9%, that their fiancé had slapped their face or another part of their body during an argument or disagreement; and approximately 3% reported that their fiancé had hit them hard in different parts of their body and had continued to hit them for several minutes. Approximately 2% reported that their fiancé had threatened them with a knife or gun but had not continued with the threat, and approximately 1% reported that their fiancé had actually assaulted them with a knife or gun at least once during the period of their engagement. In addition, the engaged women were presented with three acts that measured their experience with sexual coercion by their fiancé during the engagement. About 11% reported that their fiancé had insisted on having sexual relations against their will (but did not use physical force); approximately 5% reported that their fiancé had used physical force (including hitting and threats with a weapon) to force them to have sexual relations at least once (Haj-Yahia, 2000a).

In the second survey, among married women, the reports related to events that had taken place at least once during the 12 months prior to the survey. The findings revealed that with regard to verbal and psychological abuse by the husband, 37.2% of the women reported that they had experienced a feeling of hostility; 69.5%, that their husbands had yelled at and humiliated them; 16.6%, that their husbands had made fun of their appearance; 23.5%, that their husbands had prevented them from seeing their family, relatives, and friends; and 21.7% reported that they had been told they were worth less without their husband (Haj-Yahia, 2000b). In this survey, the women were also presented with 12 situations of violence that measured their experience with physical violence by their husband during the 12 months prior to the survey. The findings showed that 21.8% of the women reported that their husbands had pulled them by force; 18.5%, that their husbands had twisted their arm; 13.4%, that their husbands had pushed them over and continued to kick them; 11.6%, that their husbands had hit them hard with a stick, belt, chair, or similar object; 3%, that their husbands had threatened them with a knife or gun; and 2.2% reported that their husbands had assaulted them with a knife or gun. In addition, the married women participating in this survey were asked about their experience with sexual abuse by their husband. Sixteen percent of the women reported that their husbands had insisted on having sexual relations in various ways that caused them discomfort; 7%, that their husbands had used threats to force them to have sex; and 3.5% reported that their husbands had used physical force (including hitting them and threatening them with a weapon) to force them to have sex (Haj-Yahia, 2000b). In both surveys, the women were asked about their experience with economic abuse (being kept dependent on the partner, who controlled all the resources) and with violence by other people in their family, community, and society or harm by informal and formal agents when they sought assistance.

An Israeli national survey conducted in 2001 examined both the incidence of IPV against women and attitudes about the problem of violence against women in Israel. The survey sample consisted of 2,544 families from different localities and cultures in Israel. The findings indicated that in Muslim Palestinian families, the rate of violence was higher than in Jewish families. Families from both societies that reported violence against women were characterized as traditional, conservative, and religious; they had lower levels of education; the men were younger and unemployed; the women victims were unemployed; the families had more economic difficulties; and the average number of years of marriage was lower (Eisikovits, Winstok, & Fishman, 2004). These findings support the argument put forth in the professional literature that societies with relatively high rates of IPV against women, such as the Palestinian society, are characterized by, for example, a patriarchal culture in terms of gender roles; emphasis on the values of family unity; priority of the national group over the emotional and physical well-being of the individual and over human and civil rights; social exclusion; and high rates of problems such as unemployment, poverty, and community violence (Haj-Yahia & Peled, 2013; Levinson, 1989; Malley-Morrison & Hines, 2004) .Additionally, the survey findings emphasized the difficult reality that Palestinian families have experienced since the establishment of the state of Israel, as well as the inequality between Palestinian society in Israel and the majority society in the areas of education, welfare, health, industrialization, employment, mobility, housing, and law enforcement (Ghanem, 2002; Rouhana, 1997). These attributions might provide insights into why the incidence of IPV is higher among Palestinian women than among Jewish women in Israel. Moreover, Palestinian society has conservative expectations of women who face violence and sometimes even places the responsibility and blame for violence on them, whereas attitudes toward violent husbands are lenient (Haj-Yahia, 2002). It is possible that these two contexts (cultural and political) constitute risk factors that underlie the higher percentages of violence among Palestinian women and families in Israel.

In light of this situation, and as alluded to earlier, we propose additional studies that would provide more accurate measures of the problem of IPV against Palestinian women based on some of the broad definitions of the problem. Studies should also investigate additional populations of Palestinian women in Israel who are victims of violence and who have not been examined to date. These populations include young Palestinian women who have experienced violence by their boyfriend, fiancé, or partner; divorced Palestinian women who have custody of their children; older women who are victims of violence; women who are victims of violence and do not have legal status in Israel (mainly Palestinian women from the occupied territories, who are married to Palestinian men in Israel but do not have a legal status as citizens of Israel); and women living in various regions who have a variety of sociodemographic characteristics (e.g., age, education, religion, years of marriage, number of children). In addition, instruments must be developed to address the difficulties and barriers faced in the attempt to estimate the problem of violence (e.g., failure to report violence and the unique contexts of Palestinian society in Israel mentioned earlier).

Consequences of Violence against Women

Life in the shadow of violence has numerous consequences for all aspects of a woman's life (behavioral, cognitive, emotional, functional, and social). In addition, IPV has consequences for the children and for the women's family members (Iverson et al., 2013). Recent studies have emphasized that the consequences experienced by women from ethnic minorities in a country are more severe than those experienced by women from the majority group (Akyüz, Yavan, Şahiner, & Kiliç, 2012; Hamza, 2010; Iverson et al., 2013; Rafaeili, 2012). Research findings have also revealed that the women's socioeconomic status, ethnic affiliation, immigration, and cultural/political context can intensify the consequences of violence (Abu-Ras, 2007; Dutton, 2009; Edelson, Hokoda, & Ramos-Lira, 2007; Hamza, 2010; Iverson et al., 2013; Malley-Morrison & Hines, 2004; Rafaeili, 2012). Against this background, over the past decade, research has aimed to identify the factors that make some women more vulnerable to violence. Furthermore, researchers have begun to recognize the importance of understanding the sociocultural and sociopolitical context of women who are victims of violence and the reported consequences (Sabina, Cuevas, & Schally, 2012). For example, Cwikel, Lev-Wiesel, and Al-Krenawi (2003) conducted a study among Bedouin women in the Negev who had experienced physical violence to examine the mental and physical health consequences. In that study, the women indicated that the violence was directly related to poor mental health (depression, low self-esteem, helplessness, hopelessness, low social support), gynecological symptoms, and a tendency toward general morbidity. In Haj-Yahia's survey (2000b), married Palestinian women were presented with six questions about the consequences of physical violence for them. The findings revealed that 14.6% of the women reported feeling intense pain after the assault; about 3.2%, that they had suffered fractures in various parts of their bodies as a result of the physical assault; and about 4%, that they had fainted when their husband assaulted them. In addition, 46%–62% of the women indicated that IPV is often dangerous not only for the woman but also for the entire family system. They perceived the violence as having the potential to undermine family solidarity. A substantial percentage of women (47%–61%) tended to believe that IPV is often dangerous because it can harm the woman's status in the community (as a mother, housewife, woman) and cause disputes between her family of origin and her husband's family of origin.

These findings, which relate to the extent of danger as a consequence of violence, are explained by the sociocultural context of Palestinian society. In this context, emphasis is placed on family solidarity and on the sanctity of the family at almost any price, as well as on maintaining the woman's honor, status, reputation, and image vis-à-vis her children and community. In addition, women are expected to maintain their roles as mother and wife despite the violence and to maintain the relationship between the couples' families of origin. In the survey relating to the consequences among engaged Palestinian women who had experienced psychological, physical, and sexual abuse by their fiancés, the participants reported lower self-esteem and higher levels of depression, anxiety, and feelings of stress than women who had not experienced abuse by their fiancés (Haj-Yahia, 2000a).

Another study examined the consequences of violence as reflected in the experience of Palestinian mothers in Israel who are victims of IPV and how that abuse affected their children (Arda, 2006). The women participating in the study described extreme changes in their own behavior and the behavior of their children as a result of the violence perpetrated by the partner. They further indicated that these changes had brought them to the point where they hit and abused their children. The experience of motherhood was portrayed as arousing fear, anger, stress, and violence against their children. These descriptions contradict the prevailing view that motherhood is an experience of wholeness and strength that unifies and maintains the family, even in cases of domestic violence. The women in this study also indicated that their partner's violence had accompanied them since the beginning of the marriage, and they perceived it as a destructive force that harmed their motherhood, their family, and their children. The experience of violence aroused in them a sense of loneliness, mental fatigue, physical exhaustion, economic distress, and burnout in their maternal role. Those outcomes are accompanied by the social expectations of the Palestinian woman's role as wife and mother and her obligation to maintain the family, the marriage, respect, and faithfulness to the husband, and to family relationships (Arda, 2006).

Similar findings were identified in a US study that focused on the sense of stress and overload aroused by the maternal role among women who are victims of IPV. Edelson et al. (2007) compared Latino women in the United States (who had immigrated from South America or Mexico, or who were from the United States) and non-Latino women, with emphasis on the social, cultural, and political context of ethnic minorities. The study revealed that the Latino women, part of a minority group, who had experienced IPV reported more stress in their maternal roles than did non-Latino women from the majority group. The Latino women also reported higher levels of symptoms related to trauma and depression, as well as lower personal and social esteem. In addition, positive events played a less significant role in their lives (Edelson et al., 2007). These differences were associated with rigid, conservative social and cultural expectations from Latino women with regard to motherhood and responsibility to their children. In that study, the Latino women who were victims of IPV indicated that they felt a part of their family and their community. They needed to be an integral part of their society and to meet the expectations of being mothers despite the violence against them. These social expectations posed a heavy burden on the victimized women. Moreover, their status as members of a low SES minority with a limited command of the majority language (English) further intensified their sense of distress, helplessness, and hopelessness as well as the burden posed by motherhood. This might have even prevented them from seeking external assistance, although they believed that such help was suited to their needs and the needs of their children (Edelson et al., 2007).

Another qualitative study examined the practical consequences of violence against Palestinian women while focusing on women's resources and the potential importance of the sociocultural and sociopolitical context of Palestinian society to these consequences (Alnabilsy, 2013). The study findings identified damage and adverse consequences at the personal level with regard to physical, emotional, cognitive, and behavioral/functional components, as well as in other aspects of the women's lives. These included negative consequences for interpersonal relations within and outside of the family, such as the women's perceptions of motherhood and marital relations. Other consequences documented in that study related to the sociocultural context—for example, negative consequences for the woman's status and social position and being treated with contempt. The participants also described negative consequences for their daughters, for women in their extended family, and for their parents as a result of being abused. These findings highlighted the relevance of the sociocultural context of Palestinian society, where women are expected to give priority to their children, their families, their marriage, their respect, and their collective loyalty over their personal well-being.

Another aspect of Alnabilsy's (2013) study relates to the women's social context, status, and political context, which is perceived as intensifying the emotional, cognitive, and behavioral consequences of violence for them. For example, the participants described the consequences of the violence for their motherhood, as reflected in violent behavior or impatience toward their children or in attempts to compensate the children for their hard lives. These consequences highlight the unique difficulties and challenges that women who are victims of IPV face as mothers, including the damage to their parental competence owing to restriction of material, emotional, and social resources. The difficulties also include economic problems, moving to a different home, violence by people around them, humiliation, and accusations. Other implications for the victims' status as women and mothers is reflected in their fear that society or the social services and therapists will criticize their functioning as mothers and spouses. In addition to cultural and social norms that increase the stress and emotional consequences of violence experienced by Palestinian women in Israel, the sociopolitical context of these women is another factor that intensifies their distress. This context also leads them to perceive their situation as hopeless and to feel helpless not only in terms of their status in the family and the community but also in the broader context of Israeli society. All of the women participating in this study assessed their economic situation as low-to-average, and the employed women described their work conditions as difficult and unstable. The women also described their social, economic, and employment statuses and their level of education as low. This was aggravated by many years of violence in their marriage; it intensified the cycle of violence and increased the women's emotional burden as well as the consequences for their parenthood. In addition, it was more difficult for them to break the cycle of violence, fulfill themselves, function as mothers, and maintain family harmony. Three of the women participating in the study indicated that the severe violence, the social and family pressure, and the lack of external support from the state in matters such as housing, employment, and assistance for them and their children intensified their stress and emotional burden, and even led them to attempt suicide (Alnabilsy, 2013).

In light of existing studies on the consequences of IPV for Palestinian women in Israel, we have noted that there is a dearth of research on the topic, and that no studies have considered the context of Palestinian women in Israel as an indigenous national minority; nor have any studies examined the relationship of this context to the consequences of violence against these women and their family members. The review of relevant research indicates that most of the existing studies examined the consequences of violence for the women from an objective point of view and were based on a quantitative design (Haj-Yahia, 2000a, 2000b). Other studies have only examined the women's experience of violence by their husbands and its consequences (Shoham, 2012). Very few studies have examined other violence that women experience by family members, acquaintances, and their social environment and the consequences of that violence. Moreover, the studies that have been conducted did not emphasize the contribution of sociodemographic variables (age, education, income, employment, religion, place of residence) to the consequences of IPV for women. Briere and Jordan (2004) showed that variables such as age, gender, socioeconomic status, existing or previous psychological disorders, a history of family dysfunction, psychological background, and sociocultural context can intervene and affect the psychological responses of women who are victims of violence and even intensify postvictimization and psychological consequences. Some researchers in this field have highlighted the importance of conducting qualitative studies to gain further insights into the complexity of the problem and its consequences based on victims' narratives (Loxton, Schofield, & Hussain, 2006).

In the context of Palestinian women in Israel, research is needed that includes variables that have not yet been examined among Palestinian victims of IPV and that can shed light on the relationship of these variables to consequences of violence. The variables that should be examined include rates of depression, decline in functioning and work, diminished economic well-being, damage to the marital and social systems, and damage to motherhood and maternal functioning, among others. It is important to examine how duration, intensity, and type of violence are related to long-term emotional, physical, functional, social, and cognitive consequences of this violence.

Coping and Help-Seeking Strategies

The professional literature relates to three main types of strategies that women use to cope with IPV. Emotional coping strategies include coping as a victim, as a helpless person, and as a survivor (Mills, 1985; Walker, 2009; Wilcox, 2006). Cognitive strategies include redefining and restructuring reality to justify the violence (Eisikovits, Goldblatt, & Winstok, 1999) or focusing on the cause of violence by blaming oneself and others (Clements & Sawhney, 2000). Behavioral strategies include fighting back (Abraham, 2000; Dutton, 1996); seeking formal and informal help (Barnett, 2001; Haj-Yahia & Shhadi, 2005); and final or recurrent separation from the partner, leaving the partner, and divorce (Gharaibeh & Oweis, 2009; Okour & Badarneh, 2011). Today, the professional literature relates to coping as a continuous process that can change over time and throughout the woman's life with her partner. In addition, coping strategies are generally viewed along a continuum: the women who are victims of IPV use a range of strategies. The perception of the woman as coping passively with violence and as helpless is at one end of the continuum; the perception of the woman as actively resisting the violence, even resorting to the rare strategy of murdering her violent partner, is at the other end (Smith & Wehrle, 2010).

Examination of the research literature on strategies for coping with IPV among Palestinian women in Israel shows that very few studies have dealt with this issue in terms of the sociocultural and sociopolitical context, as mentioned earlier. The few studies that have actually addressed strategies for coping with IPV among Palestinian women in Israel in terms of the relevance of the sociocultural and sociopolitical context of Palestinian society to their situation include the study by Haj-Yahia and Shhadi (2005). In addition, a few studies have examined the attitudes and beliefs of Palestinian women about different strategies for coping with IPV (Haj-Yahia, 2000b, 2002, 2003a, 2003b). There are also a few studies that relate to how Palestinian women cope with IPV through the use of formal services and the Israel police. These include difficulties in seeking help from the police, lack of trust in the social services, lack of understanding, and institutional insensitivity toward the lives of Palestinian women in Israel (Eisikovits, Buchbinder, & Bshara, 2008; Shalhoub-Kevorkian, 2000, 2004).

Haj-Yahia and Shhadi (2005) discussed two theories that explain and describe how women cope with IPV: learned helplessness (Seligman, 1975); and survival theory (Gondolf & Fisher, 1988). However, these theories have not been examined in collectivist contexts such as Palestinian society in Israel (Haj-Yahia & Shhadi, 2005). Moreover, the findings of Haj-Yahia (2000b) contradict the assumption that Palestinian women cope passively with violence against them and reconcile themselves to it. In that survey, it was found that Palestinian women in Israel use various strategies and means to combat violence against them despite their isolation, the lack of suitable formal and informal resources, and the complexity of their sociocultural context. Haj-Yahia and Shhadi (2005) explained how the strategies of Palestinian women in Israel for combating and coping with violence against them are affected by their personal and environmental resources as well as by the alternatives available to them, by their cultural context, and by the sociopolitical conditions of Palestinian society. According to Haj-Yahia and Shhadi (2005) these women deal with personal and sociocultural obstacles and limitations as well as with sociopolitical structures to combat the violence.

We examined the relevance of these variables on the basis of the three types of coping strategies previously presented. The findings revealed the following: (1) At the level of personal strategies, the women tried to appease and placate their husbands, stay away from them so that the man would refrain from violent behavior, apologize to them, and not anger them. (2) The women sought help from informal agencies when they saw that the personal strategies did not stop the violence against them. At first, they tried to receive help from their families of origin; afterward, they sought help from their husbands' families, from friends, or from neighbors (the least preferred strategy). (3) The women went to formal agencies as a last resort to receive support and guidance in stopping the husband's violence, as well as assistance and guidance for the husband and family. This also included requests for protection and shelter in case the husband continued his violence. The women mentioned that when they sought formal help, they had no intention of taking revenge or belittling their husband and his family, nor did they intend to divorce. Rather, they did so in the hope of treating the problem of violence and bringing it to an end.

Examination of the strategies adopted by Palestinian women indicates that they had internalized both the traditional norms accepted by women who are victims of violence and the social expectations that they would maintain the family unit, care for the welfare of their children, preserve the institution of marriage, and maintain harmony in the family. In addition, the findings indicate that the women had internalized traditional feminine and masculine roles in Palestinian society, as they attempted to solve their problems within the family and refrained from seeking help from external formal agencies (Haj-Yahia & Shhadi, 2005).

Another study conducted by Haj-Yahia (2002) examined attitudes regarding coping strategies for dealing with IPV among Palestinian women who have not experienced such violence. The study yielded findings about variables that could provide insights into the impact of the women's sociocultural context on the beliefs previously mentioned (i.e., attitudes toward women, gender role stereotypes, and expectations relating to maintaining the family unit and the children). In addition, the study examined the relevance of these attitudes to various sociodemographic variables (age, religion, level of education). For example, older women with low levels of education believed that battered women should change their behavior to appease the violent husband and cause him to change his behavior and that they should seek informal assistance or assistance from relatives to put an end to the violence. Younger and more educated women, in contrast, believed that society was responsible for the husbands' violence and that the women should seek formal assistance to prevent and break the cycle of violence against them (Haj-Yahia, 2002). This suggests that the battered woman's age and level of education play an important role and indicates how these aspects affect the choice of coping strategies. A study conducted among women aged 55 and over who had experienced IPV throughout their marriage revealed that the participants had used cognitive coping strategies and had developed a philosophy of life to stay with their violent partners and maintain the family unit (Zink, Jacobson, Pabst, Regan, & Fisher, 2006).

In addition, research dealing with Palestinian women's preferences for coping with IPV has found that they prefer to maintain the family unit or to leave their partner for a limited time to solve the problem and put an end to the violence. However, they prefer to do this without totally breaking up the family unit or divorcing, and they seek assistance within the Palestinian community (Haj-Yahia & Shhadi, 2005; Hamza, 2010; Morse, Paldi, Egbarya, & Clark, 2012). These findings are consistent with the results of studies that have revealed that there are women who do not succumb to the violence, even if they continue to live with their partners and are aware that the social and political context they live in does not offer appropriate solutions to women who are victims of violence, and even if they are expected to use strategies that do not lead to divorce and dissolution of the family unit (Campbell, 2004; Gharaibeh & Oweis, 2009; Kanagaratnam et al., 2012; Okour & Badarneh, 2011; Rhodes & McKenzie, 1998; Zakar, Zakar, & Krämer, 2012).

The sociopolitical context of Palestinian society in Israel is another aspect that was found to be relevant to the Palestinian women's preferences and choices of strategies for coping with violence. Haj-Yahia (2002) found that at least some of the Palestinian women participating in the survey were influenced by sociopolitical factors in their choice of coping strategies. Some of them were opposed to reporting to the police and social services because they perceived those agencies as divisive; as breaking up families; as representing the oppressive establishment; as discriminating, controlling, and not providing adequate services at the level provided to the Jewish population; and as failing to respond to the needs of the woman and her family. Haj-Yahia and Shhadi (2005) argued that women who are victims of IPV perceive the existing services as threatening the unity of the family and of Palestinian society in Israel. In other studies of Palestinian women who are victims of IPV and women who are victims of sexual abuse, the participants described a similar sense of distrust and suspicion of the police and the existing services, and they were reluctant to seek help from them (Adelman, Erez, & Shalhoub-Kevorkian, 2003; Alnabilsy, 2013).

In Alnabilsy's (2013) study, the strategies that the women described for coping with violence by their intimate partners were affected by the sociocultural and sociopolitical context of Palestinian society in Israel. The study revealed that, in the initial stage of their marriage, the women highlighted the use of personal strategies to protect themselves and survive the violence. These strategies included appeasing and placating the violent husband, avoiding contact with the husband, refraining from undermining his authority, avoiding physical resistance or assault against the husband, and obtaining resources to cope with the partner's violence. In the initial stage, these resources were at the social and cultural level—for example, within the family and community. As a last resort, the women sought assistance from formal, external agencies such as social services and the police. Seeking help from formal services was the final, most desperate step, to which the women, their families, and the Palestinian community were opposed in principle. Another dimension at the interpersonal level included repeated attempts to separate from the husband and a desire to break up the family unit—but this did not include actual divorce. The victims of IPV interviewed in this study all used more than one coping strategy to protect themselves and their children from severe violence.

Despite the studies reviewed here, comprehensive research is still needed on coping strategies used by Palestinian women who are victims of violence in Israel because little is known about their coping strategies as they get to know their partners and during the engagement. Moreover, little is known about the coping strategies used by women who have left or divorced their violent husbands, by those who went to battered women's shelters with or without their children, and by women who reported to the police or took legal measures against their violent partner. It would also be relevant to conduct studies on various aspects of motherhood among Palestinian women who are victims of IPV. In addition, research is still needed that highlights the importance of other variables and their relationship to the strategies of Palestinian women for coping with violence. The variables include demographic characteristics (e.g., education, income, employment, economic independence, area of residence), the frequency and severity of violence, personality attributes (e.g., self-esteem and self-image, depression, and locus of control), cognitive and behavioral variables (e.g., attitudes and perceptions about women, learned helpless responses, and self-blame), environmental factors and resources (e.g., the availability of formal and informal services), and the suitability of those services for the needs of Palestinian women. It would be appropriate to examine the role and responses of social networks (e.g., neighbors, close friends, work colleagues) vis-à-vis women who are victims of IPV. It would also be worthwhile to examine the role of the extended family and the family of the violent partner vis-à-vis the woman, when she chooses different coping strategies. There is also a lack of research that addresses these issues in terms of their relevance to the contexts previously described.

Conclusion

In this chapter we attempt to shed light on studies that have addressed the problem of IPV against Palestinian women in Israel. We review the research literature relating to definitions of the problem of violence, to its incidence, its consequences, and to women's strategies for coping with it. In addition, we attempt to provide knowledge about the sociocultural and sociopolitical context of Palestinian women in Israel. Owing to the dearth of knowledge on this topic, we also make recommendations for future research that can provide more comprehensive insights into the problem and its characteristics. We have emphasized that if IPV against Palestinian women in Israel is examined only in relation to personal variables or in terms of the cultural context, norms, and values of Palestinian society without considering the political status of these women and the impact of the Israeli-Palestinian conflict, researchers and therapists will develop partial or mistaken perceptions of the problem. This can encourage discriminatory policies and racism in law enforcement and prevention of violence against these women (Haj-Yahia, 2011; Shalhoub-Kevorkian, 2004). Moreover, the review in this chapter shows how belonging to an indigenous national minority in a complex political context can intensify the woman's distress and vulnerability—especially when she must contend with governmental and formal institutions (such as welfare authorities, the police) that represent the establishment and identify with the Jewish majority (Eisikovits et al., 2008).

RAGHDA ALNABILSY is Researcher and Lecturer in the Department of Social Work at Ruppin Academic Center, Israel.

HANEEN ELIAS is Researcher and Lecturer in the Department of Social Work at Ruppin Academic Center, Israel.

References

Abraham, M. (2000). *Speaking the unspeakable: Marital violence among South Asian immigrants in the United States.* New Brunswick, NJ: Rutgers University Press.

Abu-Ras, W. (2007). Cultural beliefs and service utilization by battered Arab immigrant women. *Violence Against Women, 13*(10), 1002–1028.

Adelman, M., Erez, E., & Shalhoub-Kevorkian, N. (2003). Policing violence against minority women in multicultural societies: "Community" and the politics of exclusion. *Police & Society, 7*, 105–133.

Akyüz, A., Yavan, T., Şahiner, G., & Kiliç, A. (2012). Domestic violence and woman's reproductive health: A review of the literature. *Aggression and Violent Behavior, 17*(6), 514–518.

Alnabilsy, R. (2013). *The house will crumble if its women are absent: Intimate partner violence against Arab women: The impact of the sociocultural and sociopolitical context on perceptions, consequences, and patterns of coping with the problem* [in Hebrew] (Unpublished doctoral dissertation). Paul Baerwald School of Social Work and Social Welfare, Hebrew University of Jerusalem, Israel.

Arda, A. (2006). *The experience of Arab women who were abused and subsequently abuse their children* [in Hebrew] (Unpublished master's thesis). Bob Shapel School of Social Work, Tel Aviv University, Israel.

Barnett, O. W. (2001). Why battered women do not leave, part 2: External inhibiting factors—Social support and internal inhibiting factors. *Trauma, Violence, & Abuse, 2*(1), 3–35.

Briere, J., & Jordan, C. E. (2004). Violence against women: Outcome complexity and implications for assessment and treatment. *Journal of Interpersonal Violence, 19*(11), 1252–1276.

Campbell, J. C. (2004). Helping women understand their risk in situations of intimate partner violence. *Journal of Interpersonal Violence, 19*(12), 1464–1477.

Clements, C. M., & Sawhney, D. K. (2000). Coping with domestic violence: Control attributions, dysphoria, and hopelessness. *Journal of Traumatic Stress, 13*(2), 219–240.

Cwikel, J., Lev-Wiesel, R., & Al-Krenawi, A. (2003). The physical and psychosocial health of Bedouin Arab women of the Negev area of Israel: The impact of high fertility and pervasive domestic violence. *Violence Against Women, 9*(2), 240–257.

Dutton, M. A. (1996). Battered women's strategic response to violence: The role of context. In J. L. Edelson & Z. C. Eisikovits (Eds.), *Future interventions with battered women and their families* (pp. 105–123). Thousand Oaks, CA: Sage.

Dutton, M. A. (2009). Pathways linking intimate partner violence and posttraumatic disorder. *Trauma, Violence, & Abuse, 10*(3), 211–224.

Edelson, M. G., Hokoda, A., & Ramos-Lira, L. (2007). Differences in effects of domestic violence between Latina and non-Latina women. *Journal of Family Violence, 22*(1), 1–10.

Eisikovits, Z., Buchbinder, E., & Bshara, A. (2008). Between the person and the culture: Israeli Arab couple's perceptions of police intervention in intimate partner violence. *Journal of Ethnic & Cultural Diversity in Social Work, 17*(2), 108–129.

Eisikovits, Z., Goldblatt, H., & Winstok, Z. (1999). Partner accounts of intimate violence: Towards a theoretical model. *Families in Society: The Journal of Contemporary Social Services, 80*(6), 606–619.

Eisikovits, Z., Winstok, Z., & Fishman, G. (2004). The first Israeli national survey on domestic violence. *Violence Against Women, 10*(7), 729–748.

Ghanem, A. (2002). The Palestinians in Israel: Political orientation and aspirations. *International Journal of Intercultural Relations, 26*(2), 135–152.

Ghanem, H. (2011). The Nakba [in Arabic]. In N. Rohana & A. Sabag-Hori (Eds.), *Palestinian in Israel, reading in history, politics and society* (pp. 16–26). Haifa: Mada-Al Carmel: Arab Center for Applied Social Research.

Gharaibeh, M., & Oweis, A. (2009). Why do Jordanian women stay in an abusive relationship: Implications for health and social well-being. *Journal of Nursing Scholarship, 41*(4), 376–384.

Gondolf, E. W., & Fisher, E. R. (1988). *Battered women as survivors: An alternative to treating learned helplessness.* Lexington, MA: Lexington Books.

Haj-Yahia, M. M. (2000a). Patterns of violence against engaged Arab women from Israel and some psychological implications. *Psychology of Women Quarterly, 24*(3), 209–219.

Haj-Yahia, M. M. (2000b). Wife abuse and battering in the sociocultural context of Arab society. *Family Process, 39*(2), 237–255.

Haj-Yahia, M. M. (2002). Attitudes of Arab women toward different patterns of coping with wife abuse. *Journal of Interpersonal Violence, 17*(7), 721–745.

Haj-Yahia, M. M. (2003a). Beliefs about wife beating among Arab men from Israel: The influence of their patriarchal ideology. *Journal of Family Violence, 18*(4), 193–206.

Haj-Yahia, M. M. (2003b). *Beliefs of Arab women about wife beating.* Unpublished manuscript.
Haj-Yahia, M. M. (2011). Contextualizing interventions with battered women in collectivist societies: Issues and controversies. *Aggression and Violent Behavior, 16*(4), 331–339.
Haj-Yahia, M. M., & Peled, E. (2013). Guest editors' note [in Hebrew]. *Society and Welfare, 33,* 3–6.
Haj-Yahia, M. M., & Shhadi, N. (2005). Arab women's patterns of coping with violence against them. In A. Ghanem & M. Mustafa (Eds.), *Civic developments among the Palestinians in Israel II* (pp. 89–144). Tamra, Israel: Ibn-Khaldun.
Hamza, M. (2010). *A phenomenological study of the symptoms of expression of intimate partner violence in Arab women* (Unpublished doctoral dissertation). Argosy University, San Francisco, CA.
Iverson, K. M., Bauer, M. R., Shipherd, J. C., Pineles, S. L., Harrington, E. F., & Resick, P. A. (2013). Differential associations between partner violence and physical health symptoms among caucasian and African American help-seeking women. *Psychological Trauma: Theory, Research, Practice, and Policy, 5*(2), 158–166.
Kanagaratnam, P., Mason, R., Hyman, I., Manuel, L., Berman, H., & Toner, B. (2012). Burden of womanhood: Tamil women's perceptions of coping with intimate partner violence. *Journal of Family Violence, 27*(7), 647–658.
Lawson, J. (2012). Sociological theories of intimate partner violence. *Journal of Human Behavior in the Social Environment, 22*(5), 572–590.
Levinson, D. (1989). *Family violence in cross-cultural perspective.* Newbury Park, CA: Sage.
Loxton, D., Schofield, M., & Hussain, R. (2006). Psychological health in midlife among women who have ever lived with a violent partner or spouse. *Journal of Interpersonal Violence, 21*(8), 1092–1107.
Malley-Morrison, K., & Hines, D. (2004). *Family violence in a cultural perspective: Defining, understanding, and combating abuse.* Thousand Oaks, CA: Sage.
Mills, T. (1985). The assault on the self: Stages in coping with battering husbands. *Qualitative Sociology, 8*(2), 103–123.
Morse, D. S., Paldi, Y., Egbarya, S. S., & Clark, C. J. (2012). "An effect that is deeper than beating": Family violence in Jordanian women. *Families, Systems, & Health, 30*(1), 19–31.
Okour, A. M., & Badarneh, R. (2011). Spousal violence against pregnant women from a Bedouin community in Jordan. *Journal of Women's Health, 20*(12), 1853–1859.
Rafaeili, T. (2012). *Israeli and immigrant women survivors of intimate partner violence: The contribution of personal and environmental characteristics to depression* [in Hebrew] (Unpublished master's thesis). School of Social Work, Bar-Ilan University, Israel.
Rhodes, N. R., & McKenzie, E. B. (1998). Why do battered women stay?: Three decades of research. *Aggression and Violent Behavior, 3*(4), 391–406.
Rouhana, N. N. (1997). *Palestinian citizens in an ethnic Jewish state: Identities in conflict.* New Haven, CT: Yale University Press.
Sabina, C., Cuevas, C. A., & Schally, J. L. (2012). The effect of immigration and acculturation on victimization among a national sample of Latino women. *Cultural Diversity and Ethnic Minority Psychology, 19*(1), 13–26.
Seligman, M. E. (1975). *Helplessness: On depression, development, and death.* San Francisco: W. H. Freeman.
Shalhoub-Kevorkian, N. (2000). Blocking her exclusion: A contextually sensitive model of intervention for handling female abuse. *Social Service Review, 74*(4), 620–634.
Shalhoub-Kevorkian, N. (2004). Racism, militarisation and policing: Police reactions to violence against Palestinian women in Israel. *Social Identities, 10*(2), 171–193.

Shalhoub-Kevorkian, N. (2010). How should we read violence against Palestinian women in Israel? [in Arabic]. *Jadal, 6*, 1–4.

Shalhoub-Kevorkian, N., & Daher-Nashif, S. (2013). Femicide and colonization: Between the politics of exclusion and the culture of control. *Violence Against Women, 19*(3), 295–315.

Shoham, E. (2012). *A glimpse behind the walls: Violence toward women in segregated communities* [in Hebrew]. Beersheva: Ben-Gurion University of the Negev.

Smith, M., & Wehrle, A. (2010). Homicide of an intimate male partner: The impact on the woman. *Issues in Mental Health Nursing, 31*(1), 21–27.

Stover, C. S. (2005). Domestic violence research: What have we learned and where do we go from here? *Journal of Interpersonal Violence, 20*(4), 448–454.

Walker, L. E. (2009). *The battered woman syndrome* (3rd ed.). New York: Springer.

Wilcox, P. (2006). *Surviving domestic violence: Gender, poverty and agency*. Houndmills, UK: Springer.

Zakar, R., Zakar, M. Z., & Krämer, A. (2012). Voices of strength and struggle: Women's coping strategies against spousal violence in Pakistan. *Journal of Interpersonal Violence, 27*(16), 3268–3298.

Zink, T., Jacobson, C. J., Jr., Pabst, S., Regan, S., & Fisher, B. S. (2006). A lifetime of intimate partner violence: Coping strategies of older women. *Journal of Interpersonal Violence, 21*(5), 634–651.

17

ABUSE OF OLDER ADULTS AMONG PALESTINIAN CITIZENS IN ISRAEL

Social, Economic, and Family Related Factors

Samir Zoabi

A PERSON'S LIFE COMPRISES SEVERAL STAGES OF DEVELOPMENT. Most of these are characterized by growth and strengthening of both natural qualities and skills, but the last stage, old age, is characterized by loss and decline in many realms of life—social, psychological, economic, and health (Kluckhohn, 1971). These changes inevitably create a new social situation to which older persons and society must adapt. In many cases, this challenge is compounded by abuse and neglect of older people, further burdening and embittering their lives (Zoabi, 2000).

The information presented in this chapter is based primarily on two major research projects that I conducted in two different time periods between 1994 and 2000. These studies comprehensively examined the incidence of abuse and neglect of older adults in Palestinian society in Israel (Zoabi, 1994, 2000). This chapter is also based on results of other research on the dimensions and characteristics of this problem in Israel and other places in the world.

The topic encompasses all types of abuse of older adults—psychological, physiological, sexual, economic, and that of neglect. The focus is on violence and abuse that occur in the homes of older people, primarily committed by relatives, such as their children, the children's spouses, grandchildren, and other family members.

Research on the abuse and neglect of the elderly has provided a long, detailed list of risk factors that affect the development and severity of their plight. This chapter concentrates on an in-depth, integrative investigation of three groups of risk factors that earlier research on older adults in Palestinian society in Israel has identified as critical to the development of violence. Further understanding of these risk factors may also inform members of the caring professions when developing relevant and effective treatment and prevention programs.

The first group of risk factors includes the sociodemographic characteristics of older victims of abuse; the second is associated with the sociodemographic characteristics of the abusive caregivers; and the third refers to the structural and interactional characteristics of the informal social support networks of older people who are abused.

Abuse of Older Adults: A Definition

Abuse of older people is both a source of personal distress and a serious social problem. It represents the failure of the social structure and of society's mechanisms to prevent abuse and provide care of the victims of a specific age group (Govil & Gupta, 2016).

Straus, Gelles, and Steinmetz (1980) claimed that there is more violence than love in the modern family. In light of the accelerated processes of modernization experienced by the Palestinian society in Israel, family networks are unable to fulfill their traditional roles, particularly those of support and protection (Litwin & Zoabi, 2003). Khalaila and Litwin (2011) found that in some cases the social network becomes a source of injury and distress instead of support and protection.

Based on my personal experience as a professional in direct contact with older adults, some of whom suffer abusive treatment, I believe that abuse may be manifested not only in assault and visible violent behavior but also in many other types of abuse and neglect, some of which are difficult to identify and treat. Examples of these additional forms of abuse include social exclusion, psychological abuse, verbal abuse, sexual abuse, threats and fear tactics, violation of rights, economic abuse, and financial exploitation.

In other studies, the abuse and neglect of older people has been defined as active behavior that causes physical and/or mental pain, or the prevention of essential mental and/or physical services by the direct caregivers of the older victims. This definition represents an attempt to integrate several definitions that together may provide a comprehensive description of the situation and enable identification of the many aspects of the problem (Litwin & Zoabi, 2003; Lowenstein, Eisikovits, Band-Winterstein, & Enosh, 2009). Examination of the different definitions reveals a similarity in general content but differences in the internal division and categorization of the various abusive behaviors. Johannesen and LoGiudice (2013), Lowenstein et al. (2009), and Zoabi (2000) have discussed the following types of abuse:

- Physical abuse refers to causing the older person physical pain by means of physical injury, such as blows, burns, pushing, or wounding. Some researchers have included sexual abuse in this category. Many have emphasized the importance of special attention to its symptoms, which older people are seldom willing to report.
- Psychological abuse refers to actions that may cause stress and mental injury to the older person, such as yelling, humiliation, isolation, manipulation, ignoring, or treating the person like a child.

- Economic abuse indicates any activity aimed at taking control of the older person's sources of income and/or property, including exploitation of those resources for one's own financial needs.
- Neglect refers to subjecting the older person to physical and/or psychological stress by failing to provide attention and care. Neglect may be intentional or, in some cases, nonintentional.

The Informal Social Support System

Every person in modern society has informal social networks (Steptoe, Shankar, Demakakos, & Wardle, 2013). Litwin and Zoabi (2003) found that in most cases these networks provide a response to the different emotional, social, mental, and instrumental needs of the individual. Litwin (1998) described the informal social support network as a series of informal interpersonal contacts and social interactions in which the individual enjoys emotional and material support, such as a sense of belonging and identity. Thoits (1982) claimed that people receive social, emotional, and instrumental support through interactions with people in their environment and conceived of social support as a fit between the needs of the individual and the resources required to fulfill them. Similarly, Litwin (1998) perceived social support as a measure of correspondence between a person's social needs and the resources required to fulfill them.

Wethington and Kessler (1986) saw the social support system as a buffer that enables individuals to adapt to stress and physiological, health, social, and emotional problems. They differentiated between perceived support and received support. Perceived support plays a more important role than actual support received in predicting a person's ability to adjust to stress.

Mitchell (1969) and Litwin (1996) presented two main approaches regarding social support networks. The first focuses on the morphological structure of the network. In contrast, the second approach centers on the functional aspects, reciprocity, and the degree to which direct needs are fulfilled as a result of the relationship with and the presence of network members. This approach focuses on the substance and significance of the relationships within the network, the degree of reciprocity, and the frequency of interaction among members.

Along these lines, Rosenfeld (1968) noted that in Palestinian society in Israel, older people did not feel regression during the process of aging because they had strong and active family networks consisting of many people who were willing to help the elders fulfill their financial, physiological, health-related, social, and mental needs. Litwin (1997), Thoits (1995), and Lin and Dean (1984) found a strong interaction between the structural and interactional characteristics of support networks. They concluded that although little research has been invested in studying these relationships, it seems that the simplest and most reliable measure for assessment of social support is the presence or absence of close ties in a person's life (e.g., friends, lovers, confidants).

Abuse and Neglect of Older Adults:
Frequency, Discovery, and Reporting

It is difficult to estimate the scope of abuse of older people both around the world and in Palestinian society in Israel. The literature on this subject cites a long list of factors that impede effective and accurate establishment of the rate of incidence of abuse and neglect of older adults (Lowenstein, 1995; Pittaway & Westhues, 1994). Some of these factors are related to the victims of elder abuse and neglect and their abusive caregivers and others are associated with cultural and methodological factors or characteristics of the professional caregivers (Zoabi, 1994, 2000).

Zoabi (1994) studied the dimensions and characteristics of violence against older people in Palestinian society in Israel. The research participants, all social workers, were asked to report on older people under their care at the time or in the past 18 months. The findings indicated that 2.5% (434) of all older Palestinians living in the north of Israel had suffered abusive treatment of some kind—physiological, psychological, or economic abuse or intentional or nonintentional neglect. Six years later, Zoabi (2000) conducted another study of abused older people. The results showed a significant increase in the percentage of older adults who had suffered abuse and neglect, reaching 4% of the older Palestinians living in the north of Israel.

Comparison of the rates of abuse according to type of location (city, suburban village, and isolated village) found that 4.9% of all urban older people suffered abuse; in the suburban villages, 2.2%; and in the isolated villages, 1.1%. According to the research findings, this difference was explained mainly by the impact of modern living conditions and changes in the social and family support networks, a trend found to be strongest in the large cities, weaker in the suburban villages, and weakest in the isolated villages (Zoabi, 1994, 2000).

With regard to the different types of abuse of older people in Palestinian society in Israel, these studies revealed that psychological abuse is the most common: approximately 66.8% of the older people who were abused suffered psychological abuse, approximately 3.5% suffered physical abuse, about 11.5% suffered economic abuse, and 18.2% suffered neglect (Zoabi, 1994, 2000).

Research conducted in Israel has indicated a high rate of abuse among the general population of the country. The national figures have also shown a significant increase in the percentage of older people who suffer abusive treatment. Lowenstein (1995) estimated that 20,000 to 50,000 older adults in Israel (between 4% and 10% of the total older population) suffered abuse of some type—physical, psychological, economic, or that of neglect. About a decade later, a national survey revealed troubling findings that indicated a significant increase in the rate of elder abuse nationwide. This later study included 1,045 older participants who lived in their homes; 18.4% of them experienced some type of abuse (Lowenstein et al., 2009).

Family violence in general and violence against older people in particular is one of the hidden social problems in the world (Hantman, Cohen, Hroost, & Sassi, 2004). Among some families, the violence is frequent, but it is considered a family matter in which intervention by others is not acceptable. In such cases, three types of factors hinder effective and accurate detection of the occurrence of abuse: factors related to the personal attributes and practical considerations of the older victims of abuse, factors associated with personal attributes and practical considerations of the professionals involved, and cultural factors (Litwin & Zoabi, 2003; Lowenstein, 2003; Zoabi, 2000).

In my research on violence against older adults and interviews with older victims of abuse, there were clear indications of denial on the part of the victims regarding abuse, and they staunchly refused to formally report the violence exerted toward them to the relevant authorities. These older people gave a number of reasons for their unwillingness to report the violence toward them: (a) they feared revenge by the abusive caregivers; (b) they feared placement in community institutions, such as assisted-living facilities or geriatric hospital wards; (c) they feared they would lose the little attention they received; (d) they wanted to protect the abusive caregiver—often their child or another relative—from legal proceedings; (e) some of them believed that they had contributed to the occurrence of abuse; and (f) some of them saw the abuse of their son or daughter as a sign of their personal failure in child-rearing and therefore preferred to keep the abuse a secret (Litwin & Zoabi, 2003; Zoabi, 2000).

Anetzberger and Alon (2015) added another factor, functional and mental impairment of older people, arguing that such disabilities isolate them socially and reduce the chances of detection of their victimization. In quite a few cases, according to their research, abusive caregivers exploit these weaknesses and impose social isolation on their victims, forbidding them to leave the house or contact external organizations, to conceal the abuse or neglect (Holt, 1994; Pritchard, 1993). Litwin and Zoabi (2003) noted social isolation and detachment from the environment as a prominent risk factor among older people who suffer abuse and neglect in the Palestinian society in Israel.

Zoabi (1994) found that in 65% of the elder abuse cases detected in Palestinian society in northern Israel during the 18 months prior to 1994, the social workers took no measures to respond. Although the social workers were aware of the problem and understood the laws forbidding it, they lacked the professional skills and diagnostic tools to make a qualified diagnosis and provide proper intervention. The study suggested that the lack of reporting by the social workers in these cases might have stemmed from concern about their own professional image (Zoabi, 1994).

It seems that professionals also contribute to the inadequate detection of cases of abuse and neglect of older people. Some authors (Alon, 2006, 2015; Alon & Doron, 2009) showed that the extent of reporting abuse and neglect by professionals was incomplete and limited. Social workers and nurses have argued that the lack of reporting in some cases was mainly owing to the unwillingness to intervene in personal matters of the older people (Alon & Doron, 2009).

Penhale (1993) presented several factors related to caregivers that she found hindered reporting and identification of elder abuse cases: (a) lack of knowledge about abuse and neglect of older people; (b) absence of a uniform, unequivocal definition of the concept of abuse and neglect of older people; (c) the professionals' lack of financial and professional resources for investigation and intervention, including treatment techniques; (d) a desire of the social workers to protect the right to privacy and confidentiality; and (e) personal views that justified the anger of the abusive caregivers. According to Zoabi (1994), the conduct of social workers exposed to cases of violence and injury in Palestinian society in Israel is often characterized by a lack or an inadequacy of professional response to the problem. In this study, professionals said that they preferred not to intervene in such cases, based on a desire to protect the privacy of the older people and their families. They also noted that they did not feel they had the tools, knowledge, and instrumental resources (such as budgets, organizations, and the like) that would enable them to provide effective care.

The findings also indicated a statistically significant relationship between type of abuse and type of reaction of professionals to the identification of physical abuse and neglect. In cases of physical abuse, social workers tended to take legal action, but in those of intentional and nonintentional neglect, they tended to relocate the victims from their homes to community institutions. In contrast, in cases of psychological and economic abuse, no relationship was found between type of abuse and the responses of the social workers. It seems that professionals responded and tried to help older people who suffered types of violence that were more visible, but in cases of psychological and economic abuse, it was difficult for social workers to determine whether abuse was taking place, and therefore they intervened less (Zoabi, 1994).

It seems that the development of social services for older adults has increased awareness of their abuse and their willingness to report the abuse and neglect to human service providers, mental health practitioners, the criminal justice system, and even community leaders. These include a telephone hotline for older adults, visits by volunteers without specific requests, distribution of written material on the rights of senior citizens by the National Institute of Insurance (NII) and the Service for the Elderly in the Israel Ministry of Social Affairs and Social Services and community organizations, as well as the development of alternative arrangements to living at home, such as day centers and homes for older adults (Litwin & Zoabi, 2003). All these may have increased older people's awareness of possible places to turn to with complaints about abuse and neglect, introduced them to alternative residential frameworks, made a genuine contribution to their self-confidence, and encouraged them to report abusive treatment or neglect (Zoabi, 2000).

Another interesting finding is the differences in the percentage of reports by victims of different types of abuse. Reports by older victims of psychological abuse, economic abuse, or intentional or nonintentional neglect accounted for 55% of the cases exposed, compared with 88% by victims of physical abuse. It seems that the severity of physical abuse and consequent stress suffered by the victims cause them to report it more often than those who suffer other types of abuse (Zoabi, 2000).

Cultural factors, particularly in traditional societies such as the Palestinian society in Israel, are considered central in the process of exposing and reporting cases of abuse and violence against older people. It has been found that the detection of elder abuse has been affected to a great degree by the views of the professionals with regard to the rights of older people to self-fulfillment. In addition, the expectations, values, and cultural background (particularly urban or rural place of residence, age, and socioeconomic status) of the caring professional who identifies abuse were found to be relevant. Moreover, characteristics of the nonprofessional caregivers were shown to influence the professionals' assessment of the situation. Wealthy and/or young caregivers were perceived as abusive, but those who were older and not well-to-do were perceived as neglecting. In addition, exposure and treatment of abuse and neglect that took place within the home were particularly difficult to identify. It was found that social workers were reluctant to report abuse to their superiors, for fear that it would harm the image of their culture (Zoabi, 2000). This may be particularly true among Palestinians, as respect for elders has long been a source of cultural and societal pride. From the perspective of the Palestinian social worker, older people are expected to enjoy a position at the center of the family network and benefit from full attention and care. Therefore, for these professionals, reporting on older people who suffer abuse could shatter the myth of the social status of the older generation and reflect negatively on their cultural image (Sharon & Zoabi, 1997; Zoabi, 1994).

Litwin and Zoabi (2003) indicated cultural factors as a significant deterrent to the exposure and intervention in cases of abuse and neglect of older people. According to their study, in traditional Palestinian society in Israel, where religion and society demand respect and suitable care for older people, abuse is not acknowledged and therefore is not addressed appropriately by the service organizations or the media.

Sociopolitical factors may also hinder the exposure and treatment of cases of abuse and neglect of older people (Sharon & Zoabi, 1997). For instance, factors such as hostility toward the government institutions due to lack of services and the inadequate number of professional workers inhibits people in Palestinian society in Israel from utilizing professional community services. These factors significantly reduce professional involvement in the lives of older people, thus hindering the process of exposure and treatment. According to Sharon and Zoabi (1997), this is particularly prominent among older victims of abuse and neglect.

Abuse and Neglect of Older Adults: Risk Factors

The literature includes many factors that have been identified as increasing the chances of abuse and therefore warrant special attention by mental health practitioners (Alon, 2006; Alon & Doron, 2009; Cohen, Halevi-Levin, Gagin, & Friedman, 2006). This section presents a comprehensive view of the structural and interactional characteristics of the informal support network of older adults as a significant risk factor in the incidence and persistence of abuse (Zoabi, 2000).

The data provided here include in-depth consideration of three types of risk factors: (a) characteristics of older victims of abuse, (b) characteristics of abusive caregivers, and (c) structural and interactional characteristics of the informal support systems of the older people who are abused. A full understanding of these factors enhances the effective professional preventive and therapeutic responses to the problem.

Characteristics of Older Victims and Social Implications of Abuse

According to Zoabi (2000), the most common types of abuse of older people were neglect in providing care, psychological abuse, and financial abuse. The study results also found that most of the cases of abuse began before the victim became older and before the victim contacted the social services. However, only a minority of these people contacted the social services to report their experience with abuse and neglect; in most cases, they asked for other types of assistance, such as financial aid or help with health and other problems. The professionals detected abuse on average two-and-a-half years prior to the victim's report but did not report it themselves. The victims of physical abuse reported it more often than the victims of other types of abuse, and social workers also detected this type of abuse more often by means of personal observation. In most cases, other family members, particularly women and children, also suffered abuse from the same abusers.

In terms of age, the findings revealed that those who were abused were relatively old (aged 75 and older). Moreover, the probability of abuse increased with age (Zoabi, 1994, 2000). It has also been found that aging is accompanied by a higher probability of physical and psychological weakness and illness as well as economic and social decline (Litwin & Zoabi, 2003). These processes lead to increased economic, physical, and mental demands and pressures on caregiving family members. In some cases, the family caregivers also suffer personal and economic crises and stress, and sometimes they lack the means to withstand the pressure. This situation sometimes leads to violence, abuse, and neglect (Litwin & Zoabi, 2003; Sharon & Zoabi, 1997). Khalaila and Litwin (2011) described the care of an older person at home as a difficult task that requires physical and mental efforts.

Research has shown that most older victims suffer health, functional, and cognitive difficulties that create daily dependence on their caregiving relatives. There is also evidence that the greater the dependence and disabilities of the older people, the greater the chances of an abusive and neglectful incident (Sharon & Zoabi, 1997). This situation is liable to worsen in cases of social, economic, and demographic changes such as those experienced by Palestinian society in Israel and in cases where the caregivers also suffer from economic, social, and emotional problems (Khalaila & Litwin, 2011).

There are two possible ways of interpreting the potential situation in Palestinian society in Israel. On the one hand, it might be claimed that the family burden created by the dependence and disability of older people in this society is greater and more distinct from that in other places in the world because of the special characteristics of Palestinian society in Israel as a society in transition. People in this society suffer from a relative shortage of formal services for the support of older people with disabilities and support for their family networks (e.g., assisted-living facilities, day centers, sheltered housing, treatment centers). Consequently, the emotional, economic, and physical pressure on those who care for older people with disabilities is likely to be much greater than in other places in the Western world and, indeed, than in the local Jewish society. Therefore, the threshold of abuse toward older people with disabilities and dependence in Palestinian society in Israel is liable to be higher compared with other societies (Azaiza & Brodsky, 1997).

According to an alternative view, on the other hand, older people in Palestinian society in Israel enjoy a strong and extensive informal support network anchored on cultural and religious rules. This is likely to decrease the threshold of abuse in this society. A strong informal network may reduce the degree to which older people with disabilities rely on members of the network because the burden of care is divided among a large number of people (Khalaila & Litwin, 2011; Litwin & Zoabi, 2003). With respect to financial dependence, research has shown that older people who suffer abuse in Palestinian society in Israel usually do not receive financial support from their children and fund their expenses themselves. Only in a very few cases were they found to receive financial aid from their children (Zoabi, 2000).

With regard to the issue of finances, there are also two possible interpretations. One explanation is that abuse may occur when older people need financial support but their children refuse to fulfill this need. In such cases, economic dependence constitutes a stress factor and plays an important role in the development and persistence of abuse. Alternatively, older people may suffer abuse when they are financially independent but refuse to support their children who need financial assistance. In these cases, property and income may serve as a premise for their children to abuse them and take control of these resources by force (Alon, 2006; Holt, 1994; Litwin & Zoabi, 2003; Pittaway & Westhues, 1994).

Research conducted among Palestinian citizens in Israel also found that the percentage of widows and widowers among older victims was particularly high. In general, people usually lose their spouses at a late age, when the needs of the widow or widower, and thus the pressure on their caregivers, are relatively great. This is all the more so when the deceased was also the main caregiver of the older person. In these cases, bereavement is accompanied by the creation of a vacuum in the provision of services. In most cases, the burden of care falls on relatives, particularly the person's children, who are often subject to social, financial, and health-related pressures (Litwin & Zoabi, 2003).

Another reason for the high percentage of widows and widowers among the abused may be that the death of a spouse represents the older person's loss of the person closest to him or her—the individual who had protected him or her throughout their lives together. This is particularly true in the case of women who lose their husbands, as in Arab tradition and culture the latter have the primary duty to protect their wives (Litwin & Zoabi, 2003; Lowenstein, 2003).

With regard to the gender of victims of elder abuse, research has indicated that most of the abused are women because of their longer lifespan (Sharon & Zoabi, 1997). As noted, the incidence of abuse increases with age, therefore, it is reasonable to assume that older women suffer abuse more often than older men (Sharon & Zoabi, 1997; Zoabi, 1994, 2000).

Zoabi (2000) suggested that another explanation for the gender difference is associated with the strong element of patriarchy in Arab society. Traditionally, men in Arab society fulfilled instrumental roles, and their relationships with their children were based on authority. It is reasonable to assume that despite the weakening of the older person's strength with age, the authority of the father continued to influence the parent-child relationship.

In contrast, women traditionally fulfilled expressive tasks, and their ties with their children were based on emotion, not authority. With the weakening of her mental and physical strength, the ability of the woman to continue to provide these emotional needs declines considerably. Furthermore, her now-mature children require less support. This is particularly true in families of low socioeconomic status, where it seems that the practical constraints of life leave little room for emotion. As a result, older women more often become victims of abuse and violence (Zoabi, 1994).

Research has shown a difficult economic situation among older victims of abuse in Palestinian society in Israel (Zoabi, 1994, 2000). According to the findings, 74% percent of the victims were of low economic status. A review of the research in this field reflects the general consensus that this can be attributed to the more extensive involvement of professionals in the lives of people of lower status. However, these figures do not imply that abuse is nonexistent in middle and high socioeconomic groups. The contrary may be true, as people of high socioeconomic status have the social, economic, and emotional status to conceal what happens within their families (Holt, 1994; Penhale, 1993; Pritchard, 1993).

Additional interpretations have also been suggested with regard to differences in economic status. These are primarily related to the economic security that generally characterizes older people of middle and high socioeconomic status, which is expressed in ownership of land or property or in a regular fixed income, providing the person with protection and resistance to abuse and neglect in several ways (Alon, 2006). First, they may utilize their economic resources as an instrument for obtaining good care and services. An example is the payment or promise of inheritance to relatives in return for their care (Zoabi, 1994, 2000). In addition, based on the experience of professionals, financial means may enable older people to find diverse solutions when they sense the risk of abuse and neglect. These include, for example, the option of moving to their own residence, remarriage, taking advantage of day centers or assisted-living facilities that enable them a dignified life, and the purchase of services from private organizations. Thus, these relatively well-to-do older people reduce the pressure on caregiving relatives and decrease the chances of abuse and neglect (Alon, 2006).

Second, it has been found that older victims of abuse and neglect feel ashamed of what has happened to them. This often leads to detachment from their social environment, which in turn may significantly intensify the incidence of abuse (Litwin & Zoabi, 2003).

Not surprisingly, it has been found that the experience of abuse and neglect usually makes the older victims very angry and sad. Alon (2006) reported that they often direct this anger at themselves and suffer a decline in self-confidence and self-esteem as well. Alon (2006) also found that another typical characteristic in such cases was denial of the experience and an exerted effort to provide explanations, usually unrealistic and unconvincing, for the side effects that characterize abused older people. In many cases, the victims tried to explain and justify the abuse they suffered.

Characteristics of Abusive Caregivers

The findings of most research regarding abusive caregivers of older people in Palestinian society in Israel are similar to those of studies conducted in other places and among other populations in Israel (Litwin & Zoabi, 2003; Sharon & Zoabi, 1997). The only difference is the gender of the majority of abusers, which seems to be a unique feature of Palestinian society. Lowenstein et al. (2009), as well as other researchers, found that most of the caregivers in Israeli society that abuse older people are women, in most cases daughters, who are expected to care for their parents and ensure their physical, mental, and social needs. However, other research has yielded different findings, indicating that the abuse of older people in Palestinian society in Israel happens in the family, and it is usually carried out by men, especially sons (47%), followed by daughters-in-law (20%), daughters (9%), spouses (18%), relatives (4%), and others (2%) (Zoabi, 1994, 2000).

Sharon and Zoabi (1997) also found additional factors of abuse and neglect that were associated with the pressure experienced by caregivers of older people, in particular the residential patterns, family status, and occupational status of the abusive caregivers. The findings showed that in general, in all types of abuse, 45% of the abusive caregivers lived with the older victim in the same residential unit. In cases of physical abuse alone, the decisive majority of abusers (75%) lived in the same housing unit as the victim. It seems that sharing the same residence increases the chances of friction and pressure on the caregiver and, subsequently, of physical abuse. Lowenstein (2003) also found that most of the abusive caregivers in Israeli society in general were married (76%) and unemployed (40%) or housewives (25%).

Another interesting finding refers to the age range of the abusers. The majority of abusers (68%) were between 30 and 40 years old (Zoabi, 1994, 2000). According to the literature, the pressure on people of this age as breadwinners and parents is great, making the treatment of an older person at home all the more difficult

(Kosberg, 1988; Litwin & Zoabi, 2003). In comparison, the percentage of abusers under the age of 29 was relatively low (11%), likely because the caregivers of that age, especially sons, had very few other commitments and could more easily fulfill the various needs of their parents and their older relatives. The relatively high percentage of abusers who were married (75%) supports this explanation (Zoabi, 2000).

The relatively high percentage of unemployed people and housewives among the abusive caregivers (65%) also suggests that pressure is an important factor in the incidence and persistence of abuse. Unemployed people usually suffer from economic, psychological, and social pressures (Alon & Doron, 2009). Caring for an older person is a particularly difficult task for them in several respects. The high percentage of the unemployed involved in physical abuse (80%) reinforces this explanation presented by Zoabi (1994, 2000).

The examination of the relationship between abuse and neglect of older people and other patterns of abuse in the nuclear family of the abusive caregiver suggests that abuse of an older person is an indicator of different types of abuse in the family of the caregiver, and vice versa (Lowenstein, 2006). In 62% of the reported cases of abuse, the professionals also reported additional patterns of abuse in the caregiver's nuclear family (Zoabi, 2000). Research revealed that violence seems to be an accepted, legitimate behavior pattern among certain population groups, most often associated with low socioeconomic status (Eisikovits, Winterstein, & Lowenstein, 2005).

The characteristics of the abusers presented in this section provide a system perspective of the factors that promote the incidence and persistence of abuse of older people. As part of this perspective, the presence of several personal characteristics (such as addiction, mental disorders, and others, discussed next), economic factors (such as unemployment, financial problems), and family factors (such as divorce, living together with or in proximity to the older person), as well as the demands of caring for an older person with disabilities at home, are very significant factors in the incidence of abuse and neglect of older people.

Furthermore, it has been found that living with abusive parents (and thus learning abuse) plays an important role in the incidence of abuse (Lachs & Pillemer, 1995; Litwin & Zoabi, 2003). An examination of the relationship between characteristics of abusing caregivers and types of abuse has indicated that a large percentage of the caregivers responsible for physical abuse were addicted to drugs and alcohol (Zoabi, 1994, 2000). According to these findings, the use of addictive substances placed caregivers in a difficult emotional, social, and economic situation that could lead to the physical abuse of older people. In addition, the social and economic difficulties involved in drug addiction created physical and mental needs that could diminish the caregiver's mental and physical ability. It has also been found that caregivers who suffer from mental disability and are unable to assess their own behavior often become physically abusive and neglectful (Lachs & Pillemer, 1995; Lowenstein & Ron, 1999).

The Informal Social Support Network of Older Victims of Abuse

Al-Haj (1989) argued that in the modern era of traditional Palestinian society in Israel, the individual has more freedom to choose from numerous behavioral patterns, a realm previously dictated by family and social pressure and by religious requirements. In Palestinian society in Israel, the extended family is being increasingly replaced by the nuclear family, with its individual- and achievement-oriented character. This trend is causing a decline in the family's role in many social realms, among them the functioning and the characteristics of the informal social network of older people. This, in turn, has affected the attitude toward these people and their social status.

There is a dearth of research on the structural and interactional characteristics of the informal support systems of older people who suffer abuse and neglect in Palestinian society in Israel. The findings of an earlier study clearly indicated that, in general, the structural and interactional qualities of the informal networks of abused older people were much weaker than those of their counterparts who did not suffer abuse (Zoabi, 2000). Thoits (1995) and Litwin and Zoabi (2003) have called for research on the relationship between the structural and interactional characteristics of the informal support systems and different social problems.

Litwin and Zoabi (2003) assessed the degree of risk to older people of being abused according to several dimensions: sociodemographic characteristics of the older person; the degree of influence of the informal social network in modern life; the person's economic dependence, disabilities, and relationship with the formal social networks; and the structural and interactional characteristics of the individual's informal support system. In the past, research in this area focused on describing the characteristics of older people who were abused (Alon & Doron, 2009). In contrast, the consideration of risk factors in the study Litwin and Zoabi performed was integrative, and the relative predictive ability of each of the factors was examined.

The results revealed a very high rate of accurate prediction of abuse by the structural and interactional characteristics of the informal support network of the older person. The model of prediction was significant; 92% of the research population was correctly classified by using it. In addition, the degrees of prediction of each of the four steps implemented in the data analysis were found to be significant. However, all the variables up to the fifth step—namely, the sociodemographic and modern-life characteristics and disability in daily functions—were classified together correctly in only two-thirds of the population (note that 50% reflects no prediction). The informal social networks added another 18%—more than each of the other research variables—to the classification (Litwin & Zoabi, 2003).

These findings indicated that structural and interactional characteristics of the informal social network are critical factors in the incidence and persistence of the abuse and neglect of older people. Naturally, the effectiveness and influence of the network may function as therapeutic and preventive factors. It is reasonable to assume that the reconstruction, empowerment, and activation of one's social network may have a significant positive impact on the mental, physical, and social welfare and well-being of an older victim of abuse. Furthermore, it may moderate the negative impact of many factors, such as disability and dependence, modern living conditions, among others (Litwin & Zoabi, 2003; Zoabi, 2000).

These findings reinforce and emphasize the role of the informal social support network in analyzing and understanding social problems, particularly in abuse of older people. Litwin and Zoabi (2003) and Thoits (1995) suggested that the structural and interactional characteristics of the informal social networks are equally important and beneficial in the process of treating these problems.

THE STRUCTURAL LEVEL

Earlier research indicated that older people who were abused had fewer members in their support networks than people who were not abused (Zoabi, 2000). Moreover, the support networks of people who were abused usually consisted of their children, and the networks of older people who were not abused were composed in fairly equal proportions of their children and others, such as relatives, friends, and neighbors. Kosberg (1988) and Kosberg and Garcia (1995) identified a small number of members in the support system as a factor in the abuse and neglect of older people and especially of those who were disabled. Research in Palestinian society in Israel revealed that the older victims of abuse had a relatively small number of children and other relatives caring for them. Furthermore, the greater the older person's disability and dependence, the fewer friends and children functioned as caregivers (Zoabi, 1994).

These findings on structural characteristics may be understood in different ways. On the one hand, they indicate a deficiency of caregiving and social, emotional, and financial support of older victims of abuse. On the other, they reflect that these people live in a state of isolation and social detachment, which has been shown to contribute considerably to the incidence and persistence of elder abuse (Litwin & Zoabi, 2003; Lowenstein, 2006).

Zoabi (2000), in research of Palestinian society in Israel, also investigated this structural factor in order to measure the degree to which abused and nonabused older people received assistance and support. The findings revealed that fewer members of their social networks helped and supported the older abuse victims compared with older people who were not abused.

The number of caregivers in the network largely reflects the degree to which the care of older people is divided among members of the informal network. When the support network includes a large number of members, the burden of care is shared, lessening the load on each member (Khalaila & Litwin, 2011).

The more caregivers there are for older people, the less the pressure on each member of the network, the more comfortable the atmosphere, and, as a result, the lower the risk of elder abuse and neglect. In contrast, a small number of caregivers increases the pressure on each one, creating fertile ground for abuse and its persistence (Zoabi, 2000). The division of the tasks in caring for an older person with disabilities reduces the probability of abuse and neglect (Litwin & Zoabi, 2003).

Research has also examined the spread of the older person's support network (Zoabi, 2000). In an effort to map the situation in terms of this factor, interviewers asked older victims of abuse to arrange the members of their informal network according to spheres of closeness and importance, placing those most important to them in the inner circles and those less important in the outer circles. The older people who had suffered abuse had relatively small informal networks, consisting mostly of their children. It is reasonable to assume that importance is determined not only on the emotional level but is also affected and amplified by emotional, social, physiological, and economic support. This is especially true with regard to older people with disabilities who require intensive support. Importance based solely on family relationships weakens over the years (Litwin & Zoabi, 2003).

In general, the social detachment and isolation of victims of elder abuse and neglect are particularly significant in traditional societies, such as the Palestinian society in Israel, where abuse of older people contradicts social norms and religious tenets. Research has shown that the support systems of these older people usually included only their children, and, at the same time, their relationships with caregiving and community organizations were minimal. In contrast, the networks of the older people who did not suffer abuse included relatively intensive community and social activity. In addition to children, they included friends, neighbors, and other relatives. They also applied for formal services at a higher frequency compared with their counterparts who suffered abuse (Zoabi, 2000).

In a traditional society like the Palestinian society in Israel, the isolation and detachment of older victims of abuse serve the interests of the abusers and victims alike in their efforts to prevent discovery of the abuse and neglect, on account of social stigma (Zoabi, 2000).

THE INTERACTIONAL LEVEL

It has been found that older victims of abuse in Palestinian society enjoyed less support in terms of quantity and frequency of contacts than older people who were not abused. This relative paucity was true regarding all types of support—emotional and instrumental (Zoabi, 2000).

The distancing of victims of elder abuse and neglect and the location of the members of their informal support systems in somewhat distant spheres not only reflect a relatively low level of support; these factors also indicate social, emotional, and physical isolation of the older person, which in turn contribute significantly to their abuse and its persistence (Litwin & Zoabi, 2003; Zoabi, 2000).

On the basis of these findings, it was concluded that on the functional level, victims of elder abuse and neglect were often people with disabilities whose dependence on their children was very great and who required a great deal of support but who actually received very little support compared with older people who were not abused (Zoabi, 2000). Furthermore, in addition to obtaining little support from

328 | Samir Zoabi

informal systems, the older people who were abused also enjoyed very little help from formal organizations. These findings portray a dire situation in terms of social status, health, and mental state of older people suffering abuse and neglect.

Conclusions and Recommendations

This chapter offers a review of the risk factors characteristic of older victims of abuse and of abusive caregivers. Elder abuse and neglect is defined as well as the structural and interactional characteristics of the informal support networks of older people who suffer abuse. In addition, the detection and exposure of such abuse and neglect are discussed.

Disability and dependence of older people who require care constitute a heavy emotional and instrumental burden for caregivers of certain sociodemographic characteristics (those who are older, women, those of low socioeconomic status). Furthermore, burnout and stress of caregivers exacerbate the situation, particularly when the informal social networks of the older people, of which they are an integral part, lack structural and functional means. In addition, different aspects of modernization—for example, stress and alienation—also contribute to the financial, physical, and mental difficulties involved in caring for an older person. Those factors increase and perpetuate the risk of abuse (Alon, 2015; Kosberg, 1988; Kosberg & Garcia, 1995; Litwin & Zoabi, 2003).

As for the abuser, it has been found that abusive caregivers suffer from social, mental, and financial problems more often than other caregivers. It has also been found that these caregivers, and particularly those who are physically abusive, are characterized by certain personality traits (Litwin & Zoabi, 2003; Zoabi, 2000).

Furthermore, Zoabi (2000) found that the realization of the rights of older people in the community, both by the people themselves and by relatives who care for them, is only partial. Thus, professional efforts are required to make services more accessible to the older people and their relatives. In addition, Litwin and Zoabi (2003) noted that the coping patterns of caregiving relatives of elders are limited by the emotional, economic, and physical difficulties involved in caring for an older person with disabilities in the home. This should be addressed by professional guidance and supervision as well as by provision of information about the rights of older people in the community and ways to realize them. Sharon and Zoabi (1997) reported that the dependence of older people on caregiving relatives is a major factor in the development and persistence of abuse; it is therefore important to instrumentally and emotionally empower them to be as independent as possible. Among other things, this requires development, by all means possible, of access to community services for older people, particularly those with disabilities.

The findings also indicate that older people living in urban areas are at greater risk of being abused and neglected. Therefore, professionals in cities must be particularly attentive in order to detect and address cases of abuse and neglect or those at risk of abuse. The social services in Palestinian society in Israel must invest special efforts in improving the ability of professionals to identify and handle problems of abuse and neglect of older people, particularly in cities. These capabilities can be enhanced by means of relevant training and in-service courses.

With respect to reporting, a notable increase has been found in recent years in the rate of older people that report their abuse and neglect to the legal authorities and social services. Nevertheless, more work is required to encourage older people to report cases in which they are abused. It is important to raise awareness of the potential for handling such cases as well as provide alternative living arrangements rather than remaining at home with abusive caregivers. Despite the rising number of day centers and assisted-living facilities in Palestinian society in Israel, more institutions of this type are still needed to respond to the problem of older people who remain in their homes for lack of choice. Similarly, there is need for more mental health practitioners and human service providers in the field of older adults. The actual number of gerontology professionals in the field falls short of the need.

The review of the research in the field of aging in general and violence against older people in Palestinian society in Israel in particular revealed that very little academic effort has been invested in these issues. The scarcity of studies conducted on this subject compared with studies of other age groups underscores this deficiency. Moreover, the subject of violence against older people has not received much research attention relative to other types of violence and abuse. To empower therapeutic and preventative efforts, it is important to expand the research in this area as well. Importantly, the mental health impact of exposure to abuse in older age among Palestinian citizens in Israel is a pending research subject.

Against this background, it is important to note that further research is required in the social and mental aspects of the family, which may be related to the incidence of injury of elders. In addition, there is a need for research that would facilitate the identification of dominant risk factors of injury to elders, studies of the status of reporting in this field, research that enables more accurate estimation of the incidence of domestic abuse, examination of the conduct of professionals exposed to such cases, and studies that would enable more effective professional conduct in the future.

In conclusion, as this chapter shows, the field of elder abuse in Palestinian society in Israel is in need of much change and improvement, on both research and practice levels. In addition, more work is also needed on the community level and in social policy.

The recommendations presented here represent an attempt to help alleviate this situation, based on the findings of Sharon and Zoabi (1997) and Zoabi (2000) as well as those of researchers in other places in the world. It is likely that full or even partial implementation of these recommendations could reduce the risk of abuse of older people and improve the ability of practitioners to respond in cases where such abuse takes place. Furthermore, these recommendations indicate directions for improvement in the living conditions and the personal, mental, and social welfare of older people in general, including both those who suffer abuse and neglect and those who do not.

SAMIR ZOABI is Lecturer in the Department of Social Work at Tel Hai College, Israel. He is also director of counseling for elderly people in the greater Nazareth region of the National Insurance Institute, Israel.

References

Al-Haj, M. (1989). Social research on family lifestyles among Arabs in Israel. *Journal of Comparative Family Studies, 175–195.*

Alon, S. (2006). Elder abuse and neglect: Whose definition? [in Hebrew]. *Gerontology, 33*(2), 55–69.

Alon, S. (2015). Elder abuse and neglect: Dimensions and ways of coping [in Hebrew]. In D. Prilutzky & M. Cohen (Eds.), *Practical gerontology* (pp. 445–482). Jerusalem: Joint Israel.

Alon, S., & Doron, I. (2009). Elder neglect: Theoretical, legal and practical aspects [in Hebrew]. *Gerontologia, 36*(1), 69–91.

Anetzberger, G., & Alon, S. (2015). An examination and explanation of cases of elder abuse in Israel. *The Gerontologist, 55*, 572–573.

Azaiza, F., & Brodsky, J. (1997). Changes in the Arab world and development of services for the Arab elderly in Israel during the last decade. *Journal of Gerontological Social Work, 27*(1–2), 37–53.

Cohen, M., Halevi-Levin, S., Gagin, R., & Friedman, G. (2006). Development of a screening tool for identifying elderly people at risk of abuse by their caregivers. *Journal of Aging and Health, 18*(5), 660–685.

Eisikovits, Z., Winterstein, T., & Lowenstein, A. (2005). *The national survey on elder abuse and neglect in Israel* [in Hebrew]. Haifa: The Center for Research and Study on Aging, University of Haifa and the Association for Planning and Development of Services for the Elderly in Israel (Eshel).

Govil, P., & Gupta, S. (2016). Domestic violence against elderly people: A case study of India. *Advances in Aging Research, 5*, 110–121.

Hantman, S., Cohen, G., Hroost, H., & Sassi, T. (2004). Elder abuse: A review of the phenomenon and presentation of a training project for its detection and prevention [in Hebrew]. *Gerontologia, 31*(1), 33–41.

Holt, M. (1994). Elder abuse in Britain. *Journal of Elder Abuse & Neglect, 5*(1), 33–39.

Johannesen, M., & LoGiudice, D. (2013). Elder abuse: A systematic review of risk factors in community-dwelling elders. *Age and Ageing, 42*, 292–298.

Khalaila, R., & Litwin, H. (2011). Does filial piety decrease depression among family caregivers? *Aging & Mental Health, 15*(6), 679–686.

Kluckhohn, C. (1971). Notes on anthropology and the minority elderly. *The Gerontologist, 11*, 94–98.

Kosberg, J. I. (1988). Preventing elder abuse: Identification of high risk factors prior to placement decisions. *The Gerontologist, 28*(1), 43–50.

Kosberg, J. I., & Garcia, J. L. (1995). Chapter 12: Common and unique themes on elder abuse from a world-wide perspective. *Journal of Elder Abuse & Neglect, 6*(3–4), 183–197.

Lachs, M. S., & Pillemer, K. (1995). Abuse and neglect of elderly persons. *New England Journal of Medicine, 332*(7), 437–443.

Lin, N., & Dean, A. (1984). Social support and depression. *Social Psychiatry and Psychiatric Epidemiology, 19*(2), 83–91.

Litwin, H. (1996). *The social networks of older people: A cross-national analysis.* Westport, CT: Greenwood.

Litwin, H. (1997). Support network type and health service utilization. *Research on Aging, 19*(3), 274–299.

Litwin, H. (1998). Social network type and health status in a national sample of elderly Israelis. *Social Science & Medicine, 46*(4), 599–609.

Litwin, H., & Zoabi, S. (2003). Modernization and elder abuse in an Arab-Israeli context. *Research on Aging, 25*(3), 224–246.

Lowenstein, A. (1995). Elder abuse in a forming society: Israel. *Journal of Elder Abuse & Neglect, 6*(3–4), 81–100.

Lowenstein, A. (2003). Elder abuse by family member caregivers [in Hebrew]. In A. Rozin (Ed.), *Aging and the aged in Israel* (pp. 707–713). Jerusalem: Bialik.

Lowenstein, A. (2006). Intergenerational relations within the aging family [in Hebrew]. In A. Rozin (Ed.), *Aging and the aged in Israel.* Jerusalem: Joint Israel.

Lowenstein, A., Eisikovits, Z., Band-Winterstein, T., & Enosh, G. (2009). Is elder abuse and neglect a social phenomenon? Data from the first national prevalence survey in Israel. *Journal of Elder Abuse & Neglect, 21*(3), 253–277.

Lowenstein, A., & Ron, P. (1999). Tension and conflict factors in second marriages as causes of abuse between elderly spouses. *Journal of Elder Abuse & Neglect, 11*(1), 23–45.

Mitchell, J. C. (1969). *The concept and use of social networks:* Indianapolis: Bobbs-Merrill.

Penhale, B. (1993). The abuse of elderly people: Considerations for practice. *British Journal of Social Work, 23*(2), 95–112.

Pittaway, E. D., & Westhues, A. (1994). The prevalence of elder abuse and neglect of older adults who access health and social services in London, Ontario, Canada. *Journal of Elder Abuse & Neglect, 5*(4), 77–94.

Pritchard, J. (1993). Dispelling some myths. *Journal of Elder Abuse & Neglect, 5*(2), 27–36.

Rosenfeld, H. (1968). Change, barriers to change, and contradictions in the Arab village family. *American Anthropologist,* 732–752.

Sharon, N., & Zoabi, S. (1997). Elder abuse in a land of tradition: The case of Israel's Arabs. *Journal of Elder Abuse & Neglect, 8*(4), 43–58.

Steptoe, A., Shankar, A., Demakakos, P., & Wardle, J. (2013). Social isolation, loneliness, and all-cause mortality in older men and women. *Proceedings of the National Academy of Sciences, 110*(15), 5797–5801.

Straus, M. A., Gelles, R. J., & Steinmetz, S. K. (1980). *Behind closed doors: Violence in the American family.* Garden City, NY: Transaction.

Thoits, P. A. (1982). Conceptual, methodological, and theoretical problems in studying social support as a buffer against life stress. *Journal of Health and Social Behavior, 23*(2), 145–159.

Thoits, P. A. (1995). Stress, coping, and social support processes: Where are we? What next? *Journal of Health and Social Behavior, 36*, 53–79.

Wethington, E., & Kessler, R. C. (1986). Perceived support, received support, and adjustment to stressful life events. *Journal of Health and Social Behavior, 27*, 78–89.

Zoabi, S. (1994). *Violence against the elderly in the Arab section: Reality or myth* [in Hebrew] (Unpublished master's thesis). School of Social Work, University of Haifa, Israel.

Zoabi, S. (2000). *Structural and interactional characteristics of the informal support systems of Arab elders in Israel who suffer injury* [in Hebrew] (Unpublished doctoral dissertation). Hebrew University of Jerusalem, Israel.

18

SUICIDE AND SUICIDE ATTEMPTS AMONG PALESTINIAN CITIZENS IN ISRAEL

Anat Brunstein-Klomek, Ora Nakash, Nehama Goldberger,
Ziona Haklai, Nabil Geraisy, Amir A. Birani,
Ahmad Natour, and Itzhak Levav

A CULTURALLY SPECIFIC APPROACH THAT EXAMINES THE INTERRELATIONSHIP between cultural and religious affiliation, gender, and age is important to understanding suicidal behavior in a country such as Israel, given its multivariate constitution (Gal et al., 2012; Hamdan et al., 2012; Harel-Fisch, Abdeen, Walsh, Radwan, & Fogel-Grinvald, 2012; Horton, 2006; Lester, 2012; Levinson, Haklai, Stein, & Gordon, 2006; Nakash, Barchana, Liphshitz, Keinan-Boker, & Levav, 2012). Cultural/religious affiliation may provide a set of protective beliefs, a socially supportive community, and a sense of hope (Dervic et al., 2004). All these are critical factors in the assessment of suicide risk for both prevention and intervention efforts.

Israel is a unique multicultural society encompassing various ethnic and religious groups. The majority of the population is Jewish, and approximately 19% of the total population is composed of Palestinians (Israel Central Bureau of Statistics [Israel CBS], 2014). As noted in other chapters, the Palestinian population in Israel is heterogeneous: it includes Muslims who reside in urban and rural areas, Bedouins (originally nomadic tribes of the Muslim faith, most of whom live in the south of the country), Druze, and Christians (Gharrah, 2012). The Palestinian population in Israel in 2014 numbered approximately 1.6 million (of a total population of about 7.8 million). At that time, most were Muslims (84%), including Bedouins (13% of the Palestinian population), followed by Druze and Christians (each about 8% of the Palestinian population in Israel) (Israel CBS, 2014). These groups differ in many respects, including religious beliefs and practices as well as attitudes toward suicide (Gal et al., 2012; Gharrah, 2012).

In this chapter we describe the epidemiology of completed suicide and suicide attempts among the different Palestinian groups.

Attitudes toward Suicide among Ethno-Religious Groups in Israel

Attitudes toward suicide differ among the various Israeli ethno-religious groups, although all strongly disapprove of it. According to Islamic law, suicide is regarded as homicide and, as such, is forbidden and falls under the category of capital crimes (*kabaer*). Life and death are considered God's will and therefore suicide is not only a severe sin but also a shameful act. The Qur'an strongly condemns self-inflicted death: "You shall not kill yourself. God is merciful towards you" (Qur'an Surah an-Nisa [The Women] 4:29). Illness, poverty, loss, and suffering are all considered a test of one's faith (*ibtila'a*) and one should demonstrate patience in order to be rewarded (Qur'an Surah Al-Baqarah [The Cow] 2:155–157). Despair in the face of pressures and life suffering not only implies a vote of no confidence in God and his mercy, but it also crosses the limits of the Islamic faith (Qur'an Surah Yusuf [Joseph] 12:87). In sum, a person who commits suicide seals his or her fate in hell with no hope of mercy. Since collectivism is a feature of the Muslim culture (Haj-Yahia & Sadan, 2008), families of suicide victims often face ostracism within their communities (Lubin, Glasser, Boyko, & Barell, 2001; Shah & Chandia, 2010).

On the one hand, suicide rates appear to be lower among Muslims than in other religions, even in countries that have populations belonging to several religious groups (except for a few countries in the former Soviet Union) (World Health Organization [WHO], 2014). Rates of attempted suicide, on the other hand, do not appear to be lower among Muslims compared to non-Muslims (Lester, 2006). In turn, Bedouins belong to a highly collectivistic, authoritarian, and patriarchal society. Noteworthy, despite urbanization processes that have characterized the Bedouin population in Israel over the last few decades, albeit slowly, Bedouins have largely retained their traditional tribal system (Al-Krenawi & Graham, 1996).

Christian Palestinians believe that one's life is the property of God and a gift to the world. Therefore, to destroy one's life is to wrongly assert dominion over what is God's and is a tragic loss of hope (Gearing & Lizardi, 2009). Christianity, including Catholic and Orthodox churches, sees suicide as a sin that violates the sixth commandment, "Thou shalt not kill" (Exodus 20:13), and is therefore an act against God. The gravity and guilt attributed to this sin varies among the different Christian denominations and depends on the circumstances surrounding this extreme act (Gearing & Lizardi, 2009). Historically, and continuing today, civil and criminal laws are on the books in many countries founded with Christian tenets that are designed to discourage suicide. Some of these laws disallow Christian burials to persons who commit suicide and may permit the confiscation of properties and possessions of such a person as well as of the family (Gearing & Lizardi, 2009). An exception is the Greek Orthodox Church in the United States, which issued a "Pastoral Letter on Suicide" (Standing Conference of the Canonical Orthodox Bishops in the Americas [SCOBA], 2007) in which the church recognizes the scientific findings about suicide. It states that, because of the complexity of suicide, both in terms of determining causes and in terms of ministering to those most affected, the general pastoral recommendation is that a church burial and memorial services should be granted.

The Druze religion, which started as a school of thought (*madhab*), diverged from Islam in the eleventh century yet continued to maintain the Arabic language. According to the Druze faith, all human souls were created in one moment, and their number remains the same. Reincarnation (*takammuss*) is a seminal component of the faith. Believers maintain that when a member of the Druze community dies, the soul is immediately reborn in another Druze body, or reborn beyond the human realm into the next ascending realm of closeness to God (Bennett, 2006). Despite a strong belief in the eternal life of the soul through reincarnation, Druze faith maintains the absolute prohibition of suicide and sees it as a violation of the basic tenets of the faith (Morad, Merrick, Schwarz, & Merrick, 2005).

The Jewish faith regards life as a gift from God, which is valued above all (Witztum & Stein, 2012). The body is given to the person for a fixed time by God, and, therefore, people are responsible for safeguarding it. Murder is one of the three cardinal sins, and one of the commandments handed down to the Jewish people forbids it. Suicide is a form of murder according to the *Talmud* and therefore breaches the biblical commandment, "Thou shalt not kill." Religious law stipulates that Jews who commit suicide are not entitled to a full Jewish burial. Indeed, even conducting the rites of mourning such as recital of the *Kaddish* (the prayer for the dead) and sitting *shiva* (a seven-day period of mourning) for those who committed suicide are controversial in religious communities (Gvion, Levi-Belz, & Apter, 2014).

In this chapter, we report the incidence rates of completed suicide and suicide attempts among the four Palestinian groups in Israel cited earlier by age and gender. We include Israeli-born Jews as a comparison group.

Methods

Data on completed suicide rates in Israel are based on the nationwide database of causes of death maintained by the Israel CBS. This governmental body receives and codes information from death certificates filled out by physicians and supplemental data on completed suicides from other sources, such as police and army records and the Israel Pathology Institute. The data file includes age, region of residence, and national/religious affiliation, allowing calculation of rates by group for 1999–2011.

Data on suicide attempts were extracted from the Israeli National Emergency Room Admissions Database (NERAD) for 2004–2012, which includes all admissions to the emergency departments of all general hospitals. Suicide attempts were identified by an entry cause of suicide attempt and/or an emergency room diagnosis of suicide attempt.

The Israel CBS also publishes yearly population estimates by age, gender, locality, and the national/religious groups mentioned previously, which enable calculation of rates of suicides and suicide attempts for these groups. Age-adjusted rates were calculated using the 2009 total population of Israel (after the 2008 census) as standard population, aged 15 and older for suicides, and aged 10 and older for suicide attempts.

Results

Suicide Rates

Table 18.1a includes absolute numbers of suicides, total crude rates, and age-adjusted rates of suicide for the total period 1999–2011 for the five ethno-religious/national groups by age and gender. Total rates for the Muslim, Bedouin, and Christian groups are similar to each other and lower than the suicide rates among the

Table 18.1a. Suicides in the Palestinian Population in Israel by Age and Gender, 1999–2011 (Absolute Numbers and Rates per 100,000 Population)

Age group/ religion	Absolute numbers						Total crude rate	Age-adjusted rate[a]
	15–24	25–44	45–64	65–74	75+	total 15+		
Total								
Bedouin	23	14	2	0	0	39	4.4	3.2
Christian	12	14	5	3	2	36	3.3	3.3
Druze	43	39	13	0	1	96	9.8	8.7
Jewish, Israeli-born	461	850	584	91	27	2,013	6.7	7.3
Muslim	56	108	37	3	1	205	2.7	2.5
Males								
Bedouin	16	8	2	0	0	26	5.9	4.5
Christian	11	13	5	2	1	32	5.9	5.8
Druze	42	34	11	0	1	88	17.7	15.6
Jewish, Israeli-born	374	680	459	66	24	1,603	10.6	11.8
Muslim	53	84	29	3	1	170	4.4	4.1
Females								
Bedouin	7	6	0	0	0	13	(2.9)	(2.0)
Christian	1	1	0	1	1	4		
Druze	1	5	2	0	0	8	(1.6)	(1.6)
Jewish, Israeli-born	87	170	125	25	3	410	2.7	3.0
Muslim	3	24	8	0	0	35	0.9	0.9

[a] 2009 population of Israel taken as standard.

Source: Adapted from *The Minister of Health report on suicide 2018* [in Hebrew]. Retrieved from https://www.health.gov.il/UnitsOffice/HD/MTI/info/Pages/suicides.aspx

Table 18.1b. Suicide Rates in Palestinian and Jewish Population Groups in Israel by Age (under 65), 1999–2011

Age group/religion	15–24	25–44	45–64
Total			
Bedouin	6.3	(3.7)[a]	—[b]
Christian	(4.7)[a]	(3.1)[a]	(1.8)[a]
Druze	15.0	8.9	(6.8)[a]
Jewish, Israeli-born	5.1	6.2	9.2
Muslim	2.4	3.1	2.6
Males			
Bedouin	(8.5)[a]	(4.2)[a]	—[b]
Christian	(8.5)[a]	(5.7)[a]	(3.7)[a]
Druze	28.9	15.2	(11.4)[a]
Jewish, Israeli-born	8.1	9.8	14.6
Muslim	4.4	4.7	4.1

[a] Rate based on 5–19 cases. [b] Rate based on less than 5 cases.
Source: Adapted from *The Minister of Health report on suicide 2018* [in Hebrew]. Retrieved from https://www.health.gov.il/UnitsOffice/HD/MTI/info/Pages/suicides.aspx.

Druze and Jewish populations. The Druze have higher rates, particularly among males. Age-adjusted rates for Muslims were 2.5 (4.1, males; 0.9, females); Bedouin, 3.2 (4.5, males; 2.0, females); Christians, 3.3 (5.8, males; no data on females); Druze, 8.7 (15.6, males; 1.6, females); and for Jews, 7.3 (11.8, males; 3.0, females), all rates per 100,000 population.

Table 18.1b presents suicide rates by age for the total population and among males under age 65. Among females and at older ages, suicides were so rare for members of the majority of the Palestinian groups that reliable rates could not be calculated. Among males, the suicide rate for the youngest age group, 15–24, was particularly high among Druze (almost four times that of Israeli-born Jews), while the rates among Bedouins and Christians were also slightly higher for this age group when compared to older age groups (25–44 and 45–64). Young adult Israeli-born Jews (i.e., those between the ages of 25 and 44) had a higher rate than all Palestinian groups except for the Druze, for whom the suicide rate was even higher. In older adults (those between the ages of 45 and 64), Israeli-born Jews had the highest rate. Rates of suicide among Muslims were the lowest at ages 15–44 and at ages 45–64. Christians had the lowest rates of suicide.

Suicide Attempts

Suicide attempts for each ethno-religious/national group by gender and age are presented in table 18.2. The data include absolute numbers, age-specific rates, total crude rates, and age-adjusted rates of suicide attempts for 2004–2012 for the five

Table 18.2. Suicide Attempts in the Palestinian Population in Israel by Gender and Age, 2004–2012

Age group/religion	Absolute numbers						Rates/100,000 population, age 15–64			Total crude rate 10+	Age-adjusted[a]
	10–14	15–24	25–44	45–64	65–74	75+	15–24	25–44	45–64		
Total											
Bedouin	29	448	304	33	2	1	149.4	95.3	34.8	83.2	72.4
Christian	18	188	253	75	4	6	102.3	79.4	35.5	60.1	58.6
Druze	7	409	209	26	1	0	198.4	63.6	17	76.4	64.9
Jewish, Israeli-born	1,138	9,870	8,331	3,843	253	104	154.4	81	74	89	83.1
Muslim	261	3,311	2,597	508	17	17	187.6	100.5	44.1	96.3	84.8
Males											
Bedouin	7	102	84	12	1	0	66.6	53.6	(27.8)[b]	42	39.1
Christian	2	47	90	44	1	4	51	56.1	42.3	42	41.3
Druze	2	299	100	21	1	0	285.9	60.3	26.9	97.8	83.1
Jewish, Israeli-born	238	3,757	3,951	1,867	102	43	114.8	76	72.6	74.6	70.9
Muslim	58	972	985	320	14	11	107.9	74.8	55.5	66.8	62.9
Females											
Bedouin	22	346	220	21	1	1	235.7	135.5	40.8	124.1	105.5
Christian	16	141	163	31	3	2	153.8	103	29	77.8	76.2
Druze	5	110	109	5	0	0	108.4	67	(6.7)[b]	54.4	46.2
Jewish, Israeli-born	900	6,113	4,380	1,976	151	61	196	86	75.4	103.7	95.7
Muslim	203	2,339	1,612	188	3	6	270.7	127.1	32.7	126.6	107.9

[a] 2009 population of Israel taken as standard. [b] Rate based on 5–19 cases.

Source: Adapted from *The Minister of Health report on suicide 2018* [in Hebrew]. Retrieved from https://www.health.gov.il/UnitsOffice/HD/MTI/info/Pages/suicides.aspx.

groups: Muslims, Bedouin, Christian, Druze, and Israeli-born Jews. Total rates of suicide attempts were highest among Muslims and Israeli-born Jews and lowest among Christians. Male rates were lower than female rates in all groups except for the Druze.

Rates of suicide attempts among Druze males were particularly high for those between the ages of 15 and 24 (286 per 100,000 persons). This rate was approximately 2.5 times that of Israeli-born Jews (115 per 100,000). The attempted suicide rate of Druze females was the lowest of the populations studied (108 per 100,000), about half that of Israeli-born Jewish females (196 per 100,000). Female rates were highest for Muslim and Bedouin groups for those in the 15- to 24-year-old age range (271 and 236 per 100,000, respectively) compared to 196 per 100,000 for Israeli-born Jews and 154 per 100,000 for Christians. However, for individuals between the ages of 25 and 44 and 45 and 64, total rates for the Druze were lowest, while for Muslims and Bedouins the attempt rates were highest in the age range 25–44 for the total population and among females.

Israeli-born Jews in the age range 45–64 had much higher suicide attempt rates than all other groups, for the total sample and among both genders. This rate was about twice that of Bedouins and Christians for the total sample. At older ages, suicide attempts were rare among the Palestinian groups.

International Comparison

Table 18.3 shows a comparison of suicide rates in various Muslim countries in the Middle East and in the former Soviet Union in 2012 with the rates of all Israeli Muslims (including Bedouins) in 2009–2011. The total rate for Israeli Muslims is similar to that in Egypt, Jordan, Iraq, Algeria, and Azerbaijan, but the male rate is moderately higher while the female rate is slightly lower.

Discussion

In this chapter, we examine the interrelationship between ethno-religious/national affiliation, gender, and age in understanding suicidal behaviors. We report on national data presenting the incidence rates of suicide and suicide attempts among the different groups in Israel and uncovering different patterns of risk for suicide and suicide attempts as a function of these cultural groups.

Suicide

The lower rates of suicide among Palestinians including Muslims, Bedouins, and Christians compared to the Druze and the Jews in Israel confirm previous findings (Gal et al., 2012; Lubin et al., 2001; Morad et al., 2005). The difference in suicide rates between Muslims and Christians and Israeli-born Jews may be explained by social norms and religious observance, which possibly serve as protective factors against suicidal behavior. Arab culture is characterized by a strong religious belief system

Table 18.3. Age-Standardized Suicide Rates[a] of Muslims in Israel, Selected Middle Eastern Countries, and Muslim Countries in the Former Soviet Union by Gender, 2012 (Rates per 100,000 Population)

Country	Male	Female	Total
Israel, Muslims[b]	3.1	0.9	2.0
Jordan[c]	2.2	1.9	2.0
Egypt[c]	2.4	1.2	1.7
Syria[c]	0.7	0.2	0.4
Lebanon[c]	1.2	0.6	0.9
Algeria[c]	2.3	1.5	1.9
Saudi Arabia[c]	0.6	0.2	0.4
Iraq[c]	1.2	2.1	1.7
Uzbekistan	13.2	4.1	8.5
Azerbaijan[c]	2.4	1.0	1.7
Turkmenistan[c]	32.5	7.5	19.6

[a] Standardized to the WHO World Standard Population. [b] Data for Muslims in Israel are based on Israeli data for 2009–2011. [c] Low coverage registration or no vital registration.
Source: World Health Organization. (2014). *Preventing suicide: A global imperative.* Geneva: World Health Organization. Retrieved from http://apps.who.int/iris /bitstream/10665/131056/1/9789241564779_eng.pdf?ua=1&ua=1.

and spiritual coping, both factors associated with lower risk for suicidality (Stack & Kposowa, 2011). Arab culture is also highly collectivistic and characterized by strong family bonds (Peleg-Popko, Klingman, & Nahhas, 2003), whereas the Israeli Jewish subculture tends to emphasize individuality among the secular (Oyserman, Coon, & Kemmelmeier, 2002; Peleg-Popko et al., 2003). Moreover, Palestinians may feel very comfortable expressing feelings, which helps them cope more effectively with life stressors (Shechtman & Halevi, 2006). In addition, there is a possibility that Palestinian society covers up, misclassifies, or fails to report completed suicides (Bursztein & Apter, 2009).

Of note are the relatively high rates of suicide among young Druze males, probably associated with factors specific to their military service (Kohn, Levav, Chang, Halperin, & Zadka, 1997). Israeli law mandates that all 18-year-old men serve in the Israel Defense Force (IDF) for three years. Military service is mandatory for Druze men and voluntary for other Palestinian groups. Military service may increase the suicide rate among young Druze males by increasing their stress levels as well as by enabling their accessibility to firearms (Morad et al., 2005). An additional factor that may affect the rates of suicide among young Druze males could involve feelings of belonging to a minority while at the same time risking their lives for their country (Scrimin, Moscardino, & Natour, 2014).

In contrast to the Druze, and in part, to the Bedouins, who volunteer to serve in the army, an additional protective factor explaining the low suicide rate among Muslims is that they usually do not serve in the military (Katz-Sheiban & Eshet, 2008) and thus are free from cultural clashes and allegiances, environmental stresses, and access to weapons.

The relatively high suicide rate found among Bedouins aged 15–24 corresponds to an earlier study that found that the levels of depression symptoms among Bedouin youth was higher than among Jewish youth (Abu-Kaf & Priel, 2008). In a recent study among Bedouins in the south of Israel, 64% of older Bedouin adolescents (aged 18–20) reported depression scores that exceeded the clinical cutoff (Abu-Kaf & Shahar, 2017).

Suicide rates were lower in older Palestinian adults, aged 65 and over, while the comparable rates for Jews were much higher (Goldberger, Aburbeh, & Haklai, 2014). It appears likely that the importance of the extended family in Palestinian society (Levav & Aisenberg, 1989) enables them to access support from the community and be granted a high social status.

The findings that men committed suicide more frequently than women across all ethno-religious groups is consistent with results reported by many international and local studies (Gal et al., 2012; Lubin et al., 2001).

Lastly, methodological issues, particularly problems in ascertaining the cause of death, may also heighten the disparity in suicide rates of Jews compared to Palestinians. Various pressures, open or covert, may result in cases of suicide being recorded as cases of undetermined external causes. Although changes with regard to how suicidality is viewed are slowly emerging in Palestinian culture, stigmatic pressures to keep suicidal behavior hidden still remain potent among Palestinians, particularly within their small communities (Lubin et al., 2001).

Suicide Attempts

In contrast to the findings pertaining to completed suicide overall, Muslims were found to engage with a higher frequency (at younger ages) in suicide attempts. The Israel Ministry of Health (2015) reported that the rate of suicide attempts has been rising in recent years, particularly among females. The rate, which was about 1.0 per 100,000 between 1999 and 2003, increased to about 3.0 per 100,000 in 2006–2010 and has become higher than that documented among Jews (Goldberger et al., 2014). The high rates of suicide attempts among Muslims may be a reflection of the rapid social change and Western acculturation that they are experiencing in Israel. These changes may be causing a weakening in traditional values. In addition, there is limited accessibility to mental health services for young Palestinians (Mansbach-Kleinfeld et al., 2010).

The high rates of suicide attempts for those between the ages of 15 and 24 is in line with international epidemiological studies and local studies showing that suicide attempts are largely a phenomenon of adolescents and young adults (Levinson et al., 2006; Levinson, Haklai, Stein, Polakiewicz, & Levav, 2007). Developmental changes, rising levels of anxiety/depression, disparities between adolescent and parent, and intergenerational conflict create conditions that are believed to lead to adolescent suicidal behavior (Gould, Greenberg, Velting, & Shaffer, 2003). Similarly, the finding that more women than men attempt suicide (except for the Druze) at younger ages is supported by international studies (WHO, 2014).

The higher incidence of suicide attempts among Druze males may be explained by an identity crisis and/or stress or frustration (see previous discussion). The lowest rate of suicide attempts found among Christians has also been noted in earlier studies (e.g., Lester, 2006) and may be explained by the Christians' perception of mental health services as less stigmatizing (Al-Krenawi & Graham, 2011).

The high prevalence rates of attempts among Muslim and Bedouin women may be explained by the social pressure that young Palestinian women are subject to. Studies have shown that women in Palestinian communities are exposed to more stressors and difficulties because they live in a society where men have greater power and authority (Barakat, 2000). Family structure in both cultures is of a patriarchal nature. That may lead some women to resort to suicidal behavior to resolve a perceived psychosocial crisis or as a protest against oppression (Bursztein & Apter, 2009). Similarly, in a recent study, parental disconnectedness was associated with suicide attempts among Palestinian girls in Israel (Harel-Fisch et al., 2012). Another important factor that may explain the high attempt rate among women is the help-seeking characteristics of the Palestinian population in Israel in relation to treatment in general and psychiatric treatment in particular. Studies have indicated that Palestinian citizens in Israel, especially women, seek less help from professional sources compared to their Jewish counterparts (Haj-Yahia, 1995, 1997; Haj-Yahia & Edleson, 1994). Druze females, however, who are the only group to have lower suicide attempt rates than males, appear to suffer less from these problems.

The differences between Jews and Palestinians in Israel in suicide rates versus suicide attempts may be explained by the hypothesis that suicide attempts among the Palestinians may be an expression of emotional distress rather than a wish to die (Ashkar et al., 2006).

Limitations

For Bedouins, we only included the Muslims in the south of Israel. This report is incomplete as there are also Bedouins in other regions in Israel who are difficult to identify in the national records. Hence, Bedouins may have been included in the Muslim group. In addition, there are still methodological problems in determining suicide rates in general in Israel and among Palestinians in particular (Lubin et al., 2001). Moreover, we did not include data on undetermined external causes of death, although in many communities suicide is highly stigmatizing and may be recorded as death from unknown causes or undetermined intention (Bursztein & Apter, 2009). Lastly, our current analysis did not include other risk behaviors—such as history of psychiatric hospitalization—that are important when examining suicidality (c.g., Harel-Fisch et al., 2012).

Conclusion

Our findings have important implications. Knowledge about cultural and religious background is essential to understanding suicide rates among different ethnic and religious groups. These results underscore the urgent need to explore suicidality among these cultural groups while highlighting the importance of examining intersectionality among ethnicity, gender, and age in identifying suicide risk and preventing suicide. The Israel National Suicide Prevention Plan (Israel Ministry of Health, 2015) conducted a successful pilot in three municipalities in Israel, including one Arab Israeli village. As a result of this pilot, a nationwide initiative has been started.

To conclude, our chapter has important clinical and research implications for both preventive and intervention efforts. The Palestinian groups vary both in terms of their suicide attempts and suicide rates and should be targeted with unique and specific approaches. In addition, females and males differ from each other in their suicidal behavior, and therefore prevention and intervention programs should target them separately.

ANAT BRUNSTEIN-KLOMEK is a clinical psychologist and Associate Professor of Psychology at the Baruch Ivcher School of Psychology at the Interdisciplinary Center in Herzliya, Israel. She is also Adjunct Associate Research Scientist in the Division of Child and Adolescent Psychiatry at Columbia University/New York State Psychiatric Institute, New York.

ORA NAKASH is a clinical psychologist and Professor in the School for Social Work at Smith College, Northampton, MA, and Adjunct Professor at the Baruch Ivcher School of Psychology at the Interdisciplinary Center in Herzliya, Israel.

NEHAMA GOLDBERGER is Coordinator in the Health Statistics Unit, Health Information Division, Ministry of Health, Israel.

ZIONA HAKLAI is Director of the Health Information Division, Ministry of Health, Israel.

NABIL GERAISY is Deputy District Psychiatrist, Northern District, Ministry of Health, Israel.

AMIR A. BIRANI is a clinical social worker in private practice and a fellow researcher with Wahiba Abu-Rass, School of Social Work, Adelphi University, New York.

AHMAD NATOUR is Associate Professor in the Law School at the Hebrew University of Jerusalem, Israel. He is also a judge in the Sharia' Court system and President of the High Sharia' Court of Appeals of the country.

ITZHAK LEVAV is Affiliated Professor in the Department of Community Mental Health, Faculty of Social Welfare and Health Sciences, at the University of Haifa, Israel. He is editor of *Psychiatric and Behavioral Disorders in Israel: From Epidemiology to Mental Health Action*, and editor (with Jutta Lindert) of *Violence and Mental Health: Its Manifold Faces.*

References

Abu-Kaf, S., & Priel, B. (2008). Dependent and self-critical vulnerabilities to depression in two different cultural contexts. *Personality and Individual Differences, 44*(3), 689–700.

Abu-Kaf, S., & Shahar, G. (2017). Depression and somatic symptoms among two ethnic groups in Israel: Testing three theoretical models. *Israel Journal of Psychiatry and Related Sciences, 54*, 32–40.

Al-Krenawi, A., & Graham, J. R. (1996). Social work and traditional healing rituals among the Bedouin of the Negev, Israel. *International Social Work, 39*(2), 177–188.

Al-Krenawi, A., & Graham, J. R. (2011). Mental health help-seeking among Arab university students in Israel, differentiated by religion. *Mental Health, Religion & Culture, 14*(2), 157–167.

Ashkar, K., Giloni, C., Grinshpoon, A., Geraisy, N., Gruner, E., Cohen, R., . . . Ponizovsky, A. M. (2006). Suicidal attempts admitted to a general hospital in the western Galilee: An interethnic comparison study. *Israel Journal of Psychiatry and Related Sciences, 43*(2), 137–145.

Barakat, H. (2000). *The Arab society in the twentieth century* [in Arabic]. Beirut: Center for Arab Unity Studies.

Bennett, A. (2006). Reincarnation, sect unity, and identity among the Druze. *Ethnology, 45*(2), 87–104.

Bursztein, C., & Apter, A. (2009). The epidemiology of suicidal behavior in the Israeli population. In I. Levav (Ed.), *Psychiatric and behavioral disorders in Israel: From epidemiology to mental health action* (pp. 267–286). Jerusalem: Gefen.

Dervic, K., Oquendo, M. A., Grunebaum, M. F., Ellis, S., Burke, A. K., & Mann, J. J. (2004). Religious affiliation and suicide attempt. *American Journal of Psychiatry, 161*(12), 2303–2308.

Gal, G., Goldberger, N., Kabaha, A., Haklai, Z., Geraisy, N., Gross, R., & Levav, I. (2012). Suicidal behavior among Muslim Arabs in Israel. *Social Psychiatry and Psychiatric Epidemiology, 47*(1), 11–17.

Gearing, R. E., & Lizardi, D. (2009). Religion and suicide. *Journal of Religion and Health, 48*(3), 332–341.

Gharrah, R. (2012). *Arab society in Israel* (5th ed.). Jerusalem: Van Leer Jerusalem Institute.

Goldberger, N., Aburbeh, M., & Haklai, Z. (2014). *Suicidality in Israel.* Jerusalem: Israel Ministry of Health.

Gould, M. S., Greenberg, T., Velting, D. M., & Shaffer, D. (2003). Youth suicide risk and preventive interventions: A review of the past 10 years. *Journal of the American Academy of Child & Adolescent Psychiatry, 42*(4), 386–405.

Gvion, Y., Levi-Belz, Y., & Apter, A. (2014). Suicide in Israel: An update. *Crisis: The Journal of Crisis Intervention and Suicide Prevention, 35*(3), 141–144.

Haj-Yahia, M. M. (1995). Toward culturally sensitive intervention with Arab families in Israel. *Contemporary Family Therapy, 17*(4), 429–447.

Haj-Yahia, M. M. (1997). Predicting beliefs about wife beating among engaged Arab men in Israel. *Journal of Interpersonal Violence, 12*(4), 530–545.

Haj-Yahia, M. M., & Edleson, J. L. (1994). Predicting the use of conflict resolution tactics among engaged Arab-Palestinian men in Israel. *Journal of Family Violence, 9*(1), 47–62.

Haj-Yahia, M. M., & Sadan, E. (2008). Issues in intervention with battered women in collectivist societies. *Journal of Marital and Family Therapy, 34*(1), 1–13.

Hamdan, S., Melhem, N., Orbach, I., Farbstein, I., El-Haib, M., Apter, A., & Brent, D. (2012). Protective factors and suicidality in members of Arab kindred. *Crisis: The Journal of Crisis Intervention and Suicide Prevention, 33*(2), 80–86.

Harel-Fisch, Y., Abdeen, Z., Walsh, S. D., Radwan, Q., & Fogel-Grinvald, H. (2012). Multiple risk behaviors and suicidal ideation and behavior among Israeli and Palestinian adolescents. *Social Science & Medicine, 75*(1), 98–108.

Horton, L. (2006). Social cultural and demographic factors in suicide. In R. Simon & R. Hales (Eds.), *The American psychiatric publishing textbook of suicide assessment and management* (pp. 107–138). Washington, DC: American Psychiatric Association Press.

Israel Central Bureau of Statistics [Israel CBS]. (2014). *Statistical abstract of Israel, Table 2, Population, by religion* [in Hebrew]. Retreived from http://www.cbs.gov.il/reader/shnaton /templ_shnaton_e.html?num_tab=st02_02&CYear=2014.

Israel Ministry of Health. (2015). The national program for the prevention of suicidality and suicide. Retrieved from http://www.health.gov.il/English/MinistryUnits/HealthDivision /MedicalAdministration/Psychology/Pages/suicide-prev.aspx.

Katz-Sheiban, B., & Eshet, Y. (2008). Facts and myths about suicide: A study of Jewish and Arab students in Israel. *OMEGA: Journal of Death and Dying, 57*(3), 279–298.

Kohn, R., Levav, I., Chang, B., Halperin, B., & Zadka, P. (1997). Epidemiology of youth suicide in Israel. *Journal of the American Academy of Child & Adolescent Psychiatry, 36*(11), 1537–1542.

Lester, D. (2006). Suicide and Islam. *Archives of Suicide Research, 10*(1), 77–97.

Lester, D. (2012). Spirituality and religiosity as predictors of depression and suicidal ideation: An exploratory study. *Psychological Reports, 110*(1), 247–250.

Levav, I., & Aisenberg, E. (1989). The epidemiology of suicide in Israel: International and intranational comparisons. *Suicide and Life-Threatening Behavior, 19*(2), 184–200.

Levinson, D., Haklai, Z., Stein, N., & Gordon, E. S. (2006). Suicide attempts in Israel: Age by gender analysis of a national emergency departments database. *Suicide and Life-Threatening Behavior, 36*(1), 97–102.

Levinson, D., Haklai, Z., Stein, N., Polakiewicz, J., & Levav, I. (2007). Suicide ideation, planning and attempts: Results from the Israel national health survey. *Israel Journal of Psychiatry and Related Sciences, 44*(2), 136–143.

Lubin, G., Glasser, S., Boyko, V., & Barell, V. (2001). Epidemiology of suicide in Israel: A nationwide population study. *Social Psychiatry and Psychiatric Epidemiology, 36*(3), 123–127.

Mansbach-Kleinfeld, I., Farbstein, I., Levinson, D., Apter, A., Erhard, R., Palti, H., . . . Levav, I. (2010). Service use for mental disorders and unmet need: Results from the Israel survey on mental health among adolescents. *Psychiatric Services, 61*(3), 241–249.

Morad, M., Merrick, E., Schwarz, A., & Merrick, J. (2005). A review of suicide behavior among Arab adolescents. *Scientific World Journal, 5,* 674–679. Retrieved from https://www .researchgate.net/publication/7632490_A_review_of_Suicide_Behavior_Among_Arab _Adolescents.

Nakash, O., Barchana, M., Liphshitz, I., Keinan-Boker, L., & Levav, I. (2012). The effect of cancer on suicide in ethnic groups with a differential suicide risk. *European Journal of Public Health, 23*(1), 114–115.

Oyserman, D., Coon, H. M., & Kemmelmeier, M. (2002). Rethinking individualism and collectivism: Evaluation of theoretical assumptions and meta-analyses. *Psychological Bulletin, 128*(1), 3–72.

Peleg-Popko, O., Klingman, A., & Nahhas, I. A.-H. (2003). Cross-cultural and familial differences between Arab and Jewish adolescents in test anxiety. *International Journal of Intercultural Relations, 27*(5), 525–541.

Scrimin, S., Moscardino, U., & Natour, M. (2014). Socio-ecological correlates of mental health among ethnic minorities in areas of political conflict: A study of Druze adolescents in Israel. *Transcultural Psychiatry, 51*(2), 209–227.

Shah, A., & Chandia, M. (2010). The relationship between suicide and Islam: A cross-national study. *Journal of Injury and Violence Research, 2*(2), 93–97.

Shechtman, Z., & Halevi, H. (2006). Does ethnicity explain functioning in group counseling? The case of Arab and Jewish counseling trainees in Israel. *Group Dynamics: Theory, Research, and Practice, 10*(3), 181–193.

Stack, S., & Kposowa, A. J. (2011). Religion and suicide acceptability: A cross-national analysis. *Journal for the Scientific Study of Religion, 50*(2), 289–306.

Standing Conference of the Canonical Orthodox Bishops in the Americas [SCOBA]. (2007). *Pastoral letter on suicide, 5/23/07.* Retrieved from http://www.assemblyofbishops.org/news /scoba/2007-05-25-letter-on-suicide.

Witztum, E., & Stein, D. (2012). Suicide in Judaism with a special emphasis on modern Israel. *Religions, 3*(3), 725–738.

World Health Organization [WHO]. (2014). *Preventing suicide: A global imperative.* Retrieved from http://apps.who.int/iris/bitstream/handle/10665/131056/9789241564779_eng.pdf ?sequence=1.

PART V
INTERVENTIONS TO RESTORE MENTAL HEALTH

19

PSYCHOTHERAPY FOR PALESTINIAN CITIZENS IN ISRAEL

Nazeh Natur

THE CURRICULUM FOR PALESTINIAN PSYCHOLOGISTS AND PSYCHOTHERAPISTS TRAINED in Israel is based on Western theories of psychology. Some authors (Al-Krenawi, 2005; Al-Krenawi, Graham, Dean, & Eltaiba, 2004; Dwairy, 1997a, 1997b, 2006; Dwairy & Van Sickle, 1996; Sue & Sue, 2003) argue that Palestinian cultural and religious restrictions may present barriers to psychotherapy, while others (Masalha, 1999) suggest that Western therapeutic theory and techniques can be applied to non-Western clients without any modifications. In this chapter, I review the literature on psychotherapy for Palestinian citizens in Israel and discuss the application of Western psychotherapeutic practices in treating Palestinian service users.

Background

Most Palestinians in pre-1948 Israel were peasants who earned their living in agriculture. At the time, the Palestinian family was traditional in nature, authoritarian, and patriarchal and had largely maintained a tribal structure. After 1948, and with the loss of the land, the vast majority of Palestinians became laborers. Accordingly, sociocultural changes have taken place, yet the core nature of the group has nevertheless remained.

Indeed, as other chapters in this book note, Palestinian society in Israel may still be defined as traditional and collectivist. Its family structure remains authoritarian, strongly religious, and with highly valued social norms. Concomitantly, however, and over the past decades, it has been undergoing transformations in economic, social, and cultural domains, including mental health. Hence, Palestinian society in Israel may presently be characterized as a society in transition (Dwairy, 1998).

Factors affecting health are numerous and include environmental factors, such as wars and disasters; exposure to violence; lack of access to basic commodities and services; social and economic determinants (e.g., poverty and discrimination); and individual attributes and behavioral patterns, such as emotional and social intelligence (World Health Organization [WHO], 2012). Wars in particular have been found to have a significant effect on mental health (Levy & Sidel, 2008). Psychological distress, among other factors, may result from personal or collective trauma. Daoud, Shankardass, O'Campo, Anderson, and Agbaria (2012) documented lower self-appraised health, poorer socioeconomic status, and higher stress among Palestinians displaced during the Nakba of 1948 and their descendants in comparison to families who were not displaced. The mental health impact of exposure to violence on Palestinian citizens in Israel has also been documented in the work of Gelkopf, Solomon, Berger, and Bleich (2008). These authors concluded that terrorism had a differential impact on Jews and Palestinians in the civilian Israeli population and that prolonged exposure of the Palestinian minority to terrorist violence led to more severe stress symptoms than among the Jewish majority.

These findings seem to indicate that the concept of traumatic memory is worth investigating in the Palestinian context in both collective and individual aspects (Elsass, 2001). Older Palestinian citizens in Israel witnessed the trauma that began with the 1948–1949 war, and the entire population continues to live with the effects of the ongoing conflict. Recall here that during the early years of the state of Israel, the Palestinian population was under military control. Since then, Palestinians in Israel have experienced numerous violent situations, directly or indirectly, in and outside of Israel. As noted in other chapters, Nakba Day, which commemorates the day the Palestinians were displaced from their homes in 1948, continues to be observed as a watershed moment in their journey of suffering. As noted elsewhere, too, additional traumatic events endured by Palestinian citizens in Israel include the raids carried out by Israel's armed forces in the 1950s and 1960s in response to Arab guerrilla groups' attacks against Israeli forces. Of note is the Kafr Qasim massacre (1956) committed by the Israeli army, in which six women, 19 men, 23 children ages 8–17, and one unborn child were killed. At the time, the victims were violating a curfew of which they were unaware.

The 1960s and 1970s generated two major wars and significant local events that affected the Palestinian population in Israel. The 1967 Six-Day War resulted in the occupation of the West Bank, the Gaza Strip, and the Golan Heights. The 1973 October war (Yom Kippur War) was initiated by Egypt and Syria. In the interim, the population experienced three years of violence known as the War of Attrition. While these wars did not directly involve the Palestinian residents of Israel, another major event, the 1976 Land Day strike and demonstrations, did. It began on March 30, 1976, when the local Palestinian leadership planned a general strike and marches to protest the announced plan of the Israeli government to confiscate thousands of acres of Palestinian land for security and settlement purposes. During the march, six young, unarmed Palestinian men were killed by the police forces, about a hundred were wounded, and hundreds were arrested. The events of Land Day left Palestinian citizens in Israel in turmoil and anger at the state of Israel and its institutions, resulting in a deep rift. This event is still commemorated annually by Palestinians. The subsequent three decades were also eventful in terms of violence and wars, beginning with the 1982 Lebanon War, followed by the first intifada between 1987 and 1993, the second intifada between 2000 and 2005, the Second Lebanon War in 2006, the First Gaza War in 2008–2009, and the Second Gaza War in 2012.

While these armed conflicts did not take place in the Palestinian localities in Israel, Palestinians followed the unfolding events on television screens and reacted with concern and anguish for their immediate relatives residing in the West Bank and Gaza.

This review briefly touches on the scope of traumatic events, including wars and institutionalized aggression, land confiscations, home demolitions, social exclusion, economic underdevelopment, and violence, that Palestinian citizens in Israel, as a national minority, have experienced through the years.

Mental Health Services

Mental health services in Israel are included within the comprehensive health-care system and are covered by universal health insurance for all citizens. Most Palestinian localities have health-care centers, yet the accessibility and quality of mental health services in Palestinian society is relatively limited. There is a significant shortage of qualified practitioners and psychotherapeutic treatment centers. Data from the Knesset Labor, Social Welfare, and Health Committee revealed that of 140 training positions available in one of the largest health-care providers in the country (Clalit), only 16 Palestinians were accepted; additionally, only 2.5% of psychologists in Israel are Palestinian, while 90% of the Palestinians who need mental health treatment do not access it (Israel Ministry of Health, 2015). Admittedly, since the inception of the psychiatric service reform and the implementation of the psychiatric rehabilitation law in 2000, progress has been noticeable, but the changes are not yet sufficient.

Social determinants of mental health, as the following quotation indicates, are particularly relevant to the understanding of mental health among Palestinian citizens in Israel: "Inequality in mental health morbidity between and within ethnic groups is at least partly linked to income, and thus to employment and education. Tackling disadvantage and discrimination in these areas could help tackle the challenge of mental health" (Mangalore & Knapp, 2012, pp. 351).

Social and cultural barriers, such as stigma and negative attitudes toward mental health and help-seeking behavior, inhibit Palestinians from seeking mental health services. Stigma and discrimination refer to negative stereotyped beliefs, prejudice, and behaviors toward persons with mental illness. Stereotyping and prejudice in mental health act as a barrier to treatment and the use of social resources, to social inclusion, and to opportunities for recovery (Kadri & Sartorius, 2005; Wahl, 1999). As in other traditional societies, the stigma of mental health services still exists; it is more socially acceptable to approach traditional healers or to receive treatment through religious guidance and other nontraditional methods than Western-oriented psychotherapists (Al-Krenawi, 2005; Al-Krenawi & Graham, 2000).

Bedouin Palestinians in southern Israel, for example, have little knowledge of mental disorders. Most of them do not recognize the term "schizophrenia." They stigmatize those with mental disorders and are opposed to working with those suffering from mental illnesses (Al-Krenawi & Graham, 1996). In addition, one study showed that Palestinians had a less positive perception of the benefits of mental health care compared to responders not living in Palestinian localities (Struch et al., 2008). Another study showed that stigma and negative attitudes toward persons with psychiatric problems are generally higher among Palestinian responders compared to responders in localities with predominant Jewish residents (Ponizovsky, Geraisy, Shoshan, Kremer, & Smetannikov, 2007). Negative attitudes and behavior toward persons with mental illness often generate feelings of disgrace, guilt, low self-esteem, social dependence, isolation, and hopelessness in the person with the disease (Rüsch, Lieb, Bohus, & Corrigan, 2006).

Although the shift in governmental policy from treating persons with mental illnesses in psychiatric hospitals to community-based centers has increased the awareness of mental health issues in Israel as a whole (Grinshpoon, Zilber, Lerner, & Ponizovsky, 2006), this increase has yet to become fully materialized among Palestinians.

A number of scholars have examined the delivery and effectiveness of psychotherapy among Palestinians in Israel (Al-Krenawi & Graham, 2000; Dwairy, 2005; Gorkin, Masalha, & Yatziv, 1985; Masalha, 1999). Most of them have tried to clarify the cultural particularities of Palestinian society and to suggest culturally adequate approaches to enable non-Palestinian clinicians to work more effectively with Palestinian service users. Those authors believe that psychotherapy with Palestinian citizens in Israel needs to be culturally modified to ensure its effectiveness.

Help seeking is one aspect that provides a critical link between the onset of mental illness and the delivery of professional help. Help-seeking characteristics among Palestinians are similar to those among Muslim Arabs in the United States. Aloud (2004) reported that the attitudes of Muslim Arabs in Ohio toward seeking formal mental health services were most likely affected by cultural and traditional beliefs about mental health problems, knowledge and familiarity with formal services, perceived societal stigma, and the use of informal indigenous resources. Among Palestinians in Israel, 46% of study participants indicated that they preferred to turn to family doctors or other nonpsychiatric medical professionals when facing a mental health problem (Ponizovsky et al., 2007).

Psychotherapy

In general, less than 30% of nonminority therapy clients terminate their treatment after one session, while among minority service users, more than 50% terminate therapy after one session (Sue & Sue, 2003). Fischer, Jome, and Atkinson (1998) proposed four basic, essential elements for successful therapy: good therapeutic relations between service user and therapist, similarity in worldviews, belief of the service user in the counseling process, and interventions believed by both therapist and service user to lead to positive outcomes.

One reason that ethnic minority service users (such as Palestinians in Israel) are not well served is that certain assumptions of Western psychotherapy conflict with their cultural values (Sue & Sue, 2003). In essence, Western psychotherapy commenced with the emergence of individualism and the need to meet the demands of modern life while compensating for the lost systems of social support, social support that had been available prior to the rise of individualism (Dwairy, 1998). According to Western theories, the aim of psychotherapy is to help a person know him- or herself better, to alleviate emotional pain, to assist with coping strategies, and to help users deal with unresolved intrapersonal issues through the promotion of values such as self-actualization, self-efficacy, personal responsibility, and social equity, among others (Pedersen, 2002; Sue & Sue, 2003). Individualism and collectivism are important constructs that distinguish Western and non-Western cultures (Triandis, 2001), as raised by other chapters of this book. In individualistic cultures, on the one hand, individuals are autonomous and independent of their own larger groups. They give priority to their personal goals over those of the group, and behavior is primarily based on attitudes and needs rather than on group norms (Triandis, 2001). Members of collectivistic cultures, on the other hand, are interdependent; they give priority to the goals of the group, shape their behavior in accordance with group norms, and are concerned with the quality of the relationships among group members (Dwairy & Van Sickle, 1996).

Many of the values and characteristics observed in both the goals and the process of Western therapy, as presented earlier, are not shared by Palestinians in Israel as they view the world from holistic, collectivistic, and spiritual perspectives (Dwairy, 1998). Therefore, effective mental health interventions must reflect the prevailing value placed on family membership, the status of women, the stigma associated with mental health symptoms, and the preference for indigenous healing (Al-Makhamreh, Hasna, Hundt, Al-Smairan, & Alzaroo, 2012; Al-Makhamreh & Hundt, 2012; Al-Makhamreh & Libal, 2011). Furthermore, empowerment of the individual, which lies at the core of Western psychotherapy, conflicts with the role of the individual in a traditional, collectivistic society, such as that of Palestinians in Israel. Western psychotherapeutic principles and values transferred without proper adaptation to non-Western clients may lead to unfavorable results for the individual and the family.

Modes of Psychotherapy

Two widely utilized theoretical approaches to therapy, cognitive-behavioral therapy (CBT) and psychodynamic therapy, are used in the context of the Palestinian family in Israel. According to Skinner (1974) and Ellis (1989), CBT appears to be culturally neutral. Further examination of behaviorism shows that, basically, behavioral therapy aims to improve the sense of self-efficacy over the environment through assertiveness training (Ellis, 1986). It is one of the most frequently used types of therapy in the treatment of mood and anxiety disorders among adults and the young. Cognitive behavioral interventions refer to the way service users create or reframe meaning about symptoms, situations, and events in their lives, as well as beliefs about themselves, others, and the world (Beck, 2005). The cognitive behavioral interventions focus on the interaction between the individuals and their environment; it is not insight-oriented, nor does it focus on self-awareness. CBT is based on the idea that one's feelings and behavior are a consequence of one's thoughts. A therapist's goal is to increase the user's awareness of inaccurate or negative thinking and the relationship between thoughts, feelings, and behavior. As a result, the user will achieve a better understanding of challenging situations and thus be able to respond to them effectively. The focus of CBT is on the here and now; it is structured and directive. The therapist identifies the client's goals and helps the client to achieve those goals. The therapist's role is to listen, coach, and support, while the user's role is to express his or her concerns, learn, and implement what is learned between sessions. Sessions are individualized, usually time-limited, and where goals are formulated. CBT can be implemented with different cultural and ethnic groups and has proven to be successful in dealing with a large array of symptoms, mainly state anxiety, test anxiety, behavioral symptoms, and self-esteem, when treating Palestinian users (Yahav & Cohen, 2008).

Other studies on the effectiveness of CBT with Muslim minorities throughout the world suggest that this form of therapy may be relatively consistent with Islamic values, but the self-statements that are central to this modality are often packaged in secular terminology inconsistent with Islamic norms. Thus, to provide culturally relevant services, practitioners need to dismantle the secular terminology and repackage it with precepts in terminology that reflects Islamic teaching (Hodge & Nadir, 2008).

Psychodynamic psychotherapy focuses on unconscious processes as evident in human behavior. Its goal is to raise awareness of the influence of past events on present behavior and on any unresolved past conflicts that are rooted in dysfunctional relationships as a result of abuse or unfulfilled desires. Psychodynamic therapy, while it can be brief, usually lasts six months or longer and is less structured than CBT. It focuses on the here and now as well as on the user's past. It places importance on the patient-therapist relationship as the focus of therapy. Hodge and Nadir (2008) found that psychodynamic approaches may not be as effective as cognitive approaches when dealing with Muslim service users. The difficulty in adopting this type of therapy with Palestinians stems, as noted earlier, from the fact that most of them are traditional, are members of patriarchal/hierarchal structured families, and may reject liberal individualistic values.

Barriers in Western Psychotherapy for Palestinians

Research on the effectiveness of Western-based psychotherapeutic principles among Palestinian clients is scarce. Cultural constructs such as individualism/ collectivism, worldview, cultural standards of therapy and their relationship to individualistic values, views and attitudes toward mental health, personal versus family well-being, self-disclosure, and acculturation are just a few of the cultural constructs that require examination and should be addressed to achieve effective therapy with non-Western clients.

The Palestinian family is characterized by a collectivistic authority structure in which the father leads the family according to traditional collectivistic norms and values (Dwairy, 1998). In the West, individualistic authority has replaced collectivistic authority. The heads of the family, father and/or mother, share authority in the family, and decision making is usually democratic and cooperative. The continuing transition of Palestinian society from traditional values and norms to Western values and way of life has brought positive and negative developments. Among others, it is accompanied by intergenerational conflicts (Al-Issa, 1990, 1995) and by the absence and/or perceived absence of governmental agencies to provide services; it is the family unit, neither fully traditional nor fully Westernized, that fills that void (Dwairy, 1998). Historically, Palestinians were colonized by the Ottoman Empire, the British Empire, and now, as some believe, the state of Israel. Conventional psychological interventions often lack congruence with native traditional practices and beliefs, and thus another form of colonization comes into being (McIntyre, 1996). I posit that rapid social change and the adverse determinant cited earlier has had a negative effect on the belief system and family structure of the Palestinians.

Negative attitudes toward mental health care as well as other characteristics emerging from the collectivist nature of the Palestinian society in Israel (e.g., shame, family honor, privacy, reputation and loss of face, in addition to problem solving only within the family unit) impinge on the willingness of persons in need among the Palestinians in Israel to seek therapy and to disclose personal information to strangers outside the family (Haj-Yahia, 1994; Sue & Sue, 2003).

Western psychotherapy focuses on the individual and the importance of individualism, autonomy, personal responsibility, taking control over one's own choices, and planning and working toward achieving personal goals (Triandis, 2001). As such, the goal of psychotherapy is to help a person develop his or her own unique identity (Sue & Sue, 2003). In contrast, for many Palestinians, the development of an identity independent from the family is not supported. Family honor and status are fundamental values, and the need for individual happiness separate from the well-being of the family is not an appropriate goal (Erickson & Al-Timimi, 2004).

In collectivist cultures, self-esteem in essence means getting along with others rather than getting ahead, and decisions are often made by family members as a group (Triandis, 2001). It is vital that when service user and therapist belong to different cultures (collectivist/individualist) the therapist is aware of the importance of the decision-making process in order to develop a healthy therapeutic relationship with the user. Because of the stigma associated with mental illness, Palestinian families prefer to approach other specialists rather than psychologists or psychiatrists. In traditional societies, individuals do not talk about personal issues outside the family unless it is for prescriptive purposes. Seeking therapeutic treatment is usually the last resort after consulting the family physician and the traditional healer.

Religion and Psychotherapy

Islam is the main religion in the Middle East and the fastest-growing religion in the world (Jenkins, 2015). For the last 1,400 years, it has ruled as the major official religion in the Islamic world. Its values and norms became Arab values and norms to the point that intellectual Christians in the Middle East would define themselves as Christians with an Islamic culture and education. A vast majority (83%) of Palestinians in Israel are Muslims and share Islamic values.

The Islamic concept of mental health focuses on abnormal behavior and is seen as a deviation from the path of health. In Islam, physical health is stressed through the sayings of the Prophet: "The strong believer is better and more beloved to Allah than the weak believer" (Sahih Muslim 2664, Book 46, Hadith 52). Historically, medieval Islamic physicians reported treating patients with illness of the mind (Paladin, 1998). Muslim scholars such as Ahmed ibn Sahl al-Balkhi (850–934) were among the first to discuss disorders related to both the body and the mind, arguing that "if the psyche gets sick, the body may also find no joy in life and may eventually develop a physical illness" (as cited in Deuraseh & Abu Talib, 2005, p. 77). Other Muslim scholars, including Alkendi (801–873), Abu Bakr Al-Razi (864–923), Ibn Hazm (994–1064), Al-Ghazali (1058–1111), Fakhr-al-Din al-Razi (1149–1209), Ibn Taymiyyah (1263–1328), and Ibn al-Qayyim (1292–1350), could be considered cognitive-behavioral theorists. In their psychotherapeutic treatment, they focused on changing the negative thoughts and beliefs of the patient on the grounds that one's ideas and beliefs do affect one's behavior.

A major component of the Islamic belief system is determinism with its external locus of control. Determinism, for a Muslim, is the inability to change what has been decreed or written in the Qur'an. External locus of control, which is characteristic of authoritarian societies in general, is the belief that all events and occurrences are transmitted to the individual from God—from a higher external power—and must be attributed to forces outside the self that therefore has no control over them.

Rotter (1966) coined the concept "locus of control," which refers to the individuals' belief as to where the forces are located that can control events that affect their lives. One's locus is conceptualized as either internal, in which the individual believes he or she is able to control his or her own life, or external, in which a person believes that his or her life and decisions are controlled by external factors that cannot be influenced or controlled by the person. An external locus of control may lead to feelings of helplessness and weaken the perception that one is shaping his or her own destiny (Rotter, 1966). Research on various aspects of mental health and locus of control has shown significant correlations between locus of control and some aspects of psychopathology (Pancer, Hunsberger, Pratt, & Alisat, 2000). For example, one study found a pervasive influence of both internal and external locus of control on mental health and adjustment among adolescent female university students in India (Jain & Singh, 2015). In Arab-Islamic culture, mental as well as physical illness is often attributed to what has been decreed by God. This characteristic of Arab culture in Israel and elsewhere stems from the desire to be a good Muslim. The belief in divine will and decree (*al-Qadar*) is one of the pillars of faith in Islam. *Al-Qadar* means that God has ordained all things from eternity. God knows when and how they will happen, and events have been decreed—"written"—according to God's will. Everything happens according to what God has decreed: "And you cannot will unless [it be] that Allah wills[,] the Lord of the 'Aalameen [mankind, jinn, and all that exists]" (Qur'an Surah At-Takwir [The Overthrowing] 81:29).

The belief in divine will and decree has also been stated by the Prophet: "Believe in Allah, His angels, His Books, His Messengers and the Last Day, and believe in *al-Qadar* (the divine decree) both good and bad." Culturally, Palestinians, Muslims, and some Christians share the common belief that one's fate or *al-Qadar* is predestined (*musayyar*), while many Muslim scholars believe that the person is given the choice (*mukhayyer*) to think, to select from many options, and to act accordingly. A believer must believe in "*al-Qada' wa'l-Qadar*" (fate), otherwise he or she has not fulfilled one of the requirements for being a believer (Al-Mahmoud & al-Rahmaan, 1418 Hijri).

Regardless of their accuracy, these and similar interpretations of Qur'anic verses and quotations from the Prophet form the basis of the cultural attribute of locus of control and determinism that characterizes Arab culture. External locus of control has a stronghold when it comes to mental illness. In a traditional authoritarian society, religion is central to the perception of mental illness as a God-given decree. Palestinians tend to attribute mental illness to external factors, and as long as this illness does not manifest itself in shameful behavior, it can be tolerated (Al-Krenawi & Graham, 1996; Dwairy, 1998). Palestinians also attend to the needs of the body, to physical illness, and are more oriented toward pharmaceutical rather than psychotherapeutic means of treatment.

As already stated, effective mental health interventions in the Middle East should reflect the prevailing value placed on family membership, status of women, stigma associated with mental health symptoms, and the preference for indigenous healing (Al-Makhamreh & Hundt, 2012; Al-Makhamreh & Libal, 2011). For example, Western psychotherapy was found to be ineffective with Muslim women mainly because it is individualistic and fragmented, while their cultural beliefs are holistic and spiritual (Carter & Rashidi, 2004). Sabry and Vohra (2013) have suggested that therapy is most effective with the integration of spirituality and religiosity. For example, listening to rhythmic Qur'anic recitation was found to be effective among a group of depressed patients, resulting in a significant decrease of depression symptoms (Poura, Rajabi, & Pishgar, 2012).

My experience confirms the benefit of integrating culturally accepted practices and religious beliefs in therapy. The following case illustrates one example:

> A couple expressed their unhappiness and their wish to expel an elderly parent living with them after the man's wife had passed away. Citations from the Qur'an as well as the sayings of the Prophet, together with recognition of a possible negative response from the community for neglecting an older parent, led them to reconsider their decision. Once they decided to keep him in the home, they asked for practical methods to alleviate the burden of caring for the elderly parent. Workable, socially accepted proposals were offered and accepted, such as dividing the daily care of the elderly man among members of the family.

Therapy with Palestinians

Among Palestinians, psychotherapeutic help seekers are multiplying, but the number of Palestinian psychotherapists is not increasing sufficiently to cover the needs. In their study that investigated the relationship between delay in treatment seeking and cultural barriers to health care, Ponizovsky et al. (2007) reported that Palestinian clients in Israel showed a twofold delay in their initial treatment contact compared to Jewish patients. One explanation was related to the Palestinians' negative attitudes toward mental health care. The delay was also associated with lower formal education, nonpsychiatric attribution of mental symptoms, and a more pessimistic attitude regarding the successful treatment of mental disorders both in general and in one's own situation.

When considering nonpsychiatric attribution of mental symptoms, it should be noted that Palestinian citizens in Israel do not generally attribute mental illness to intrapsychic causes; they tend not to pathologize behavior (Dwairy, 1998). Similar to other traditional societies, the Palestinian society attributes mental illness to external factors, some of which are person-related, such as poisoning, and some that are related to paranormal and mystical powers, such as evil spirits or the evil eye (Dwairy, 1997a, 1997b; Timimi, 1995). In addition, Palestinians in general tend not to seek help through psychotherapy because they do not believe that personal or family conflicts are associated with psychopathology (Al-Krenawi, 2005; Dwairy, 1998). Help from formal mental health agents is usually sought only when psychological anguish is unbearable (Dwairy, 1998; Okasha, Saad, Khalil, El Dawla, & Yehia, 1994). In addition, many Palestinians approach a therapist after visiting a physician, a traditional healer, and/or a religious figure (a sheikh) (Ponizovsky et al., 2007). Usually, referrals to mental health clinics are made by general practitioners who could not find any biomedical explanation for the user's symptoms (Al-Krenawi, Maoz, & Reicher, 1994). In their fundamental worldview, Palestinians believe that everything positive and negative, comes from outside, a result of fate or Allah's will (Al-Krenawi, 1992).

Among Palestinian Bedouins who seek treatment, therapy is perceived as a method or procedure used by highly qualified professionals who have the power to liberate clients from their illness. Medical and pharmacological treatments (especially injections) are usually well accepted because they come from an authoritarian external locus. Al-Krenawi (1992) suggests treating Palestinian Bedouin clients through alternative psychotherapeutic methods. In addition to the pharmacological treatments, the therapist should develop a brief strategic approach based on the client's life history; on the description of the present life situation of the patient and the family; as well as on the systemic potential for change via the family, cultural beliefs, and the environment. Historically, males tend to seek psychotherapy more often than females. However, I have found that the number of females seeking help is on the rise; females more often use their children as an excuse to come to the clinic for the first time. Because of their cultural characteristics, most clients from traditional, authoritarian, and collectivistic societies prefer an instant cure—short-term therapy that is directive and very structured (Dwairy, 1998; Gorkin et al., 1985). They also prefer treatments from male doctor therapists rather than from female specialists (Dwairy, 1998).

Psychotherapy in a Sociopolitical Context

In addition to cultural and religious factors, some scholars have discussed the sociopolitical factors involved in interventions with Arabs and Muslims. Erickson and Al-Timimi (2004) touched on the mistrust and apprehension among Arab American clients treated by US therapists, identifying the therapist with the US government's policy in the Middle East, a mistrust that stems from the traditional political alliance between the United States and Israel. Roysircar (2003) suggested that in working with Muslim American clients, therapists have a responsibility to understand the political forces and events that affect them. Inayat (2007) and Guru (2010) touched on Islamophobia and its role in disrupting therapeutic relationships with Muslim clients.

In Israel, Palestinian therapy seekers can either pursue treatment with a Palestinian therapist or an Israeli Jewish therapist. Treatment in either case may be hindered because of the implementation of Western cultural and theoretical aspects in therapy. Approaching an Israeli Jewish therapist poses a greater challenge to the success of therapy, however. In this situation, client and therapist come from different ethnic, cultural, religious, and language backgrounds. The success or failure of therapy may be determined by power differentials as the therapist and client are members of opposing sides of an ongoing violent political conflict. When treating clients, therapists must be aware of the background of this intractable conflict (Baum, 2007).

Baum (2011) identified three features that characterize the Palestinian client who is seeing a Jewish therapist: presence of the enemy mistrust, and guilt. Therapy is affected by the presence of one's opponent in the consulting room, where both the therapist and the client share feelings of antagonism when sitting opposite the enemy. The therapist feels mistrust toward the client as a representative of the opposing group, yet trust is an essential element in therapy. Studies consistently show that large numbers of the Jewish Israeli population believe that Palestinian citizens in Israel hate them and desire the destruction of the state (Oren, 2003) and that many Jews view Palestinians as a hostile minority (Mahameed & Guttmann, 1983) and as the enemy (Bar-Tal & Teichman, 2005). For example, the issue of mutual therapist-patient trust was raised by the majority of a group of in-training Jewish clinicians when they were told they would be assigned a Palestinian service user (Baum, 2010). Jewish Israeli therapists treating Palestinian clients may feel guilty owing to their belief that Israel has caused harm to its Palestinian citizens and thus either try to compensate the client or, alternatively, show feelings of aggression and other negative interactions with the client. Gorkin (1987) described a vicious cycle of guilt leading to aggression that led to more guilt and then to further attempts to compensate. Baum (2011), in his recommendations to mental health workers treating Palestinians, suggested that they be aware of the client's cultural and political background and take the time and effort to build trust with the service user. In addition, the therapist should be aware of his or her own feelings and learn to distinguish countertransference responses (i.e., therapist's emotional reaction to patient) that stem from the client's behavior because of his or her membership in an enemy group.

Proposed Solutions to Improve Effectiveness of Psychotherapy with Palestinian Citizens in Israel

Some of the literature suggests that clients prefer therapists with similar values and worldviews (Atkinson, Wampold, Lowe, Matthews, & Ahn, 1998; Dwairy & Van Sickle, 1996). In multicultural counseling, it is imperative to use theoretical principles rooted in the clients' culture, religion, and values. These principles help therapists establish credibility, especially with patients from a non-Western background. Credibility can be achieved through the conceptualization of a problem that is harmonious with the clients' belief system, by proposing culturally acceptable solutions, and by adopting clearly shared goals for treatment (Sue & Zane, 1987). In addition, speaking the client's language and understanding his or her values and belief systems, worldviews, and social and political reality are also important (Dwairy, 2006).

Therapists should pay attention to cultural issues such as clients arriving on time for their appointment, since being on time is not an important value in Middle Eastern cultures. Ending the session must be well planned in advance, for it may be culturally impolite to end the session just because the allocated time is up. The waiting room presents an issue that is closely associated with stigma. The best clinics have a separate entrance and exit, as Palestinian clients do not want to be seen coming in and out of a mental health clinic, and it is appropriate not to have service users running into each other.

Mental health professionals should make room for contextual knowledge and sensitivity (Al-Krenawi et al., 1994). By focusing on appreciation of the culture and working within the power structure of the extended family, Al-Krenawi et al. (1994) reported achieving various degrees of success in treatments for depression, post-traumatic symptoms, and conversion disorder, partly depending on collaborative work with family members.

While all Western therapeutic approaches are individually correct, "they fail to tell the whole rich story of the human being" (Dwairy, 1998, p. 165). Failing to address the whole person in his or her own environment, with attention to psychological, physical, social, and familial aspects, may be harmful rather than beneficial. Thus, therapists should initiate interventions that cause changes in the family and the social context only with the approval of the head of the hierarchy—the father. Changes in the role, status, and life of the patient not only affect the individual, as it may seem initially, but may also affect the entire family unit. A young woman is not free to do whatever she wants; the entire family, society, and village are guarding, watching, and having a say in what she is socially allowed or forbidden to do. Psychotherapy thus should be tailored to treat the body and the psyche within the social context of the client.

Conclusion

In this chapter, I describe the current status of psychotherapy for Palestinian citizens in Israel. The discussion focuses on the effectiveness of therapy for Palestinians, whether Western-oriented therapy can be applied to minorities in general and to Palestinians in particular, or whether the principles of therapy as suggested by the West should be modified to address culturally diverse clients. The vast majority of scholars recommend modifying therapy when working with a population that is ethnically, culturally, religiously, and politically diverse. The Palestinian minority in Israel faces many barriers that affect therapy. Some of these barriers are in part institutional, such as the lack of treatment centers and infrastructure, and in part cultural, such as stigma and reasons for delay in seeking help. In addition, it is possible that the prolonged exposure of the Palestinians to wars and violence has affected their mental health. Palestinian society is defined as a society in transition, facing rapid social change, high levels of unemployment, relatively high rates of mental disorders, and political discrimination. The society is still traditional and collectivistic but is moving toward a more individualistic nature—a process that has yet to be completed and may continue for a significant period of time.

Psychotherapy with Palestinians can be useful when modified culturally and carried out in a holistic familial way. For example, the therapist should be aware of the family structure, the importance of tradition, and the status of women. For the majority of Muslims, the integration of religiosity and spirituality in psychotherapeutic treatment can be effective. The lack of qualified Palestinian professional mental health providers can lead Palestinian clients to seek help from Jewish Israeli therapists. In the current sociopolitical situation, both the Jewish therapist and the Palestinian service user may face issues of mistrust and feelings of guilt, issues that are problematic for successful therapy. The therapist must be aware of his or her own feelings and biases in order to distinguish countertransference responses that stem from the client's behavior and from belonging to the "enemy" group.

In sum, establishing credibility and fostering awareness of cultural issues, family structure, tradition, interdependency, and religion are essential to successful therapy for Palestinians in Israel.

NAZEH NATUR is Dean of Students and Senior Lecturer in the Department of Psychology at Al-Qasemi Academic College of Education, Baqa, Israel.

References

Al-Issa, I. (1990). Culture and mental illness in Algeria. *International Journal of Social Psychiatry, 36*(3), 230–240.

Al-Issa, I. (1995). *Handbook of culture and mental illness: An international perspective.* Madison, CT: International Universities Press.

Al-Krenawi, A. (1992). The role of the dervish as a mental health therapist in the Negev-Bedouin society: Clients' expectations from these treatments and the extent of materialization [in Hebrew] (Unpublished master's thesis). Hebrew University of Jerusalem, Israel.

Al-Krenawi, A. (2005). Socio-political aspects of mental health practice with Arabs in the Israeli context. *Israel Journal of Psychiatry and Related Sciences, 42*(2), 126–136.

Al-Krenawi, A., & Graham, J. R. (1996). Social work and traditional healing rituals among the Bedouin of the Negev, Israel. *International Social Work, 39*(2), 177–188.

Al-Krenawi, A., & Graham, J. R. (2000). Culturally sensitive social work practice with Arab clients in mental health settings. *Health & Social Work, 25*(1), 9–22.

Al-Krenawi, A., Graham, J. R., Dean, Y. Z., & Eltaiba, N. (2004). Cross-national study of attitudes towards seeking professional help: Jordan, United Arab Emirates (UAE) and Arabs in Israel. *International Journal of Social Psychiatry, 50*(2), 102–114.

Al-Krenawi, A., Maoz, B., & Reicher, B. (1994). Familial and cultural issues in the brief strategic treatment of Israeli Bedouins. *Family Systems Medicine, 12*(4), 415.

Al-Mahmoud, Abd-al-Rahmaan. (1418 Hijri). Fate in light of the Qura'an and the Sunnah and its application by the people. [in Arabic]. Alriyad, Saudi Arabia: Dar Al-watan.

Al-Makhamreh, S., Hasna, F., Hundt, G. L., Al-Smairan, M., & Alzaroo, S. (2012). Localising social work: Lessons learnt from a community based intervention amongst the Bedouin in Jordan. *Social Work Education, 31*(8), 962–972.

Al-Makhamreh, S., & Hundt, G. L. (2012). An examination of social work interventions for use with displaced Iraqi households in Jordan. *European Journal of Social Work, 15*(3), 377–391.

Al-Makhamreh, S., & Libal, K. (2011). The Middle East: Expanding social work to address 21st century concerns. In K. Lyons, M. C. Hokenstad, N. Huegler, & M. Pawar (Eds.), *Handbook of international social work* (pp. 451–465). London: Sage.

Aloud, N. (2004). *Factors affecting attitudes towards seeking and using formal mental health and psychological services among Arab-Muslim population* (Doctoral dissertation, Ohio State University). Retrieved from https://etd.ohiolink.edu/rws_etd/document/get /osu1078935499/inline.

Atkinson, D. R., Wampold, B. E., Lowe, S. M., Matthews, L., & Ahn, H.-N. (1998). Asian American preferences for counselor characteristics: Application of the Bradley-Terry-Luce model to paired comparison data. *The Counseling Psychologist, 26*(1), 101–123.

Bar-Tal, D., & Teichman, Y. (2005). *Stereotypes and prejudice in conflict: Representations of Arabs in Israeli Jewish society.* Cambridge: Cambridge University Press.

Baum, N. (2007). Social work practice in conflict-ridden areas: Cultural sensitivity is not enough. *British Journal of Social Work, 37*(5), 873–891.

Baum, N. (2010). Jewish Israeli social work students' attitudes to the prospect of being assigned an Israeli Arab client. *Journal of Ethnic & Cultural Diversity in Social Work, 19*(2), 143–170.

Baum, N. (2011). Issues in psychotherapy with clients affiliated with the opposing side in a violent political conflict. *Clinical Social Work Journal, 39*(1), 91–100.

Beck, A. T. (2005). The current state of cognitive therapy: A 40-year retrospective. *Archives of General Psychiatry, 62*(9), 953–959.

Carter, D. J., & Rashidi, A. (2004). East meets West: Integrating psychotherapy approaches for Muslim women. *Holistic Nursing Practice, 18*(3), 152–159.

Daoud, N., Shankardass, K., O'Campo, P., Anderson, K., & Agbaria, A. K. (2012). Internal displacement and health among the Palestinian minority in Israel. *Social Science & Medicine, 74*(8), 1163–1171.

Deuraseh, N., & Abu Talib, M. (2005). Mental health in Islamic medical tradition. *International Medical Journal, 4*(2), 76–79.

Dwairy, M. (1997a). A biopsychosocial model of metaphor therapy with holistic cultures. *Clinical Psychology Review, 17*(7), 719–732.

Dwairy, M. (1997b). *Personality, culture, and Arabic society* [in Arabic]. Jerusalem: Al-Noor.

Dwairy, M. (1998). *Cross-cultural counseling: The Arab-Palestinian case.* New York: Haworth.

Dwairy, M. (2005). Culturally sensitive counseling and psychotherapy: Working with Arabic and Muslim clients. New York: Teachers College Press.

Dwairy, M. (2006). *Counseling and psychotherapy with Arabs and Muslims: A culturally sensitive approach.* New York: Teachers College Press.

Dwairy, M., & Van Sickle, T. D. (1996). Western psychotherapy in traditional Arabic societies. *Clinical Psychology Review, 16*(3), 231–249.

Ellis, A. (1986). Effective self-assertion [cassette recording]. Washington, DC: Psychology Today Tapes.

Ellis, A. (1989). Thoughts on supervising counselors and therapists. *Psychology: A Journal of Human Behavior, 26*(1), 3–5.

Elsass, P. (2001). Individual and collective traumatic memories: A qualitative study of post-traumatic stress disorder symptoms in two Latin American localities. *Transcultural Psychiatry, 38*(3), 306–316.

Erickson, C. D., & Al-Timimi, N. R. (2004). Counseling and psychotherapy with Arab American clients. In T. B. Smith (Ed.), *Practicing multiculturalism: Affirming diversity in counseling and psychology* (pp. 234–254). Boston: Allyn & Bacon.

Fischer, A. R., Jome, L. M., & Atkinson, D. R. (1998). Back to the future of multicultural psychotherapy with a common factors approach. *Counseling Psychologist, 26*(4), 602–606.

Gelkopf, M., Solomon, Z., Berger, R., & Bleich, A. (2008). The mental health impact of terrorism in Israel: A repeat cross-sectional study of Arabs and Jews. *Acta Psychiatrica Scandinavica, 117*(5), 369–380.

Gorkin, M. (1987). *The uses of countertransference*. Northvale, NJ: Jason Aronson.

Gorkin, M., Masalha, S., & Yatziv, G. (1985). Psychotherapy of Israeli-Arab patients: Some cultural considerations. *Journal of Psychoanalytic Anthropology, 8*(4), 215–230.

Grinshpoon, A., Zilber, N., Lerner, Y., & Ponizovsky, A. M. (2006). Impact of a rehabilitation legislation on the survival in the community of long-term patients discharged from psychiatric hospitals in Israel. *Social Psychiatry and Psychiatric Epidemiology, 41*(2), 87–94.

Guru, S. (2010). Social work and the "war on terror." *British Journal of Social Work, 40*(1), 272–289.

Haj-Yahia, M. (1994). The Arab family in Israel: A review of cultural values and their relationship to the practice of social work [in Hebrew]. *Society and Welfare, 14*(3–4), 249–264.

Hodge, D. R., & Nadir, A. (2008). Moving toward culturally competent practice with Muslims: Modifying cognitive therapy with Islamic tenets. *Social Work, 53*(1), 31–41.

Inayat, Q. (2007). Islamophobia and the therapeutic dialogue: Some reflections. *Counselling Psychology Quarterly, 20*(3), 287–293.

Israel Ministry of Health. (2015). *Determination of incentives to train clinical psychologists and clinical social workers responding to needs in implementing the mental health reform in the* Arab sector [in Hebrew]. Jerusalem: Israel Ministry of Health, Committee of Labour, Welfare and Health. Retrieved from http://main.knesset.gov.il/Activity/committees/Labor/Pages/CommitteeAgenda.aspx?tab=3&ItemID=569299.

Jain, M., & Singh, S. (2015). Locus of control and its relationship with mental health and adjustment among adolescent females. *Journal of Mental Health and Human Behavior, 20*(1), 16–21. Retrieved from http://www.jmhhb.org/text.asp?2015/20/1/16/164803.

Jenkins, P. (2015). The world's fastest growing religion: Comparing Christian and Muslim expansion in the modern era. In S. Brunn (Ed.), *The changing world religion map.* Springer, Dordrecht. Retrieved from https://doi.org/10.1007/978-94-017-9376-6_93.

Kadri, N., & Sartorius, N. (2005). The global fight against the stigma of schizophrenia. *PLoS Med, 2*(7), e136. Retrieved from https://doi.org/10.1371/journal.pmed.0020136.

Levy, B. S., & Sidel, V. W. (2008). *War and public health* (2nd ed.). New York: Oxford University Press.

Mahameed, H., & Guttmann, J. (1983). Autostereotypes and heterostereotypes of Jews and Arabs in different contact situations. *Psychology and Counseling in Education, 16*, 90–108.

Mangalore, R., & Knapp, M. (2012). Income-related inequalities in common mental disorders among ethnic minorities in England. *Social Psychiatry and Psychiatric Epidemiology, 47*(3), 351–359.

Masalha, S. (1999). Psychodynamic psychotherapy as applied in an Arab village clinic. *Clinical Psychology Review, 19*(8), 987–997.

McIntyre, M. P. (1996). Counselling and native healing. *Asian Journal of Counselling, 5*(1), 87–100.

Okasha, A., Saad, A., Khalil, A., El Dawla, A. S., & Yehia, N. (1994). Phenomenology of obsessive-compulsive disorder: A transcultural study. *Comprehensive Psychiatry, 35*(3), 191–197.

Oren, N. (2003, July). *Major societal events and social beliefs of conflict change.* Paper presented at the annual meeting of the International Society of Political Psychology, Boston, Massachusetts.

Paladin, A. V. (1998). Ethics and neurology in the Islamic world. Continuity and change. *The Italian Journal of Neurological Sciences, 19*(4), 255–258.

Pancer, S. M., Hunsberger, B., Pratt, M. W., & Alisat, S. (2000). Cognitive complexity of expectations and adjustment to university in the first year. *Journal of Adolescent Research, 15*(1), 38–57.

Pedersen, P. B. (2002). Ethics, competence, and other professional issues in culture-centered counseling. In P. Pedersen, J. G. Draguns, W. J. Lonner, & J. W. Trimble (Eds.), *Counseling across cultures* (5th ed.; Vol. 5, pp. 3–27). Thousand Oaks, CA: Sage.

Ponizovsky, A. M., Geraisy, N., Shoshan, E., Kremer, I., & Smetannikov, E. (2007). Treatment lag on the way to the mental health clinic among Arab- and Jewish-Israeli patients. *The Israel Journal of Psychiatry and Related Sciences, 44*(3), 234–243.

Poura, S., Rajabi, S., & Pishgar, A. (2012). Investigating the rate of Quran reciting by Persian language and literature students in comparison with students of other fields and its effect on depression, anxiety and stress. *Journal of Language Teaching and Research, 3*(5), 1004–1008.

Rotter, J. B. (1966). Generalized expectancies for internal versus external control of reinforcement. *Psychological monographs: General and applied, 80*(1), 1–28.

Roysircar, G. (2003). Religious differences: Psychological and sociopolitical aspects of counseling. *International Journal for the Advancement of Counselling, 25*(4), 255–267.

Rüsch, N., Lieb, K., Bohus, M., & Corrigan, P. W. (2006). Brief reports: Self-stigma, empowerment, and perceived legitimacy of discrimination among women with mental illness. *Psychiatric Services, 57*(3), 399–402.

Sabry, W. M., & Vohra, A. (2013). Role of Islam in the management of psychiatric disorders. *Indian Journal of Psychiatry, 55*(6), 205–214.

Skinner, B. F. (1974). About behaviorism. New York: Vintage.

Struch, N., Levav, I., Shereshevsky, Y., Baidani-Auerbach, A., Lachman, M., Daniel, N., & Zehavi, T. (2008). Stigma experienced by persons under psychiatric care. *Israel Journal of Psychiatry and Related Sciences, 45*(3), 210–218.

Sue, D. W., & Sue, D. (2003). *Counseling the culturally diverse: Theory and practice* (4th ed.). New York: Wiley.

Sue, S., & Zane, N. W. S. (1987). The role of culture and cultural techniques in psychotherapy: A critique and reformulation. *American Psychologist, 42*(1), 37–45.

Timimi, S. B. (1995). Adolescence in immigrant Arab families. *Psychotherapy: Theory, Research, Practice, Training, 32*(1), 141.

Triandis, H. C. (2001). Individualism-collectivism and personality. *Journal of Personality, 69*(6), 907–924.

Wahl, O. F. (1999). Mental health consumers' experience of stigma. *Schizophrenia Bulletin, 25*(3), 467–478.

World Health Organization [WHO]. (2012). *Risks to mental health: An overview of vulnerabilities and risk factors.* Retrieved from http://www.who.int/mental_health/mhgap /risks_to_mental_health_EN_27_08_12.pdf.

Yahav, R., & Cohen, M. (2008). Evaluation of a cognitive-behavioral intervention for adolescents. *International Journal of Stress Management, 15*(2), 173–188.

20

FROM PSYCHOANALYSIS TO CULTURE-ANALYSIS

Culturally Sensitive Psychotherapy for Palestinian Citizens in Israel

Marwan Dwairy

I N 1978 I OPENED THE FIRST PSYCHOLOGICAL SERVICES center among the Palestinian community in Nazareth, the largest Palestinian city in Israel. I had just graduated, having been trained according to Western approaches to psychology. The major experience I recall from that period is the feeling of frustration because the people of Nazareth did not respond properly to my interventions. They did not seem to fit the theories and tools I had learned and believed were universal. They did not open up and share their personal lives and feelings, especially toward their family members; they wanted miracle solutions or advice to halt their suffering; they considered the conversation, our major medium for therapy, as useless; and they were not ready to attend more than a few therapeutic sessions. For some years I insisted on applying psychodynamic therapy and tried to educate them to make them fit my theories. Here I present a case vignette from those culture-ignorant years that exemplifies the problem:

> Najwa, an Arab Muslim woman, 32 years old, came to my clinic with her husband because of daily vomiting. The medical examination did not reveal any explanation for it. They both said that everything in their lives was perfect but for the vomiting problem. They had seven healthy children, the husband earned good money, and their extended families were respected and considered honorable. Because of the patriarchal control over women in the Palestinian society, it was not easy to convince the husband to allow several personal therapeutic sessions with his wife. At the early meetings with her alone, she

continued to describe how satisfied she was in her life and how supportive her husband and their families were. She merely described how she had daily meals with her parents and family who lived across the road. The only conflictual issue she brought up was that after her marriage she had decided to wear religious clothes with *hijab*, against the will of her husband and family, who were secular Muslims. Only after several sessions did she start to disclose some distressing experiences. She said that her marriage had been arranged by the two families without her consent, when she was 17 years old. For that reason, she had given up her plans for higher education, and at age 18 she had become a mother.

She recalled that her father had hit her badly when she tried to oppose the marriage. For him it was considered as rebellion against the "word" he had already given to the other family. At later stages of therapy, she reported several physical and sexual abuses by her husband, especially during the first year of marriage, when she was not ready yet for pregnancy. At that stage of her marriage, she suffered from severe muscular tension during sexual intercourse, a somatic sign of rejection of the marriage.

To explain her experience during the oppression and abuses she had endured in her marriage, she said more than once, *"ma qdertish ablaa' hada alwadea"* [I couldn't "swallow" that situation]. Gradually, she became more and more aware of her frustration and anger. My interpretations of her physical symptoms (muscular tension and vomiting) helped her to realize that the symptoms expressed what she had avoided articulating consciously and openly. However, this analysis required her to face two sorts of resistance: internal guilt and external punishment. Internal guilt came from her Muslim belief system that prevented her from expressing anger to her parents based on the verse in the Qur'an: "Say not to them [so much as], 'uff,' and do not repel them" (Qur'an Surah Al-Isra [The Night Journey] 17:23). She also feared punishment by her husband, family, and society once she confronted them and expressed her anger. Repeatedly interpreting the resistance in various ways did not help to sustain her conscious frustration. She continued to be overwhelmed by her vomiting rather than her frustration and eventually terminated therapy with only partial improvement of the vomiting.

This case vignette exemplifies several typical aspects of the psychology of Palestinian Muslim women: the client experienced severe, unbearable patriarchal oppression and abuse but identified with the oppression and denied her anger and pain. This enabled her to live with the oppression as well as with her distress, which was expressed in physical symptoms. Needless to say, this vignette exactly fits the conversion cases discussed in psychoanalysis in which repressed drives are expressed through physical symptoms. But, why didn't my psychodynamic therapy help this woman?

Assumptions of Western Psychotherapy Unsuitable for Palestinian People

Despite the process of modernization and exposure to Western individualistic culture, Palestinian culture, as noted in other chapters, tends to be more collective, authoritarian, and patriarchal compared to the West (Barakat, 1993, 2000; Dwairy, 2006; Ghanem, 2001; Neydell, 2012). In this transitional period, some sectors of the Palestinian community, such as adolescents and educated people, adopt some individualistic Western values and practices, but in general, Palestinians remain closer to their collective traditional culture (Dwairy, 2006). The following three major assumptions of Western psychotherapy do not hold true for them:

1. individuals are independent entities and possess autonomous selves or personality;
2. intrapsychic processes and conflicts explain and predict behavior and symptoms; and
3. psychotherapy helps generate new intrapsychic order by bringing repressed unconscious content to consciousness. This new order enables self-control and self-actualization (Monte and Sollod, 2008; Rogers, 1961; Wedding, & Corsini, 2013).

The reasons these presuppositions do not hold true for Palestinians are described next.

Interdependent Identity

Western theories of development share the idea that the normal track of development leads to independent identity and autonomous personality after adolescence (Bigner, 1994; Mahler, Bergman, & Pine, 1975). This process of separation/individuation became possible in the West by virtue of the nation-states in Europe that function as states for their citizens (Dwairy, 2006, 2015). This functioning enabled the individual to rely on state institutions for survival, and thus the connection with the family became elective. In most non-Western countries, where states do not secure the needs of their citizens, individuals remain dependent for survival on their families. Therefore, the self or personality remains collective rather than autonomous. This situation holds true for Palestinians living in Israel, where the state does not secure all their needs for survival. It is the family that secures work, housing, protection, and child day care for its members (Dwairy, 2006).

Intrafamilial Processes Override Intrapsychic Processes

The main tension in people's lives in collective cultures, including that of Palestinians in Israel, is in the familial domain rather than in the self or the personality. Familial values, norms, expectations, and attitudes explain and predict the individual's behavior and feelings much more than internal constructs (self or ego) or processes (conflicts or defense mechanisms) within the personality that are in some way not autonomous. The well-known rule in collective cultures is that individuals should deny their personal needs and self-fulfillment and instead fulfill the family will, needs, values, and norms. By doing so, they receive support, approval, and protection in return. Individuals who are approved of and supported by their families are satisfied, whereas those who are disapproved of or rejected may suffer from psychological problems. Psychotherapy that targets mainly the intrapsychic processes to restore order within the personality misses the major conflict that, as mentioned, is intrafamilial (Dwairy, 2002, 2006).

Bringing Unconscious Content to Consciousness May Be Counterproductive

Most Western psychotherapy addresses the intrapsychic domain to bring unconscious content to consciousness in order to help clients lead self-fulfilling lives. However, in the Palestinian community in Israel, accessing and expressing unconscious content is typically forbidden by the family and condemned by the community. Therefore, revealing such content and facilitating its expression may bring about a difficult confrontation with the family. As noted in Najwa's case, bringing her frustration and anger toward her family to consciousness was met by twofold resistance: internal and external. In a traditional and religious society such as that of the Palestinians, individuals are raised to obey and respect their parents and to avoid any sexual behavior before or outside the marriage. Therefore, any expression of anger toward parents or taboo sexual feelings typically generates a sense of guilt. Besides this internal source of resistance, individuals are held under the control of the family and community, which are still capable of punishing any forbidden behavior. If psychotherapy makes the client conscious of anger toward parents and family—or of her sexuality—and the client initiates overt expression of this forbidden content, one can expect a confrontation with the family in which the client is the weak party. Inability of the client to express and resolve these issues leaves her with an open wound and may turn the problem into depression characterized by sadness, helplessness, hopelessness, and loneliness (Dwairy, 2006, 2015).

Culture-Analysis

Culture-analysis (Dwairy, 2006, 2015) is an approach and technique that directs therapists to employ the client's culture to bypass internal and external resistance and facilitate change while avoiding confrontation with the family. It is based on the understanding that culture is not static but rather dynamic, and that includes internal conflicts and inconsistencies. The values of each culture are anchored in collective wisdom that has been accumulated through the experiences of a group of people over time and through many different circumstances. Because each value has been inducted during a single circumstance, the accumulated values are a product of a variety of circumstances and thus include discrepancies, inconsistencies, and/or contradictions. Thus, culture is a field of inconsistent values. The values in the holy books have also been accumulated through a variety of circumstances; therefore, they include inconsistent values and directives (Dwairy, 2015).

Examples of Inconsistencies from the Qur'an

Should Muslims show kindness to disbelieving parents?

One should accompany and show kindness to parents, even if they are disbelievers. (Qur'an Surah Al-Isra 17:23–24; Surah Luqman 31:14–15; Surah Al-'Ankabut [The Spider] 29:8)
One should not show any love or friendship to those who oppose Muhammad, even if they are your parents. (Qur'an Surah Al-Mujadila [The Pleading Woman] 58:22)
Believers are asked not to take their fathers and brothers as protectors if they are disbelievers. (Qur'an Surah At-Tawbah [The Repentance] 9:23)

Who is responsible for bad actions?

All actions, good or evil, come from God. (Qur'an Surah An-Nisa [The Women] 4:78)
Good comes from God while evil comes from humans (Qur'an Surah An-Nisa 4:79)

Who has to be blamed for the wrongs done?

It is Allah who has to be blamed for all the misguidance. (Qur'an Surah Fatir [Originator] 35:8; Surah An-Nahl [The Bee] 16:93; Surah Al-Muddaththir [The Cloaked One] 74:31; Surah Al-Baqarah [The Cow] 2:142)
Man himself is responsible for the wrongs done. (Qur'an Surah Ar-Rum [The Romans] 30:9; Surah An-Nisa 4:79)

Examples of Inconsistencies from the New Testament

What is the correct attitude toward anger?

Turn the other cheek. Love your enemies. (Matthew 5:38–44; Luke 6:27–29)
Anger is a sin. (Matthew 5:22)
Jesus says that he is gentle [meek] and humble [lowly]. (Matthew 11:29)
Anger is not necessarily a sin. (Ephesians 4:26)
Jesus curses the inhabitants of several cities who did not repent at seeing his mighty works. (Matthew 11:20–24; Luke 10:13–16)
Jesus curses a fig tree when it fails to bear fruit out of season. (Matthew 21:19; Mark 11:12–14)
Jesus looks around "with anger." (Mark 3:5)
Jesus makes a whip of cords, drives the moneychangers from the temple, overturns their tables, and pours out their coins. (John 2:15)
Justice requires a life for a life, an eye for an eye. (Exodus 21:23–25; Leviticus 24:20; Deuteronomy 19:21)

What is the correct attitude toward family?

Whoever hates his brother is a murderer. (1 John 3:15)
If anyone claims to love God but hates his brother, he is a liar. (1 John 4:20)
Honor your father and your mother. It is one of the Ten Commandments
and was reinforced by Jesus. (Exodus 20:12; Deuteronomy 5:16;
Matthew 15:4, 19:19; Mark 7:10, 10:19; Luke 18:20)
Jesus says to call no man on earth your father. (Matthew 23:9)
Jesus says that he has come to divide families; that a man's foes will be
those of his own household; that you must hate your father, mother,
wife, children, brothers, sisters, and even your own life to be a disciple.
(Matthew 10:35–37; Luke 12:51–53; Luke 14:26)

Examples of Inconsistent Proverbs

Respond immediately: *Hit the iron while it is hot.*
Withhold your reaction: *Slow is safe hurrying is regretful.*
Don't judge things based on first impression: *Not all what glitters is gold.*
You can judge things based on the first impression: *The book is known from it's title.*

Comparing Culture-Analysis and Psychoanalysis

If culture or religion includes inconsistent or contradicting directives, how do people manage these contradictions? Each member in a culture selectively and unconsciously adopts some aspects of the culture and neglects others. The chosen values
constitute his or her belief system or superego and are part of the building blocks
of the conflict or problem. When a client reaches an impasse in coping with a certain psychological problem or symptom, the values and attitudes the client has em-
braced during his or her life must be modified before revealing unconscious drives
that typically negate the values selected out of the culture (Dwairy, 2015).

I have coined the term "culture-analysis" to harmonize such an approach together with psychoanalysis (Dwairy, 2006, 2015). Because a collective people adopt
a collective self, the main analysis should focus on the client's culture before entering the psychological domain. In addition, the term indicates the similarity between the two approaches—both look for content of the unconscious mind that is
remote from the client's consciousness or awareness: psychoanalysis looks for repressed drives, needs, and wishes within the client, while culture-analysis looks for
neglected, overlooked, or rejected values and attitudes within the client's culture.
In both cases, bringing new content to consciousness initiates a process of change.

One major difference between the two approaches is that in psychoanalysis
the new content typically causes resistance within the client and conflicts with her
family, while in culture-analysis no resistance takes place and no confrontations
with the family are expected; rather, culture-analysis may pave the road for bringing unconscious drives to consciousness after altering the client's beliefs that may
resist these drives. Still, there are many other significant differences between the

two approaches (Dwairy, 2015). For example, while psychoanalysis reveals intrapsychic conflicts and looks for repressed drives and needs, culture-analysis reveals inconsistencies in the client's culture and looks for ignored values or attitudes within the client's belief system and his or her culture. Furthermore, while from a psychodynamic perspective, revealing unconscious content typically escalates intrapsychic and familial conflicts, from a culture-analysis perspective, revealing ignored values enriches the client's perspective with no escalation of conflicts.

Four Stages of Culture-Analysis

Understanding the Client's Belief System

The culture-analyst does not need to thoroughly know the client's culture to apply culture-analysis. Empathy, sensitivity, and openness to understanding and learning about the client's culture are required. Collecting information about the significant events in the client's family clarifies the values and norms that direct his or her behavior and that of the family. The therapist may ask questions such as "How is it in your culture? How do your people look at this?" In the era of the internet, therapists may easily learn about any culture or look for applicable proverbs or scripture verses from any religion. They may seek advice from a religious leader, such as a sheikh, priest, pastor, or rabbi. Sometimes it may be helpful to suggest that the client get some advice from a recognized religious leader. Therapists should keep in mind that the core of most religions is similar. For instance, most religions include belief in God's will and call for accepting and appreciating God's actions and have ways or rituals for atoning for bad deeds or sins. Many proverbs are universal and based on the shared collective experience of humankind. At this stage, therapists need to pay attention to contradicting values within the client's belief system to utilize these contradictions in the second stage.

Bringing Contradictory Values to the Client's Attention

A culture-analyst does not confront the client with the therapist's values or theories but rather with values from the client's culture or religion that he or she neglects or ignores. Therapists at this stage need to understand the values that directed the client's behavior and dominated his or her feelings such as: "Say not to them [so much as], 'uff,' and do not repel them" (Qur'an Surah Al-Isra 17:23). These values are typically responsible for repressing the unconscious drives or feelings, and, as such, they cause resistance to bringing these contents to consciousness. The challenge is to find alternative values from within the client's culture that contradict the dominating values. If the client believes that God is a punishing entity, the therapist may present scripture verses saying that God is an entity of mercy and forgiveness. If the client believes that as a Sunni Muslim he or she should follow the written rules literally, with no questioning, the therapist may present verses in which God encourages people to think and learn from their experience. If the client believes that as Christian he or she must turn the other cheek, the therapist may guide his or her attention to the times when Jesus expressed anger and fought his enemies.

Revising and Enriching the Client's Belief System

Once the client has become aware of alternative values to those that had caused the impasse, the client may start revising and altering his or her belief system. This modification is usually contextual and enriches the repertoire of his or her values and makes the client more flexible in dealing with a variety of situations. If, for instance, a Christian client feels guilty for not doing enough good deeds in his or her life, the therapist may show many biblical verses saying that people are justified by faith, not by works (John 3:16; Romans 3:20–26; Ephesians 2:8–9; Galatians 2:16), which then may help the client to feel better about him- or herself. If a Muslim client feels guilty because of certain actions, the therapist may show him or her several verses in the Qur'an indicating that God is responsible for the good and bad actions of man (Qur'an Surah An-Nisa 4:78; Surah Fatir 35:8; Surah An-Nahl 16:93; Surah Al-Muddaththir 74:31; Surah Al-Baqarah 2:142) and that God could have prevented these bad acts. The therapist also may emphasize that God is an entity of mercy for those who redirect themselves (i.e., those who repent). Culture-analysis enriches the client's value system to become more flexible and allows variations in coping in diverse situations and contexts.

Cognitive, Emotional, and Behavioral Change

Enriching the client's belief system with alternative values encourages flexibility in dealing with his or her conflicts. The client becomes able to understand, feel, and cope differently and resolve the impasse. This change may occur with or without the client becoming conscious of repressed needs or drives. Sometimes the new value or directive enables the client to overcome internal resistance (guilt) and feel better about a certain attitude or action that has disturbed him or her before; at other times it paves the way for bringing a repressed need or drive to consciousness, and then the client may deal with it, express it, and feel empowered to confront the external resistance (family oppression). Therefore, sometimes culture-analysis can be used as a standalone method and may help the client feel better, but most of the time it is a preliminary stage that empowers the client to express him- or herself and face the oppression of the family.

Implementing Culture-Analysis

Culture-analysis is the best choice for clients who are not individuated enough from their families, those who do not have enough strength to confront their families, or those who live in strict, collective families. The more the client is individuated and has the fortitude to confront his or her family, the more likely it is that culture-analysis will lead to psychoanalysis that reveals unconscious drives and helps the client express them.

In reconsidering the predicament of Najwa, we note that she adopted a dependent, collective, unindividuated personality with low ability to face her strict, abusive family and husband. Therefore, she was unable to sustain contact with her repressed anger and express it. Culture-analysis could have mitigated her reluctance to express any sort of anger by helping her differentiate between not saying so much as "*uff*" to parents and using other moderate forms of expression. Apparently, the only protest she was able to make without guilt was her insistence on wearing religious cloths and a *hijab*. In fact, this kind of protest fits the idea behind culture-analysis because it is backed by values within her Islamic culture denied by her family. It may also have been possible to encourage her to express her anger passively by ceasing the daily meals with her parents. This passive-aggressive expression of anger might not have provoked her guilt and may have aroused only a mild, bearable reaction on the part of her parents. In fact, the passive-aggressive reactions were associated with her vomiting and with her complaints of not being able "swallow" the situation. Ceasing the family meals could be assumed to have altered the vomiting symptom.

A Culture-Analysis Case Vignette: Treating Anxiety and Nervousness by Moderating Extreme Islamic Values

The following case study illustrates how culture-analysis can help a client discover neglected values to deal with anxiety and nervousness.

Hakeem is a 24-year-old Palestinian student. In the last two years, he changed his major and his college three times because of failure and anxiety. Each time, he restarted with much enthusiasm and success, then after two or three months, he would become anxious and abandon his studies. When he came to therapy with his father, he had just terminated his studies at a teacher training college. He described his anxiety before and during presentations in class where most of the students were women. He was afraid of not satisfying the instructor and the female classmates. He also described difficulties in breathing.

He and his father reported nervous behavior and inexplicable loud quarrels with his sister over of her behavior. Hakeem was angry when she behaved immodestly. He interfered with her dress, her verbal behavior, and her communications with males in the college. Hakeem also clashed with his father and brothers when they missed prayers or when they interfered to restrain his nervous, controlling attitude toward his sister.

As a child, Hakeem had been hyperactive and impulsive and had had difficulty delaying satisfaction. As a result, he was punished severely in the family. Apparently, he suffered from ADHD; he was not treated properly, but rather the family dealt with it through harsh punishments. A noticeable change occurred in his life at age 10. He started praying and going to the mosque. At age 11, he memorized the whole Qur'an and won a contest based on memorizing it. After this, his behavior improved, and he became obedient to family expectations and adhered to his religion's teachings.

He described how he had been a troublemaker and aggressive as a child. He recalled how he had repeatedly abused a handicapped child in the neighborhood. Today, Hakeem regretted these actions. He attributed his improved behavior to the punishments that "helped" him control himself. He added that religion and praying helped him control his sexual desires and avoid relationships with women and relinquish masturbation.

Apparently, the combination of punishments and religion brought him to where he could control his impulsivity and hyperactivity and repress his frustration and sexuality, especially during presentations in front of the women in class. It seemed that he repressed his aggression and sexuality through identification with his oppressive family and through the defense of reaction formation—that is, expressing religious values rather than aggression and sexuality. As a result, his anxiety during presentations was related to his repressed desire to communicate with women. His nervous behavior toward his sister, father, and brother was related to his reaction formation defense mechanism, which was a way to displace his aggression. This displacement enabled him to fight with his family in the name of God rather than as a person with self-control difficulties.

From the whole clinical picture, it is obvious that Hakeem had low ego-strength: he managed to control himself by empowering his superego rather than his ego. He was emotionally dependent on his family to the extent that he behaved as if they should follow his way of life and their sins were also his sins. Based on this, it was clear to me that he would not be able to deal with his anger and sexuality without negotiating his religious belief system (superego) and moderating it first, which would necessitate culture-analysis. Therefore, I needed to find references from within his religion to moderate these irrational beliefs.

As stated before, Hakeem's religious beliefs are, in fact, selected beliefs out of the pool of Islamic teachings and beliefs. Here is part of the conversation in which his Islamic beliefs were explored and overlooked beliefs were brought to his attention in order to change his behavior.

> Therapist: It sounds as if you have taken the role of God in controlling your sister's behavior.
> Hakeem: No, it is the will of God to make girls behave and dress modestly.
> Therapist: Yes, I understand that, but did he assign to you the responsibility for making your sister behave accordingly?

Hakeem: Yes, of course, "Men are in charge of women . . ." [a well-known
sentence from a Qur'anic verse, Al-Nisa 4:34, that is commonly used
to justify the control of women by men].

Therapist: But you are trying to control your father and brothers, too, when
they miss prayers. It seems you are competing with God in his role.

Hakeem: No, God forbid.

Therapist: Then why don't you leave this task to God? Of course, if he
wants them to fulfill his will, he can achieve this easily.

I was helped by Google to find a Qur'anic verse to alleviate his desire to
control his family's behavior. I found some verses on dealing with unbeliev-
ers, such as a call to care for and show kindness to parents, even if they are
disbelievers (Qur'an Surah Al-Isra 17:23–24; Surah Luqman 31:14–15; Surah Al-
'Ankabut 29:8). When I brought these teachings to his attention, he revised
his control over his family members. However, he still needed to displace his
anger toward them and therefore had to address this anger. At the early stages
of therapy, he used to justify his parents' punishments and attributed them to
love and care for him. Later, he became able to touch the pain and frustration
he had felt at being punished because of his inability to control himself. He
then described a period when he had been full of aggression and rage against
everything and had abused several weak children.

Parental punishments and guilt feelings prevented him from coming to
terms with his rage and his sexual desires. Some Islamic values of tolerance
had to be brought to his attention to perhaps alleviate his feelings of guilt.

Therapist: It seems that you do not forgive yourself for any rage toward
your parents or any expression of your sexual desires.

Hakeem: Yes, it is forbidden. God orders us to respect and obey our parents. [He cited some verses on this issue.]

Therapist: But despite your heroic attempts to be kind to your parents,
sometimes you lose control and become nervous and clash with them.

Hakeem: (In a sad voice and helplessly) Yes, I know . . . I do not know what
to do.

Therapist: While you are trying to make your family adhere to God,
you become nervous and angry with them, which does not fit God's
teachings.

Hakeem: Yes, that is so. I am afraid that I am doing the wrong thing.

Therapist: You are trying to be perfect in your faith, behavior, and studies
and do not succeed, and now you are afraid you are doing the wrong
thing.

Hakeem: (Sad and thinks again)

Therapist: Does God order you to be perfect?

Hakeem: (Energized and provoked) No, "Perfection is only for God" [a well-known religious proverb].

Therapist: Then why do you require yourself to be perfect? As a human being you are expected to be imperfect, and God may understand that.

Hakeem: Yes, "He is forgiving and merciful." [He cited some verses supporting that God is forgiving.]

These ideas of flexibility and mercy were discussed and elaborated on in several sessions, and this helped Hakeem to revise his rigid values that had prevented him from addressing his rage toward his family and expressing his sexual desires.

Later he told me that he had asked a sheikh for advice concerning masturbation and that he was told that masturbation is recommended when it substitutes for or prevents adultery or illicit sexual intercourse.

Therapist: How do you feel about his advice?

Hakeem: I am hesitating whether to allow myself or not.

Therapist: What are you afraid of?

Hakeem: Nothing. The issue is that I avoided masturbation for two or three years, and I am afraid to become addicted to it.

Therapist: It sounds as if you had the power to avoid it for two or three years.

Hakeem: (Wondering)

Therapist: Do you think it would be more difficult for you to control the frequency of masturbation than to avoid it altogether?

Hakeem: I am not sure.

Therapist: Anyway, you proved that you have the power to avoid it when you want to.

Hakeem: (Hesitating) Is it bad for my health, doctor?

Therapist: It is safe as long as you do not overdo it.

Hakeem: The sheikh told me that once or twice a week is allowed.

Therapist: Yes, this frequency sounds safe.

Hakeem became gradually aware of many memories of insults and abusive punishments he had received as a child on a daily basis. At some moments he expressed rage, which he was able to calm down by taking a forgiving attitude, such as: "This is the way they knew" or "God forgives them."

Culture-analysis brought to Hakeem's awareness ideas of flexibility, helped him understand that nobody is perfect except for God, and led him to feel forgiveness and mercy, which were drawn from his Islamic references. Eventually, these new values were endorsed by Hakeem and altered the former rigid values that both repressed his anger and his sexuality and justified his nervousness and control over his sister and family. This alteration of values helped him to be in touch with his anger and sexuality and find moderate ways to express them. This change was accompanied by relief from anxiety and nervousness. As for his college studies, he decided to quit academic studies and work in a supermarket owned by the family.

Without this change in values, Hakeem could not have become conscious of his rage and sexual tension. In terms of client-centered therapy, this alteration enabled him to actualize his authentic self, and in terms of cognitive therapy, these values replaced his irrational rigid thoughts.

Conclusion

Psychotherapy that intends to reveal unconscious content, content that is typically forbidden expression, and to facilitate self-actualization may be counterproductive when it is applied with Palestinian clients. This Western therapy encounters internal (guilt) and external (punishments) resistance. Culture-analysis utilizes the internal inconsistency within the client's value system and brings to his or her awareness some neglected values that may help in facilitating change and in generating a new order in his or her life.

Culture-analysis is based on the assumption that all cultures or religions contain contradictions and inconsistencies. Each individual unconsciously makes a personal selection from his or her cultural belief system and neglects other values and beliefs. The Palestinian culture, too, contains many inconsistencies, and each Palestinian selects his or her personal cultural and religious beliefs that constitute part of the conflict. Resembling the way psychoanalysis reveals unconscious wishes, feelings, and drives, culture-analysis reveals unconscious or neglected values that may help in reaching a new order and new coping methods in the client's family and community. This bypasses internal resistance and mitigates external rejection and punishments.

MARWAN DWAIRY is Professor at Oranim Academic College, Israel. He is author of *From Psycho-Analysis to Culture-Analysis: A Within-Culture Psychotherapy.*

References

Barakat, H. (1993). *The Arab world: Society, culture, and state.* Los Angeles: University of California Press.

Barakat, H. (2000). The Arab society in the 20th millennium [in Arabic]. Beirut: Markaz Derasat Alwehda AlA'rabia.

Bigner, J. J. (1994). *Individual and family development: A life-span interdisciplinary approach.* Englewood Cliffs, NJ: Prentice Hall.

Dwairy, M. (2002). Foundations of psychosocial dynamic personality theory of collective people. *Clinical Psychology Review, 22*, 343–360.

Dwairy, M. (2006). *Counseling and psychotherapy with Arabs and Muslims: A culturally sensitive approach.* New York: Teachers College Press.

Dwairy, M. (2015). *From psycho-analysis to culture-analysis: A within-culture psychotherapy.* London: Palgrave Macmillan.

Ghanem, A. (2001). *The Palestinian-Arab minority in Israel, 1948–2000.* New York: State University of New York Press.

Mahler, M., Bergman, A., & Pine, F. (1975). *The psychological birth of the infant: Symbiosis and individuation.* New York: Basic Books.

Monte, C. F., & Sollod, R. N. (2008). *Beneath the mask: An introduction to theories of personality.* Danvers, MA: Wiley.

Neydell, M. K. (2012). *Understanding Arabs: A contemporary guide to Arab society.* Boston: Nicholas Brealey.

Rogers, C. R. (1961). *On becoming a person.* Boston: Houghton Mifflin.

Wedding, D., & Corsini, R. J. (2013). *Current psychotherapies.* New York: Cengage Learning.

21

PSYCHIATRIC REHABILITATION IN THE CONTEXT OF PALESTINIAN CITIZENS IN ISRAEL

David Roe, Paula Garber-Epstein, and Anwar Khatib

PSYCHIATRIC REHABILITATION (PsR) IS THE ADAPTATION AND APPLICATION OF rehabilitation principles and practices used with a variety of disabilities to help people with serious mental illness (SMI) (Roe, Lachman, & Mueser, 2009). It focuses on helping them learn and practice strategies—and gain support—for better coping and management of their illness. As a result, PsR helps shift the focus from symptoms and deficits to personal strengths and goals.

Over the last decade, PsR has been influenced by efforts to promote recovery-oriented services and evidence-based practices (EBPs). The recovery movement stresses helping people with SMI acquire equal rights and opportunities to live a personally meaningful life in their community of choice, despite the limitations of their illness (Anthony, 1993; Deegan, 1993). The EBP movement emphasizes the importance of identifying and implementing interventions that have been found to lead to desirable outcomes (Drake et al., 2001). Notable examples of EBPs for PsR include supportive employment (helping people with SMI acquire competitive jobs in integrated community settings, emphasizing preference, rapid placement, and job coaching), illness management and recovery (IMR) (which helps teach and practice illness management skills while setting personal goals to work toward recovery), and family psychoeducation (which focuses on forming a working alliance with family members of people with SMI and learning and practicing helpful skills). It is important to keep these global influences in mind while attempting to understand the development of PsR in Israel and specifically in the context of the Palestinian communities in Israel.

The development of PsR services in Israel reached a milestone in 2000 with the approval of the Rehabilitation in the Community of Persons with Mental Disabilities

Law (Aviram, Ginat, & Roe, 2012). This legislation specifies a set of services to be provided to people with SMI that address the key disadvantages often faced by service users in areas such as employment, education, and residence and that implement practices emphasizing social skills, case management, and family psychoeducation.

The task of implementing innovative practices in established social systems, even practices known to be effective, is far from simple. Service delivery occurs within complex systems and social contexts. Services need to be adapted and delivered with sensitivity if they are to be perceived as relevant and helpful to people who vary considerably in their cultural background, religious beliefs, and physical and social environments. Consequently, service providers face the challenge of developing and implementing PsR services that are both loyal to their core values as well as flexible and sensitive to the relevant social context and culture. Some studies argue that the vision of recovery and the practice of PsR might not be suitable for ethnic minorities, immigrants, and refugees (Hasnain et al., 2011; Tobin, 2000). These groups, despite their need and potential to benefit from such services, might have the least access to them owing to a broad range of barriers including cultural, institutional, structural, environmental, economic, political, and societal obstacles (Balcazar, Suarez-Balcazar, Taylor-Ritzler, & Keys, 2010).

The objective of this chapter is to discuss unique challenges in implementing PsR services and interventions among Palestinian citizens in Israel and possible ways to overcome these challenges. We begin with a brief, general overview of the Palestinian population in Israel and its culture in the context of our subject matter, followed by this group's patterns of health service use. We then describe possible barriers to the use of PsR services, which were identified during a year-long effort to disseminate IMR in this Palestinian population and work in a focus group with key Palestinian PsR stakeholders in Israel. Finally, we make some recommendations for future research and clinical and mental health policy implementations.

Palestinian Citizens in Israel: Cultural Characteristics and Service Use

As noted in previous chapters, Israel is a multicultural and pluralistic society consisting of two major ethno-national groups, Israeli Jews and Palestinians, who differ in many aspects including their religion, culture, language, values, and social constructs. Religion differentiates Israeli Jews from Palestinians as the latter group includes Muslims, Christians, and Druze. Concerning cultural values, to make a gross generalization, Palestinian citizens in Israel are often referred to as belonging to a traditional, collectivistic culture, whereas Israeli Jews have been described as living in a modern, individualistic, Western culture. In terms of social constructs, Arab societies are often characterized by patriarchy and primary group relations with an emphasis on the collective over the individual, in contrast to modern secular Israeli society. With regard to mental health service utilization, data have consistently revealed large gaps, with much higher use among the Jewish population (Levav, Ifrah, Geraisy, Grinshpoon, & Khwaled, 2007). Similarly, lower rates of PsR utilization have been identified among the Palestinian population. According to the Israel Central Bureau of Statistics, although Palestinians constitute almost 20% of the population, only 7% of PsR service users in Israel are Palestinians (Diab & Sandler-Loeff, 2014).

Various reasons have been suggested for the infrequent use of mental health services among the Palestinian population. These include lack of information and knowledge about services, inaccessibility to services, language barriers, stigma, and a preference for religion-based remedies and rituals over conventional medical treatment methods.

Methods

In an attempt to identify barriers to the use of PsR services among Palestinian citizens in Israel, we analyzed data from two sources. The first consisted of summaries written by five practitioners who implemented IMR groups. This was a widely used PsR intervention attended weekly by 13 Palestinian service users in various geographical regions over a 10-month period, from 2011 to 2013. The mental health practitioners comprised four women and one man. Four were Muslim, one was Bedouin, and their ages ranged from 25 to 35 years. The second source was a verbatim transcription of a recorded two-hour focus group attended in 2015 by 10 key PsR stakeholders, all Palestinians, who were invited by the Psychiatric Rehabilitation Division at the Israel Ministry of Health because of their seniority and considerable experience. Seven participants were women and three were men, nine were Muslim, one was Christian, and their ages ranged from 25 to 45 years. Four were PsR providers, two were service directors, and four were policy makers.

The data reduction was based on grounded theory and strategies outlined by Strauss and Corbin (1990) pursuing the following stages: (a) open-coding case analysis, (b) axial coding, (c) identifying changes, and (d) creating a synthesis. The first stage, open-coding case analysis, included reviewing all the data and analyzing, examining, and comparing the data for similarities and differences and giving instances names or conceptual labels that best captured their essence. During the second stage, axial coding, analysis focused on revealing the connections between conceptual labels and categories, conditions that gave rise to it, the context in which it was embedded, the strategies by which it was handled, and the consequences of those strategies. The third stage, identifying changes, focused on process by identifying points at which changes had occurred. Stage four focused on creating a synthesis, which included preserving the individual stories and their meaning from the participants' point of view while seeking patterns of regularity in the data.

Results

Several central themes emerged from the qualitative analysis of the reports from the IMR groups, whose participants were all from the Palestinian sector, and from the rehabilitation workers' focus group transcription. These themes must be addressed when examining the degree of relevance of the recovery approach and the rehabilitation principles in operation in the Western world and, hence, in Israeli society. The following discussion includes participants' comments to help illustrate the themes.

Family Focused Rehabilitation: The Family's Place in the Life of the Individual in the Context of PsR

Palestinian society in Israel is presented as a collectivistic society, where individuals are seen as an inseparable part of the group to which they belong. Hence, people's social context and their group belonging have a definitive impact on their rehabilitation process, which holds its origins in Western culture, emphasizing individuality and personal goals:

> "As we are a collectivistic and not an individualistic culture, it is impossible to make a separation [between the family and the individual]. It is impossible . . . there's nothing you can do about it." Another participant added, "In our society, when someone starts coping with a mental problem, the family pulls together, pulls together with all its might. It's part of the tradition, part of our mentality."

The society perceives the family and the individual as one entity, especially when coping with a crisis. The traditional values that guide the way members of the society manage a crisis has an impact on the coping strategy: "When someone in the family is ill, the whole family pulls together to help him/her over the crisis."

The family does not always appreciate the assistance provided to service users with SMI, and the proposed solutions might even contradict the family's worldview. Therefore, the professional help is sometimes seen as incongruent with the family's values: "You come along and say, 'I want to help, let's take him out, say, remove him from home into assisted living or to a hostel.' What? Have you gone crazy? It's as if you want me to throw him out."

Viewing the family as an integral part of the process and understanding the importance of the family members' involvement is manifested initially in the individuals' desire to determine personal goals as part of the group vision. Thus, for example, service users often include the family when setting these personal goals:

> "R. said that one of her goals was that her brother would get married and start a family." "B. said that she and her mother did household chores together, and that she thought that this could explain how she defined her goals when her mother was a significant part of these goals."

A gap between the family's understanding of the problem and solution and the plans and services offered may create a barrier to the rehabilitation process if the latter does not include appropriate societal and familial values. To advance suitable work processes, constant communication with family members is necessary to convey and integrate information in the process:

> "When working with the families—the parents, the siblings—we explain that we are taking her out, taking the young woman with us, and we are in telephone contact with you the whole time to reassure you that everything is all right. She arrived at the service and has had the treatment. She's absolutely fine; she is coming home."

The Perception of Illness, Mental Health, and Treatment Modalities

How family members perceive the illness dictates the model they adopt to understand and give meaning to what the person with SMI experiences. Some see the illness as a "sin or as a *jinn* [genie] that possesses the person." Others see the illness as "bewitchment, and people attribute all kinds of supernatural explanations to the illness because it is not perceived as an illness." Others explain it this way: "With people with SMI . . . they say that it is because of him, because of what he did, because of his sins, because he was possessed by a *jinn*."

These explanatory models have an impact on the modes of help the family seeks when the medical model (e.g., psychopharmacology, psychotherapy) has been rejected:

> "C. spoke about her mother taking her to the sheikh [indigenous healer] at the start of her illness." "P. said she remembers that when her illness first broke out, the medication was shameful, and so it wasn't suggested as treatment immediately, but they used other methods such as rituals and visiting sheikhs."

The perception of mental illness as a type of sorcery or as a punishment for the afflicted person's sins dictates the treatment methods sought because the family desires the approval of their religious leaders. Indeed, turning to religious leaders as a preferred course of action when the illness is first diagnosed appears in reports by both rehabilitation workers and people with SMI.

Some families transition from religion-based explanations to acceptance of a medical model and begin to perceive of the family member's condition as an illness. Exposure to the mental health recovery model, which emphasizes the consumer's active involvement in the recovery process, can be confusing for family members:

> "A lot of families . . . respond with the statement . . . flat-out . . . 'don't ruin it for us now. We have reached the stage that he is ill. We want him to be ill, we want him to get the treatment, to receive a response; it is very reassuring for us. We are at a stage where we don't want the "consumer" definition.'" "A lot of families actually want the status of the illness, a 'patient,' and they fight for that.

'Leave it as it is; don't touch that. We know that he is ill and it is very legitimate in Palestinian society to be ill. The ill status is very much accepted; and the consumer, in rehabilitation—that is a very strange concept.'"

As evident in the preceding reactions, the recovery orientation, which is promoted in the rehabilitation services, might generate unique challenges among Palestinian population groups in Israel. Many have experienced the positive impact of shifting from a religion-based explanation to a medical model of illness. In this context, the introduction of recovery-oriented language and ideology can be experienced as threatening and destructive:

"It is a great help to convince the person with SMI to take medication, to come for a check-up . . . after many failures with him, after many years of grievance. So it is sometimes important for the families to say that the illness exists in spite of that. Don't say rehabilitation, don't say consumer. Don't drive me nuts! Don't, in fact, destroy what I have achieved after so many years."

The family's need to preserve the diagnosis of mental illness as an attempt at acceptance and coping conflicts with the rehabilitation staff's wish to present options for achieving recovery and rehabilitation. Differences in perception apparently lead to the creation, at times, of two contradictory explanatory models, using different concepts, which might disrupt the rehabilitation process and the degree of cooperation. In these cases, rehabilitation workers will, once again, find themselves striving to implement a health-care model that is irrelevant to the population.

The stigma involved with mental illness and fear of exposure also influence the perception of the illness, the act of help seeking, and how the rehabilitation process is conceived. Rehabilitation workers describe their encounters with the stigma of mental illness:

"A lot of families in this sector still keep this secret of mental illness within the family. However, there is distress and they want a response. They want to keep it confidential and don't want the exposure. They know that if [they] go into a specific clinic at a specific location, or go to a particular social club, [they] have exposed [themselves], and they don't want this, they avoid it." "A lot of families . . . and consumers don't want to go to . . . a social club or a rehabilitation center that is labeled as belonging to the group. So they prefer to receive services that demand less exposure."

According to the descriptions of the IMR facilitators, the consumers' encounter with the stigma also takes place within the family:

"C. told me that her family mocks her and laughs at her when she opens the [IMR] booklet. They say to her: 'Take your medicine and nothing more; there's no need to read books to care for yourself!' C. said that this makes her feel embarrassed to open the booklet and read."

The lack of acceptance of the illness and the shame felt by some family members are also barriers to seeking suitable treatment for people with SMI. These following comments illustrate what some people with SMI experience as a result of this stigma:

> "She told me that she ran away from home to a psychiatric hospital, and only told her parents of her whereabouts when she regained her mental balance. Her father visited her, slapped her, and insulted her, and said: 'Your being in the loony bin has put me to shame.'"
>
> "My father used to come with me to the doctor and on our way to the office, he always asked me not to tell the doctor about my thoughts and the voices I hear, so as not to embarrass him. He always managed the consultation, and sometimes I didn't even understand what they were talking about. I needed him to come to the office because it's a long way from home. I can't take a bus because it is not common for a woman to ride a bus on her own."

The need to avoid exposing the mental illness to the community also leads to confrontations within the family unit. The wish to keep the illness a secret is explained, additionally, as a fear of the implications of disclosure to other members of the family who may suffer social sanctions:

> "Because exposure in the [Palestinian] sector carries a very heavy price, it can damage a whole family. It's not specific to the person with the illness, it's not only the exposure of that individual, but I have exposed an entire family. If it's a woman . . . then her chances of marriage . . . let's say, this can be harmful to women in the family. The whole family pays a very heavy price."

The perception of the illness by the individual, the family, and the community illustrated in the comments in this section creates the sociocultural context that must be considered when developing a rehabilitation model. This model must be tailored to the society's perception of the illness while facilitating the individual's integration into that society, either together with or notwithstanding the illness. As apparent from the text and according to the perceptions of both the family and Palestinian rehabilitation workers, the issue of exposure carries a heavy burden with multiple consequences.

Economic Status and Poverty as Barriers to Utilizing Rehabilitation Services in the Palestinian Sector

The economic status of many of the people with SMI who seek help also emerges as a significant factor that may serve as a barrier to seeking and utilizing rehabilitation services. For example, while social and recreational services are not consumed, employment services are more attractive:

"There, they earn money and it motivates them, together with the sense of receiving social legitimization." "There is room to increase the employment services, more so specifically in this sector. Because it actually improves the economic status in the home . . . something that spurs people on, and we really have a lot of success stories with supported employment."

Utilization of services is, to a certain extent, related to the social roles that are accepted and valued in the society. This is one reason for greater utilization of the employment services, mainly supported employment, which assists individuals' inclusion in the open market. In addition, their integration into work and their ability to earn a salary enhances their contribution to the family's income.

Importantly, the individual's and family's economic situation must be seen within the larger context of the lack of infrastructure in the Palestinian villages that appears to prevent some potential consumers from taking advantage of existing services. In particular, accessibility to services seems vital: "Accessibility to services is one of the problems. There is one framework that is utilized by close to one hundred consumers, or even a little more, just because it is accessible. Rides to the social club are provided. They have transportation that brings people from the villages, and it is thanks to this that they are included." Good transportation, which allows for mobility and accessibility, also enables people to travel to work.

In most of the villages, the public transportation infrastructure is not well developed and limits accessibility to services: "There is a problem with the infrastructure for public transportation. A bus goes past almost every half hour, but people don't use it. The internal public transportation is something new, but it is still hardly ever used. People already got used to the fact that it doesn't exist."

The lack of economic resources at both individual and community levels is one of the potential barriers to receiving and using appropriate services. Thus, economics, together with the aforementioned barriers, complicates the creation of a rehabilitation model tailored to Palestinian society.

Discussion and Recommendations

The findings presented in this chapter report on the perspective of Palestinian rehabilitation workers and society stakeholders and indicate the importance of creating a unique rehabilitation model for this sector in light of the gaps between the existing model and the desired sociocultural-based model. The characteristics of the society and the family's perception as a focus for intervention emerge as central, as opposed to the place of the individual in Western-based treatments. In addition, the society's perception of the illness, the significance of mental illness, and fear of its exposure are described as contributing to the individual's and family's attitude toward the rehabilitation processes and their acceptance of the illness. In the focus groups, rehabilitation workers noted several strategies learned from their own experience that contributed to creating a meaningful relationship that advanced the rehabilitation process, and they viewed the family as a resource in any discussion regarding the development of a rehabilitation plan. Palestinian society's perception of mental illness and its accompanying stigma, the fear of exposure that both the individual coping with SMI and the family feel, and the anxiety over potential consequences of that exposure seem to influence the individual's rehabilitation process. Alongside the characteristics of the society and the perception of the illness, poverty emerges as an additional barrier with possible implications for utilization of rehabilitation services and the perception of them as irrelevant by members of the society.

These findings address the challenge of how to adapt the potentially positive aspects of a recovery-oriented ideology and empirically supported interventions to Palestinian citizens in Israel, whose culture differs greatly from the Western culture on which this orientation is based.

In light of these findings, a reformed approach that takes into account the different cultural characteristics while creating a tailored rehabilitation model is needed. To provide effective treatment that will advance the goals of the individual and the family, we suggest a model that draws mainly on interpersonal communication and insists on acquaintance with the language, values, beliefs, and traditions of the target group.

Some promise comes from the recent review by Hasnain et al. (2011) that reported evidence from several studies that culture plays an important role in client-level rehabilitation outcomes. They reported that culturally adapted interventions improve rehabilitation outcomes for minority and immigrant individuals with a wide variety of disabilities, especially in three major areas: disability-related symptoms; client knowledge of their disability; and psychosocial outcomes of well-being, self-efficacy, and quality of life. These findings suggest that culturally adapted interventions can play a useful role in reducing service disparities and improving rehabilitation outcomes for culturally diverse individuals with disabilities. Future research could explore the critical components or mechanisms that make cultural adaptations work.

For example, a successful implementation of interventions in the Middle East must consider the overriding value placed on family membership, the role and status of women, stigma associated with mental health symptoms, a preference for indigenous healing, and the lack of formal mental health interventions (Al-Makhamreh & Libal, 2011). In this culture, similar to other conservative populations, symptoms and mental health disorders are often perceived to have external or supernatural causes, such as the will of God, divine punishment, and others (Al-Krenawi, Graham, Ophir, & Kandah, 2001). In addition, families of individuals with mental illnesses risk a damaged reputation or diminished social status in the community. Young women in particular are affected by the stigma of having a mental health disorder that might damage marital prospects or affect current marital relationships (Shalhoub-Kevorkian, 2005).

The experience of shame and the motivation to hide the illness is common, of course, not only in the Palestinian population. Western society, however, shows some signs of a shift, with notable examples including a new program entitled

Coming Out Proud (Corrigan, Druss, & Perlick, 2014). This change is based on the belief that there is nothing shameful about mental illness and that people with influence, such as caregivers, need to convey this message to empower others. In the Palestinian society in Israel, however, the trend appears to be active discouragement against revealing mental illness and encouragement to hide the illness, fostering feelings of shame and perpetuating the stigma.

In sum, to benefit successfully from the Western body of knowledge in implementing PsR services for the Palestinian population, it is important to explore and engage with local cultural beliefs and values for more effective adaption of mental health treatment. We strongly recommend increasing public awareness of mental illness and stress the importance of incorporating strategies to reduce stigma. Health service systems should work closely with primary health services, understand local religious and cultural beliefs, and build local support from key community leaders. The involvement of local stakeholders and community leaders in the adaptation process is critical for successful adaptation.

Similarly, there is a clear need to focus on partnership with local practitioners who are familiar with the regional cultural norms. Intervention protocols must be adapted to local customs and languages, and concerted efforts have to be made for active involvement and incorporation of family, if this is part of the culture. At the same time, culturally congruent empowerment is needed.

DAVID ROE is a clinical psychologist and Professor in the Department of Community Mental Health at the University of Haifa, Israel, and Adjunct Professor at Aalborg University, Denmark. He is author (with Patrick W. Corrigan and Hector W. H. Tsang) of *Challenging the Stigma of Mental Illness: Lessons for Advocates and Therapists*, and author (with Abraham Rudnick) of *Serious Mental Illness: Person-Centered Approaches*.

PAULA GARBER-EPSTEIN is a clinical social worker and Lecturer at the Bob Shapell School of Social Work, Tel Aviv University, Israel.

ANWAR KHATIB is a clinical social worker and Lecturer in the Department of Community Mental Health at the University of Haifa and Department of Social Work of Zefat Academic College, Israel.

References

Al-Krenawi, A., Graham, J. R., Ophir, M., & Kandah, J. (2001). Ethnic and gender differences in mental health utilization: The case of Muslim Jordanian and Moroccan Jewish Israeli outpatient psychiatric patients. *International Journal of Social Psychiatry, 47*(3), 42–54.

Al-Makhamreh, S., & Libal, K. (2011). The Middle East: Expanding social work to address 21st century concerns. In K. Lyons, M. C. Hokenstad, N. Huegler, & M. Pawar (Eds.), *Handbook of international social work* (pp. 451–465). London: Sage.

Anthony, W. A. (1993). Recovery from mental illness: The guiding vision of the mental health service system in the 1990s. *Psychosocial Rehabilitation Journal, 16*(4), 11–24.

Aviram, U., Ginat, Y. & Roe, D. (2012). Mental health reforms in Europe: Israel's rehabilitation in the community of persons with mental disabilities law: Challenges and opportunities. *Psychiatric Services, 63*(2), 110–112.

Balcazar, F. E., Suarez-Balcazar, Y., Taylor-Ritzler, T., & Keys, C. B. (2010). *Race, culture and disability: Rehabilitation science and practice.* Boston: Jones & Bartlett.

Corrigan, P. W., Druss, B. G., & Perlick, D. A. (2014). The impact of mental illness stigma on seeking and participating in mental health care. *Psychological Science in the Public Interest, 15*(2), 37–70.

Deegan, P. E. (1993). Recovering our sense of value after being labeled: Mentally ill. *Journal of Psychosocial Nursing and Mental Health Services, 31*(4), 7–9.

Diab, S., & Sandler-Loeff, A. (2014). Mental health and people with mental illness in Arab society in Israel [in Hebrew]. Retrieved from http://www2.jdc.org.il/sites/default/files/NifgaeiNefesh.pdf.

Drake, R. E., Essock, S. M., Shaner, A., Carey, K. B., Minkoff, K., Kola, L., . . . Rickards, L. (2001). Implementing dual diagnosis services for clients with severe mental illness. *Psychiatric Services, 52*(4), 469–476.

Hasnain, R., Kondratowicz, D. M., Borokhovski, E., Nye, C., Balcazar, F., Portillo, N., . . . Gould, R. (2011). *Do cultural competency interventions work? A systematic review on improving rehabilitation outcomes for ethnically and linguistically diverse individuals with disabilities* (FOCUS Technical Brief No. 31). Austin, TX: SEDL, National Center for the Dissemination of Disability Research.

Levav, I., Ifrah, A., Geraisy, N., Grinshpoon, A., & Khwaled, R. (2007). Common mental disorders among Arab-Israelis: Findings from the Israel national health survey. *Israel Journal of Psychiatry and Related Sciences, 44*(2), 104–113.

Roe, D., Lachman, M., & Mueser, K. T. (2009). The emerging field of psychiatric rehabilitation. *Israel Journal of Psychiatry and Related Sciences, 46*(2), 82–83.

Shalhoub-Kevorkian, N. (2005). Disclosure of child abuse in conflict areas. *Violence Against Women, 11*(10), 1263–1291.

Strauss, A. L., & Corbin, J. (1990). *The basics of qualitative analysis: Grounded theory procedures and techniques.* Newbury Park, CA: Sage.

Tobin, M. (2000). Developing mental health rehabilitation services in a culturally appropriate context. *Australian Health Review, 23*(2), 177–184.

INDEX